Diagnostic Techniques in Equine Medicine

Diagnostic Techniques in Equine Medicine

A textbook for students and practitioners describing diagnostic techniques applicable to the adult horse

FGR Taylor BVSc PhD MRCVS

MH Hillyer BVSc CertEP CertEM (Int. Med.) MRCVS

Department of Clinical Veterinary Science
University of Bristol
Bristol, UK

WB SAUNDERS COMPANY LTD
London Philadelphia Toronto Sydney Tokyo

WB Saunders Company Ltd

24–28 Oval Road
London NW1 7DX

The Curtis Center
Independence Square West
Philadelphia, PA 19106-3399, USA

Harcourt Brace & Company
55 Horner Avenue
Toronto, Ontario, M8Z 4X6, Canada

Harcourt Brace & Company, Australia
30–52 Smidmore Street
Marrickville
NSW 2204, Australia

Harcourt Brace & Company, Japan
Ichibancho Central Building
22-1 Ichibancho
Chiyoda-ku, Tokyo 102, Japan

A catalogue record for this book is available from the
British Library

ISBN 0-7020-1663-2

Typeset by Wyvern Typesetting Ltd, Bristol
Printed and bound in Great Britain by The Bath Press, Bath

Contents

Diagnostic techniques

Post-mortem investigations

A colour plate section appears between pages 294–295

Contributors

ARS Barr, MA VetMB PhD DVR CertSAO DEO Dip ECVS MRCVS, University of Bristol, Department of Clinical Veterinary Science, Langford House, Langford, Bristol, UK.

Chapter 13: Musculoskeletal diseases

SM Crispin, MA VetMB BSc PhD DVA DVOphthal Dip ECVO MRCVS, University of Bristol, Department of Clinical Veterinary Science, Langford House, Langford, Bristol, UK.

Chapter 15: Ocular diseases

GB Edwards, BVSc DVetMed MRCVS, University of Liverpool, Department of Veterinary Clinical Science, Leahurst, Neston, Wirral, Merseyside, UK.

Contribution to Chapter 2: Examination of the alimentary tract per rectum

TS Mair, BVSc PhD MRCVS, The Bell Equine Veterinary Clinic, Mereworth, Maid-stone, Kent, UK.

Chapter 12: Respiratory diseases

MW Patteson, MA VetMB DVC PhD Cert VR MRCVS, Vale Veterinary Group, Bushy Farm Equine Clinic, Breadstone, Berkeley, Gloucestershire, UK.

Chapter 9: Cardiovascular diseases

ED Watson, BVMS MVM PhD FRCVS, Department of Veterinary Clinical Studies, Royal (Dick) School of Veterinary Studies, Veterinary Field Station, Easter Bush, Roslin, Midlothian, UK.

Chapter 7: Genital diseases, fertility and pregnancy

Acknowledgements

The authors gratefully acknowledge the contributions from their colleagues listed on page vii. They are also indebted to Jane Craig MRCVS, and John Conibear for advice and help with the illustrations and photography. Vicki Martin BVSc, is warmly thanked for providing the line drawings.

Preface

This book is a response to the many telephone calls we receive from practitioners requesting either detailed information about a diagnostic technique, or an indication of the tests which might narrow down a list of differential diagnoses. Diagnosis is fundamental to the appropriate treatment and well-being of the equine patient, yet despite the many excellent clinical texts that are now available, few seem to explain in sufficiently precise terms which clinicopathological tests are appropriate and how particular techniques are performed. The aim of this book is to provide an illustrated practical guide to the various diagnostic techniques in equine medicine. It covers the adult horse and is intended for students, recent graduates and those veterinary practitioners who do not specialize in equine work and may be unfamiliar with some of the diagnostic approaches.

We have tried to ensure that the instructions are sufficiently detailed to allow completion of a procedure by following the text. Where appropriate, the advantages and disadvantages of a technique receive brief comment, together with a guide to the interpretation of results. For the purpose of practicality the techniques are grouped by chapter on an organ system basis.

In addition, a number of chapters have appendices which indicate applications of the described techniques to a given set of clinical circumstances such as anaemia, polyuria/polydipsia, nasal discharge, etc. It is emphasized throughout that clinical pathology and other diagnostic techniques are complementary to rather than a substitute for thorough clinical examination. The importance of recognizing clinical signs is paramount and these are given when relevant. Some of the specialized techniques made possible by recent advances in technology, such as nuclear scintigraphy and Doppler echocardiography, are beyond the scope of this book since they are not yet available to most practitioners. However, their diagnostic usefulness is indicated where appropriate so that their value in referring a patient to a specialist centre is appreciated. Each chapter concludes with suggested texts for further reading, the majority of which are easily accessible to the practitioner.

We hope that this book will prove useful to practitioners, and beneficial to their patients. We would welcome comments, suggestions and constructive criticisms.

FGR Taylor and MH Hillyer

Disclaimer

Every effort has been made to check the drug dosages given in this book. However, as it is possible that dosage schedules have been revised, the reader is strongly urged to consult the drug companies' literature before administering any of the drugs listed.

1 Submission of samples and interpretation of results

I. Submission of samples

Clinical pathology should be used either to confirm a diagnosis or to assist in the systematic deduction of a diagnosis. Laboratory investigations are not a substitute for a thorough history and clinical examination; they are complementary in that they provide further information.

Routine clinicopathological investigations include the following:

- Haematology
- Biochemistry of serum/plasma or other fluid
- Microbiology
- Histopathology

Many practices have established or are developing their own laboratory facilities, but in many cases it will be necessary to forward samples to a veterinary laboratory. One of the major limitations to test quality is the suitability of the sample which is received by the laboratory. Before submitting material, several factors should be considered:

- The choice of test
- The suitability of the sample for the intended test
- The information which should accompany the sample
- The suitability of packaging for postal or other delivery

Choice of test

The chosen test must be relevant and provide information concerning the implicated organ system. One of the purposes of this book is to indicate the range of clinicopathological tests that can be applied to the different organ systems of the horse. From these guidelines the clinician must select the laboratory tests most likely to confirm or refute a diagnosis based upon the history and clinical examination. A batch of ill-chosen tests will provide little or no information at considerable expense.

Suitability of the sample for the intended test

A sample can only be suitable if an adequate volume is collected into an appropriate container and submitted to the laboratory as quickly as possible. For evaluation of blood, serum, plasma and other fluids, a small volume is usually sufficient (no more than 2 ml), but this will obviously depend upon the number of additional tests required. Blood samples which are haemolysed or lipaemic are usually unsuitable for assay procedures and those taken from dehydrated animals will produce spuriously high biochemistry results.

Table 1.1 shows the samples and containers that are appropriate to particular tests, but the specific requirements of individual laboratories should always be checked. Many will supply their own preferred containers, pack-

Table 1.1. Appropriate samples and containers for clinicopathological tests

Test	*Sample*	*Container/medium*
Haematology		
Blood count +/- differential	Whole blood	EDTA
Plasma fibrinogen	Labs vary:	
	Whole blood (heat precipitation)	EDTA
	Plasma (thrombin coagulation)	Sodium citrate
Coagulation tests PT/PTT	Whole blood	Sodium citrate
Blood enzymes		
Most enzymes	Labs vary:	
	Serum usually preferred	Plain glass
	Plasma possible	Heparin
Glutathione peroxidase	Whole blood	Heparin
LDH	Serum	Plain glass
Blood electrolytes		
Serum electrolytes	Serum preferred	Plain glass
	Plasma electrolytes possible	Heparin

Table 1.1. Appropriate samples and containers for clinicopathological tests (*continued*)

Test	*Sample*	*Container/medium*
Other biochemistry		
Urea	Serum (preferred) or plasma	Plain glass or heparin
Creatinine	Serum (preferred) or plasma	Plain glass or heparin
Total protein	Serum	Plain glass
Albumin (and globulin)	Serum	Plain glass
Protein electrophoresis	Serum	Plain glass
Glucose	Plasma	Oxalate–fluoride
Total bilirubin	Serum (preferred) or plasma	Plain glass or heparin
Total serum bile acids	Serum	Plain glass
Serum triglycerides	Serum	Plain glass
Blood hormones		
Cortisol	Serum (preferred) or plasma	Plain glass or heparin
Thyroxine	Serum (preferred) or plasma	Plain glass or heparin
Triiodothyronine	Serum (preferred) or plasma	Plain glass or heparin
Progesterone	Serum (preferred) or plasma	Plain glass or heparin
Testosterone	Serum (preferred) or plasma	Plain glass or heparin
Oestradiol	Serum (preferred) or plasma	Plain glass or heparin
Oestrone sulphate	Serum (preferred) or plasma	Plain glass or heparin
PMSG	Serum	Plain glass
Blood culture		
Aerobic/anaerobic	Whole blood	Aerobic and anaerobic bottles or single system
Serology		
Bacterial/viral antibody	Serum	Plain glass
Urine		
Urinalysis	Urine	Clean non-leak container
Urinary fractional excretion of electrolytes	Urine plus serum (preferred) or plasma	Clean non-leak container plus plain glass or heparin
Culture	Mid-stream	Sterile non-leak container
Oestrogens (Cuboni test)	Urine	Clean non-leak container
Body fluids		
Cytology	Fluid	EDTA
Biochemistry	Fluid	Plain glass
Culture	Fluid	Plain sterile container
Faeces		
Faecal egg count	Faeces	Clean non-leak container
Larval count	Faeces	Clean non-leak container
Culture	Faeces	Clean non-leak container

aging and labels on request. It is well worth developing a working rapport with a veterinary laboratory which is reasonably close to the practice.

Haematology samples

The most suitable anticoagulant for haematological investigations is ethylenediamine tetra-acetic acid (EDTA). Heparin tends to cause 'clumping' of leucocytes and alters their staining properties. Plasma fibrinogen estimation can also be undertaken using an EDTA sample, but only if the laboratory employs a heat precipitation technique. The thrombin coagulation technique for fibrinogen estimation requires plasma to be submitted in sodium citrate. Blood coagulation studies (e.g. prothrombin time; partial thromboplastin time) require whole blood to be submitted in sodium citrate.

Blood samples should be collected at rest from the large free-flowing jugular vein. If possible, the horse should not be excited, but if this seems likely the first sample taken should be the one submitted for haematology, in order to minimize the effect of splenic contraction. The most convenient technique is the use of evacuated glass tubes ('Vacutainer': Becton-Dickinson, UK) containing EDTA. These are also available in unbreakable plastic but the vacuum life is shorter. Some laboratories prefer the use of polypropylene tubes for safe carriage in the post, but these are not evacuated and require filling from a syringe. In either case the tubes should be filled to capacity and gently mixed by several inversions.

When using a needle and syringe to collect blood before transfer into a container with anticoagulant, the following precautions must be observed:

- Blood must not be kept in the syringe for more than 90 seconds, otherwise clots form.
- The needle must be removed from the syringe before transferring blood into the sample tube, otherwise haemolysis may occur.
- The sample tube must be filled to the indicated line, otherwise the working concentration of EDTA will be incorrect. An increase causes changes in red cell size and inaccurate results, whereas a decrease predisposes clot formation.
- The blood must be mixed with the anti-coagulant by immediate, gentle inversion.

Haematology samples are best processed immediately, but this is often impractical and for short-term storage the tube should be kept cool or, if possible, refrigerated at 4° C. Ideally, an air-dried smear should always be prepared soon after the sample is taken. The reason is that prolonged contact of EDTA with cells can alter their morphology and the leucocytes become difficult to identify. The smear does not need to be stained for several days and can be dispatched to the laboratory in the unstained state, together with the blood sample. Special slide holders can be supplied by the referral laboratory for this purpose (Fig. 1.1).

Preparation of a blood smear

The glass slides used for smear preparation must be scrupulously clean and free from finger marks. Ideally, they should be stored in spirit and wiped dry with a tissue before use. The sample is well mixed by gentle inversion and a drop of blood is placed towards the end of a horizontal slide by pipette. The short edge of a second slide is used as a spreader and is placed

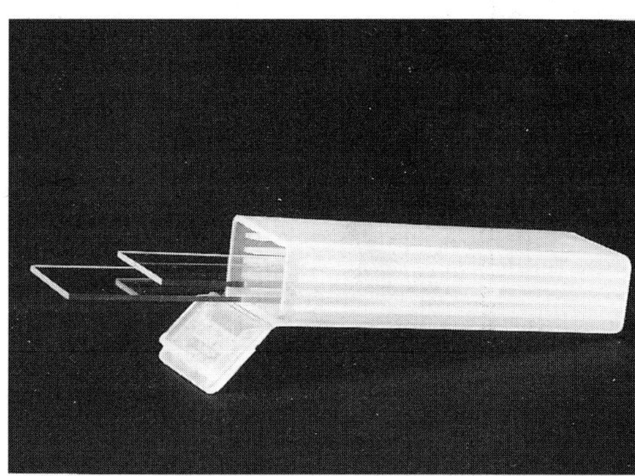

Figure 1.1   Polypropylene slide holder suitable for sending blood smears (courtesy of Grange Laboratories, UK).

in front of the drop of blood at an angle of about 40° (Fig. 1.2). It is first drawn gently backwards to make contact with the drop, which is immediately distributed along the spreading edge by capillary action. Once evenly distributed along this edge, the blood is then smeared along the length of the slide by a single, steady, forward movement of the spreader. The prepared smear is then dried quickly by waving it rapidly in air. The slide can be identified by writing across the centre of the dried smear with a pencil; this will not interfere with subsequent staining or the differential count.

The technique of smear preparation is easily acquired but requires a little practice. Poor smears are produced by one or more of the following mistakes:

- Using dirty slides and/or a chipped spreader
- Using a drop of blood that is too large
- Using a spreader angle that is insufficiently acute
- Using a forward movement that is too fast
- Using a slow, jerky forward movement

Biochemistry samples

Samples submitted for biochemistry may be of serum, plasma, or other fluid. *Serum is preferred by most laboratories for blood biochemistry and is essential for certain tests such as serology (antibody titration) and protein electrophoresis.* Although a perceived advantage of plasma is that it is easily

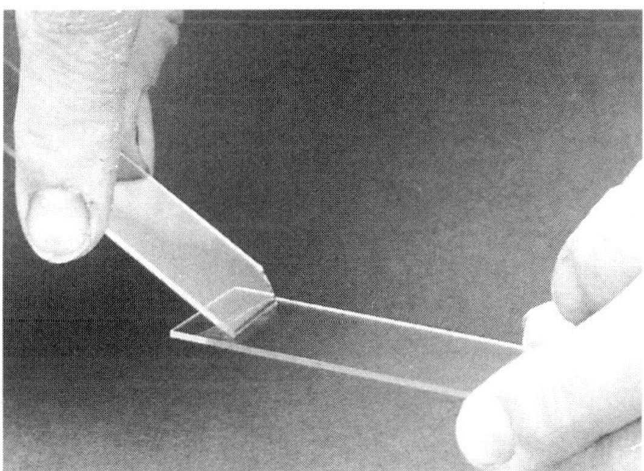

Figure 1.2   Preparing a blood smear.

separated from whole blood by standing or centrifuging prior to dispatch, it is unsuitable for some electrolyte and enzyme estimations and it does not store satisfactorily. Where plasma is acceptable, the blood should be collected into heparin anticoagulant. Common container requirements are shown in Table 1.1.

Whether clotted or heparinized samples are used, the serum or plasma should be separated from red cells as soon as possible to avoid interactions between the two. The worst extreme, haemolysis, results in red cell constituents interfering with the measurement of enzymes, electrolytes and minerals. Haemolysis can be minimized by using clean dry equipment, avoiding perivascular blood sampling and by not traumatizing the sample during or after collection. Postal samples of whole blood sent during extremes of hot or cold weather are particularly prone to haemolysis.

Serum separation

An optimal serum yield can be obtained by collecting blood into a plain evacuated glass tube ('Vacutainer': Becton-Dickinson, UK) and leaving it to stand in a warm room, or a 37° C incubator, to allow optimal clot formation. Once the clot has formed, it can be freed from the sides of the container with a length of sterile swab stick and left to retract fully from the glass surface. The serum can then be decanted into a clean container or, ideally, centrifuged to sediment the clot and cells. Many laboratories now recommend the use of unbreakable polypropylene tubes for safe transit of samples in the post.

If this separation procedure is not possible, the whole blood sample should be kept cool (4° C) until dispatch in order to decrease the rate at which enzymes, metabolites, electrolytes and minerals are exchanged between the cells and fluid.

For practices having a centrifuge, special serum-gel tubes ('Monovette': Sarstedt, UK) are available, which permit a one-step separation of serum in a clotted sample. Venous blood is drawn by syringe and transferred to the tube. Subsequent centrifugation interposes an inert gel between the cells and serum, thus ensuring good results after transit.

Microbiology samples

Where possible, samples should be collected before the use of antibiotics and due care should be taken to avoid contamination. Appropriate precautions are given in the relevant sections of this book.

Sufficient quantities of material should be submitted in sterile containers. *Sample volume and transport conditions directly influence the prospect of obtaining positive results.* If a fluid sample can be obtained, it should be submitted in a container and not absorbed onto a swab. The identification and interpretation of culture results can be helped by preparing and fixing a smear (for subsequent Gram stain) at the time of sampling.

In some instances swabs may provide an inadequate sample for culture and unless submitted in an appropriate transport medium they will certainly dry out and the microorganisms will die. Swabs can be used to obtain specimens from the conjunctivae, freshly ruptured skin pustules, deep wounds and soft tissue infections. The selection of a suitable transport medium depends upon the suspected organism(s) and should be discussed with the referral laboratory, which will probably supply the media and appropriate packaging material. These considerations are particularly important to the successful isolation of viruses from nasopharyngeal swabs.

In general, the ideal samples for culture are aseptically collected pus, exudate or tissue fluid. These are best collected into sterile containers with airtight screw-caps. Fluids that are normally sterile such as blood, and pleural, peritoneal and synovial fluids, should be aspirated by syringe since the risk of contamination is then minimized and larger volumes are made available for culture. Faeces should also be submitted in a screw-cap bottle; containers with push-on caps are to be avoided.

For the culture of anaerobes, samples must be protected from air because most clinically important obligate anaerobes cannot survive more than a brief exposure to atmospheric oxygen tensions. This can be achieved by placing a swab in a suitable transport medium, or filling a container with the sample in order to minimize the air gap.

Antibiotic sensitivity tests

For all practical purposes it is usually necessary to begin antibiotic treatment before the results of sensitivity testing are available. In such cases antibiotic choice is dictated by clinical judgement based on experience. However, it is important that a sample for isolation of the causative organism should be taken before treatment begins. In the laboratory, some bacteria which are recognized by Gram stain and culture may have predictable sensitivity patterns and therefore testing is not always necessary. Others, such as Gram-negative facultative anaerobes (*E. coli*, *Salmonella* spp. etc), do not have predictable sensitivity patterns and warrant testing.

Referral laboratories may offer a range of antimicrobial sensitivity tests but most commonly employ direct antibiotic sensitivity testing, in which an antibiotic disc is placed on the surface of a plate which has been cultured or subcultured from the original sample. Although this technique offers a relatively quick result, the information obtained is empiric and less useful than the more sophisticated dilution techniques which provide information on the minimum inhibitory concentration (MIC) of an appropriate antibiotic. The likely significance of an isolate and its supposed sensitivity pattern should be discussed with the microbiologist if it is not indicated in his/her report.

Histopathology samples

Specimens for histology should be fully representative of the lesion and should usually include the junction between normal and abnormal tissue. Samples should be fixed in 10% formol-saline and be of a sufficiently small size to allow rapid penetration of the fixative. As a guide, a diameter of no more than 1 cm, and a thickness of no more than 5 mm, are ideal dimensions; but not all specimens will permit this. The volume of tissue to fixative should be no more than 1:10 and both should be placed in a sturdy, wide necked container which can be sealed (the wide-neck facilitates specimen removal).

Special fixatives are sometimes required for certain procedures such as endometrial biopsy, cytology or immunofluorescence. These should be discussed with the referral laboratory, which will probably be able to supply them.

Information which should accompany the sample

Most laboratories supply their own request forms indicating the type of information required. Some detailed clinical history is essential, particularly in the case of histopathology which is expected to produce a diagnosis. In most cases a tentative differential diagnosis is also useful to the laboratory; it helps with the interpretation of findings and/or suggests further tests.

Packaging for postal or other delivery

In general, most tests are not significantly affected by a postal transmission period of up to 48 hours, but samples sent late in the week will inevitably be subjected to delivery and processing delays. Some samples are of sufficient bulk or urgency to warrant a courier delivery service. If the laboratory is within travelling distance, the client may be willing to deliver the specimen personally. However, he/she should understand that discussion of the results and their implications must, in the first instance, be between the laboratory and the referring veterinary surgeon.

For most samples postal delivery services are acceptable, but the onus is on the sender to ensure that the packaging complies with legal requirements and that the sample will not expose anyone to danger. In the UK, the Royal Mail's conditions for sending samples must be observed, otherwise they may be destroyed and the sender made liable to prosecution. For packaging requirements in other countries, check with the appropriate postal service. As a guide to packaging, the Royal Mail approves the following procedure:

- *Primary containers.* A sealed container, such as an evacuated glass or polypropylene blood tube, should be wrapped in sufficient absorbent material to contain all possible leakage. This is then sealed in a leak-proof plastic bag. Any container must not exceed 50 ml capacity, but special multi-specimen packs are approved; providing that each primary container is separated from the next by sufficient absorbent packing (Fig. 1.3).
- *Secondary containers.* The primary package must be placed in either: a strong cardboard box with a full depth lid; a grooved two-piece polystyrene box sealed with self-adhesive tape; a cylindrical light metal container with a screw-top lid, or a polypropylene clip down container (Fig. 1.4).
- *Outer packaging.* The complete package is then placed in a padded bag. These are available in various standardized sizes (Fig. 1.5).
- *Labelling.* The label must clearly declare that the package is a 'PATHOLOGICAL

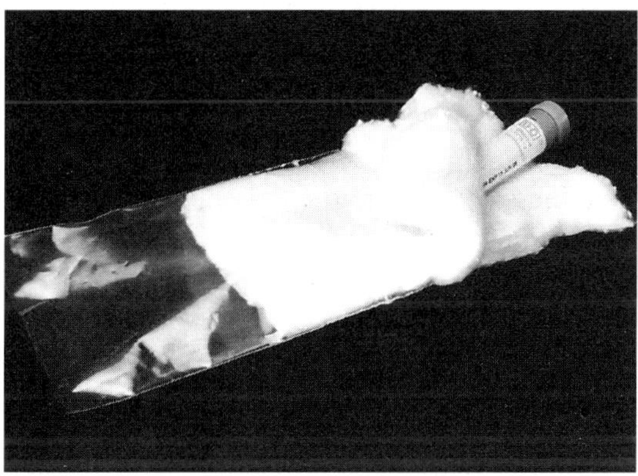

Figure 1.3   Primary package. The sample tube is wrapped in absorbent material and sealed in a leak-proof plastic bag.

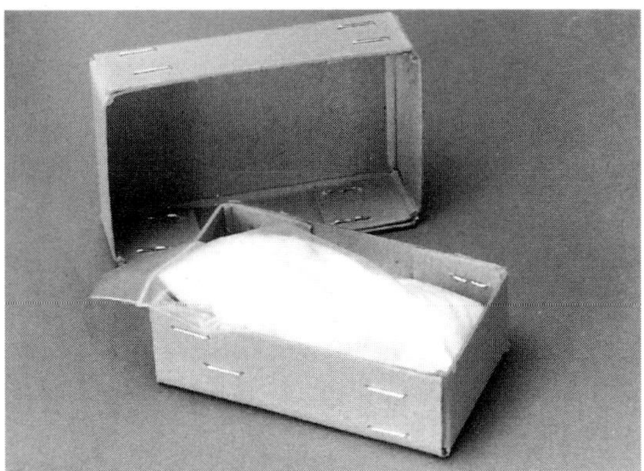

Figure 1.4   The primary package is placed in a secondary container – in this case a cardboard box with a full depth lid.

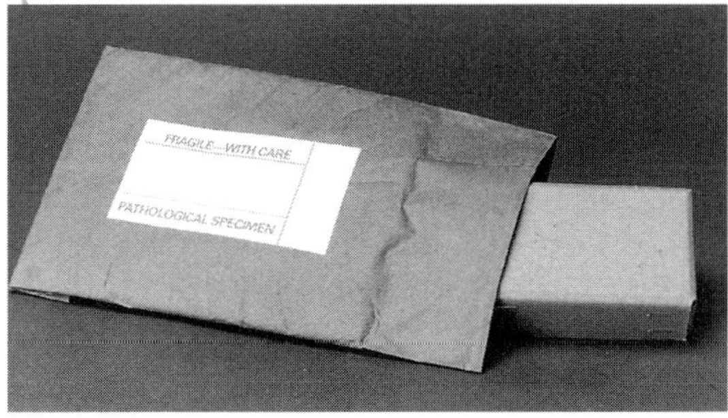

Figure 1.5   The complete package is placed in a padded bag bearing a clear hazard warning address label.

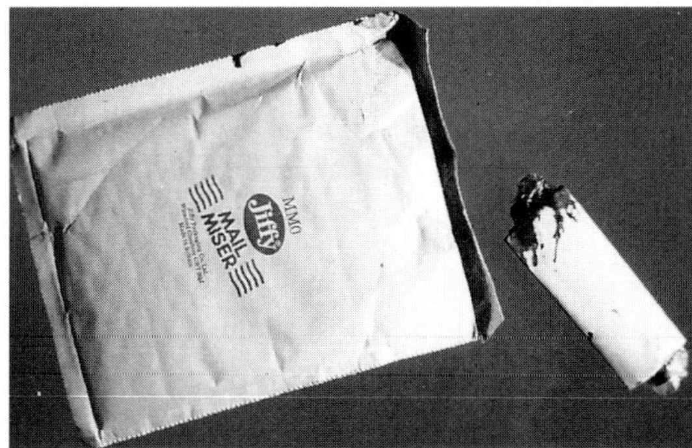

Figure 1.6   Smashed blood tube and soiled packaging due to inadequate packing precautions. The tube was wrapped in the referral notes which were rendered unreadable.

SPECIMEN' and must bear the warning 'FRAGILE — WITH CARE' (Fig. 1.5). As well as the laboratory address, the package must bear the name and address of the sender.

Figure 1.6 shows an example of unsatisfactory packaging in which the primary container has no absorbent wrap or secondary container. The padded bag failed to protect the sample from destruction and exposed those handling it to pathological material.

II. Interpretation of results

A disease process is dynamic and has a beginning, a middle and an end. However, a solitary test result obtained somewhere along this time course can only reflect the situation at a fixed point, and this limits its interpretation. By analogy, it is like attempting to uncover the plot of a movie from a single frame. It is often more informative to have the results of several sequential samples, but the costs may be unacceptable. The purpose of this section is to act as a guide to the interpretation of haematology and blood biochemistry reports.

In many instances the clinical history and examination that led to the selection of a test will lend weight to its interpretation. Where a marginal abnormality is reported, a repeat submission at a later time will confirm or refute a significant trend. *One of the traps to avoid in evaluating laboratory data is overinterpretation of scant or inconclusive information.* However, pathological situations are most usually associated with dramatic and recognizable changes.

Normal laboratory ranges

Before any tentative interpretations can be made, the normal laboratory range for a parameter must be considered. In general terms, a result will be reported as below, within, or above its accepted range. However, normal ranges invariably differ between laboratories. In some cases this is due to inherent differences in analytical procedure and is most marked in the quantitation of serum enzyme activity; in this instance the same tests on the same sample will produce different results in different laboratories. *In consequence, haematology and biochemistry results must always be interpreted in the context of the normal range given by the referral laboratory.*

Normal ranges for clinical pathology data are usually derived from the mean values ($\pm$ 2 standard deviations) of a healthy horse population. However, this concept excludes 5% of samples from the normal range; that is, 2.5% of normal samples will predictably be above the upper normal range and 2.5% will be below the lower normal range. In consequence, it is difficult to be certain that the result of a single sample, obtained from an unfamiliar patient, is a reliable indicator of disease; unless the parameter value is extreme.

Interpretation of haematology

Haematology profiles display marked differences between breeds and crossbreeds (see below), but are usually fairly consistent between laboratories. Some differences will occur as a result of laboratory operator technique and subtle differences in the settings of automated counters. However, this does not usually affect the interpretation of obvious changes or trends in haematology.

Erythrocyte parameters

It is important to realize that adult equine erythrocyte parameters are subject to a number of physiological variables which will influence laboratory results. These include breed, current fitness, and activity or excitement at the time of sampling.

- *Breed.* The 'hot-blooded' breeds (light horses, Arabians and Thoroughbreds) have higher erythrocyte parameters in terms of packed cell volume (PCV), red blood cell count (RBC) and haemoglobin concentration (Hb), than 'cold-blooded' breeds (native ponies and draught horses). Interbreeds, such as hunter types, lie somewhere in between. Table 1.2 illustrates this point by showing typical erythrocyte ranges for the different groups.
- *Fitness.* Fit horses show a higher PCV, RBC and Hb than those that are resting or unfit. Fit racing Thoroughbreds therefore have the highest of these parameters. A result in a fit horse which is at the low end of a normal range should be regarded as abnormal.
- *Activity or excitement.* Recent exercise, or excitement at the time of sampling, will significantly increase the PCV, RBC and Hb as a result of splenic contraction.

In a healthy horse it is usual to find day-to-day variations in red cell parameters, but these should all be within the normal range indicated for the breed. In an unhealthy horse, an increase in parameters above the normal range suggests dehydration. Decreases below the normal range suggest anaemia (see 'Anaemia' in Chapter 8: 'Blood disorders').

Table 1.2. Typical erythrocyte parameter ranges* for different groups of adult horse.

Parameter	Thoroughbred	Hunter	Pony
PCV%	40–46	35–40	33–37
RBC x 10^{12}/l	7.2–9.6	6.2–8.9	6.0–7.5
Hb g/dl	13.3–16.5	12.0–14.6	11.0 –13.4
MCHC g/dl	34–36	34–36	33–36
MCV fl	48–58	45–57	44–55
MCH pg	14.1–18.1	15.1–19.3	16.7–19.3

*Adapted from data supplied by the Clinical Pathology Diagnostic Service, Department of Clinical Veterinary Science, University of Bristol.

Packed cell volume (PCV)

The PCV is a measure of the volume percentage of red cells in whole blood. It is easily determined by centrifuging a column of whole blood to separate the cellular elements from the plasma. The volume occupied by packed cells is then expressed as a percentage of the total volume (PCV%). Being easily determined, it is the most useful monitor of dehydration (haemoconcentration) during a disease process.

Red blood cell count (RBC)

The red cell count is expressed as the number of red cells per litre of whole blood (RBC x 10^{12}/l).

Increases over the normal range are consistent with haemoconcentration, whereas decreases are consistent with anaemia.

Haemoglobin (Hb)

The haemoglobin content of whole blood is expressed as the concentration per 100 ml (Hb g/dl). Increases over the normal range are consistent with haemoconcentration, whereas decreases are consistent with anaemia.

Mean corpuscular haemoglobin concentration (MCHC)

The MCHC is an index of the haemoglobin concentration per 100 ml of *packed red cells* expressed as g/dl. It is obtained by multiplying the haemoglobin concentration of whole blood (Hb g/dl) by the packed cell factor (100 divided by PCV%).

Mean corpuscular volume (MCV)

MCV is an index giving the average volume of each erythrocyte in femtolitres (fl). It is calculated by dividing the volume of red cells per litre (PCV% x 10), by the number of red cells per litre (RBC x 10^{12}/l). Depending upon the reported volume, the cells may be variously described as microcytic, normocytic or macrocytic. However, unlike in other species, these features are not useful in interpreting regenerative or non-regenerative types of anaemia in the horse since equine erythrocytes mature within the bone marrow rather than in the circulation, even during intense erythropoiesis. In consequence, the MCV is seen to progressively increase or decrease over time, but it usually remains within a normal range. The best indicator in the horse of whether an anaemia is regenerative or non-regenerative is a bone marrow aspirate or biopsy (see Chapter 8: 'Blood disorders').

Mean corpuscular haemoglobin (MCH)

This index is an expression of the average haemoglobin content of a single cell in picograms (pg). It is obtained by dividing the concentration of haemoglobin in a litre (Hb g/dl x 10) by the number of red cells in a litre (RBC x 10^{12}/l). An increase above the normal range is consistent with haemolysis.

Leucocyte parameters

As with erythrocytes, the white blood cell parameters are also subject to physiological variables. These usually take the form of a leucocytosis which can be induced by apprehension, stress, or recent exercise.

White blood cell count (WBC)

In the healthy adult the white cell count is usually between 6–12.0 x 10^9/l, and the resting ratio of neutrophils to lymphocytes is about 60:40. Small numbers of monocytes and/or eosinophils may be present, but each will not normally exceed 5% of the total count.

Leucopenia is a depression of the WBC below normal limits and is a feature of endotoxaemia and/or septicaemia. It therefore occurs in gut catastrophes associated with toxaemia or in the early stages of any severe bacterial disease (e.g. pleuropneumonia; peritonitis; salmonellosis).

Leucocytosis is an elevation of the WBC above normal limits and is a feature of acute and chronic inflammatory disease. Leucopenia, which is associated with the early stages of a bacterial disease, invariably progresses to a state of leucocytosis over 2–3 days.

Neutrophils

Neutrophilia occurs in response to inflammation (often but not invariably associated with infection), stress, or the concurrent use of corticosteroids. Acute inflammatory leucocytosis features a neutrophilia and, if severe, juvenile band forms appear ('left shift'). In protracted states of toxaemia, the cytoplasm fails to complete its maturation and is reported as 'foamy'.

Lymphocytes

Lymphopenia occurs during the early stages of viral infection and is attributed to lymphocyte sequestration in lymphoid tissues. The count recovers within a few days. The lymphocyte count can also be depressed by stress and the concurrent use of corticosteroids.

Monocytes

In health, monocytes hardly feature in the differential count and they are depressed in acute disease. However, chronic inflammatory leucocytosis is usually accompanied by a monocytosis.

Eosinophils

In health, the eosinophil portion of the differential count is low. Eosinophilia may be provoked by hypersensitivity responses and in some instances this could be associated with the early stages of active parasite migration. However, in the authors' experience eosinophilia cannot be interpreted as pathognomonic of parasitism; neither do heavily parasitized horses necessarily show an eosinophil response.

Basophils

Basophils rarely feature in the differential count of healthy horses. In other species they are regarded as circulating mast cells, but the role associated with their appearance in the circulation of sick horses is undefined.

Platelets

The normal platelet count of horses is low compared with other domesticated species. An abnormally low count may be an artefact of 'platelet clumping' in EDTA. If thrombocytopenia is suspected on clinical grounds, a sample for platelet count should be submitted in sodium citrate rather than EDTA.

Plasma fibrinogen concentration

Estimation of the plasma fibrinogen concentration is not usually part of a haematology profile. However, some laboratories employ a heat precipitation technique using whole blood in EDTA, so that it may be convenient to report it with a haematology profile. Other laboratories use a thrombin coagulation technique which requires a plasma sample submitted in sodium citrate.

Plasma fibrinogen is an acute phase protein, the circulating concentration of which increases to a peak within 48–72 hours of the onset of an inflammatory process. *It is a sensitive indicator of septic inflammation in the horse and in the authors' experience is a more reliable monitor of disease progression than blood leucocyte counts.* It is particularly useful in monitoring the response to antibiotic treatment. A persistently raised fibrinogen concentration is consistent with an ongoing bacterial inflammation, despite any apparent normality of the WBC and its differential count.

Interpretation of blood biochemistry

Table 1.3 shows typical blood biochemistry ranges for the adult horse, but excludes serum enzyme activities. Serum enzyme concentrations (international units per litre) are estimated using commercial kits which are optimized for different reaction temperatures. Different laboratories may use different kits, and the results and normal ranges may differ accordingly. For this reason the authors do not attempt to provide normal enzyme activity ranges. It is preferable for the clinician to interpret the significance of an enzyme result against the normal range for the referral laboratory. It is the responsibility of that laboratory to ensure, through quality control procedures, that the results accurately reflect a comparison with their own normal ranges. Non-enzymic blood constituents that have absolute concentrations, such as g/l or mmol/l, are relatively unaffected by analytical conditions but even so, variations occur. *When communicating or discussing test results, the clinician should always be prepared to quote the laboratory's normal range.*

Table 1.3. Typical blood biochemistry ranges* for the adult horse.

Content	Range
Total protein	60–70 g/l
Albumin	30–40 g/l
Globulin	20–35 g/l
Urea	3.2–5.2 mmol/l
Creatinine	128–188 µmol/l
Glucose	3.5–6.0 mmol/l
Total bilirubin	11–49 µmol/l
Sodium	135–145 mmol/l
Potassium	3.3–5.0 mmol/l
Chloride	93–103 mmol/l
Calcium	2.86–3.06 mmol/l
Magnesium	0.6–1.0 mmol/l
Inorganic phosphorus	0.81–1.21 mmol/l
Triglycerides	<1.0 mmol/l

*Adapted from data supplied by the Clinical Pathology Diagnostic Service, Department of Clinical Veterinary Science, University of Bristol.

The various chapters in this book that deal with the different organ systems give specific indications for clinical biochemistry, together with the interpretation of results. The notes below serve as a brief collective reference to the interpretation of blood biochemistry in the horse.

Serum proteins

The total serum protein (g/l) is a measure of the combined concentration of albumin and globulins in the serum. A gradual increase in the total protein over days/weeks usually reflects an increase in the globulin component as a result of infection and/or inflammation. Sudden increases probably reflect dehydration. However, many diseases associated with progressive dehydration may also be accompanied by albumin loss (e.g. gastrointestinal crises), and in these instances total protein is not a sensitive indicator of dehydration. Because of this, sequential PCV determinations may be preferable indicators of patient dehydration.

Albumin

Albumin is synthesized in the liver. Increases in serum concentration may be associated with dehydration, but decreases are most usually associated with a *protein losing enteropathy* and therefore reflect alimentary disease. A less likely cause of hypoalbuminaemia in the horse is loss to effusion (e.g. peritonitis; pleuritis), and least likely causes are glomerulonephropathy or liver failure.

Globulin

Apart from dehydration, total globulin concentrations may also be increased by:

- Acute inflammatory processes causing increases in acute phase protein concentrations
- Chronic inflammatory processes causing increases in immunoglobulin concentrations
- Strongyle parasitism causing increases in $IgG_{(T)}$ concentration
- Liver failure resulting in decreased catabolism of globulins

Some veterinary laboratories offer an assay of serum $IgG_{(T)}$ concentration. If raised above the normal range it is evidence of active strongyle migration, but it is not pathognomonic.

Albumin/globulin (A/G) ratios

In health, the A/G ratio approximates to 1.0 or more. Shifts in the ratio may occur in a number of pathological states, but the information lacks specificity. A fall in the ratio, owing to a decrease in albumin and an increase in globulin, may be a feature of either inflammatory bowel disease, exudative effusion (e.g. peritonitis; pleuritis), strongyle parasitism, or liver failure. Any chronic inflammatory process in which the globulin concentration increases will also cause the ratio to fall, even if the albumin concentration remains normal.

Serum protein electrophoresis

Agarose gel electrophoresis separates equine serum proteins into four fundamental bands, which are characterized in order of their electrophoretic mobility. These bands are stained and identified as albumin with subdivisions of alpha, beta and gamma globulins. Once the total protein concentration is known, the laboratory can determine the individual protein concentrations within each band by densitometer. However, the results of electrophoretic analysis of horse serum are not always comparable between laboratories because of differences in the separative technique. As a result there are conflicting data regarding the 'normal' concentration ranges of the various protein fractions. Clinicians are therefore advised to interpret protein shifts as empirical increases or decreases, rather than absolute values. Table 1.4 shows an empiric interpretation of protein shifts.

Serum enzymes

In health, the circulation contains low levels of most intracellular enzymes derived from normal cell turnover. In disease, there is a release of enzymes from damaged cells, which increases their circulating concentration. Depending upon organ specificity, these enzymes may be used diagnostically to identify the diseased organ or cell type. The major drawbacks to interpretation are the ubiquitous nature of some enzymes and the poor stability of others. Poor stability results in a rapid loss of activity between collection and assay.

Alkaline phosphatase (SAP or ALP)

ALP may be released following damage to the intestinal epithelium, the hepatobiliary tract, or bone. Many laboratories can narrow these differentials by estimating the concentration of the isoenzyme *intestinal alkaline phosphatase (IAP)*. Increases in ALP concentration are either associated with gut damage (parasites or other inflammation), biliary obstruction, or increased bone metabolism. Serum ALP has good stability in transit.

Amylase

In health, amylase concentrations in the circulation of horses are very low. The concentration is significantly increased in serum, peritoneal fluid and urine during pancreatic necrosis. This is a very rare condition in the horse which presents as acute intractable colic. However, because of its rarity, it is unlikely that a differential of pancreatitis would be pursued in cases of acute colic and the diagnosis usually follows post-mortem examination. Amylase is very stable in serum.

Aspartate aminotransferase (AST or AAT)

This was formerly designated glutamine oxaloacetate transaminase (GOT) and is still found as such in the literature. The enzyme is released following cell disruption in a number of soft tissues including the liver, skeletal muscle, and cardiac muscle. When the concentration is found to be

Table 1.4. Empiric interpretation of serum protein shifts as revealed by electrophoresis.

Disease	Albumin	Alpha	Beta	Gamma
Acute infection	Normal	++ (APPs)	Normal	Normal
Chronic infection	Normal	+ (APPs)	+ (IgG$_{(T)}$)	++ (Igs)
Viral infection	Normal	Normal	+ (IgG$_{(T)}$)	++ (Igs)
Intestinal parasitism	Low (PLE)	++ (APPs)	++ (IgG$_{(T)}$)	Normal
Hepatic failure	Low	Normal	Normal	+++ (Igs)

Abbreviations: PLE = protein losing enteropathy; APPs = acute phase proteins; Igs = Immunoglobulins; IgG$_{(T)}$ = Immunoglobulin G (subclass T).

increased, a cross-check on the serum concentration of a muscle-specific enzyme, most conveniently *creatine phosphokinase*, will indicate whether or not the likely origin is muscle. A slight increase above normal range is usual after exercise. Serum AST in transit will lose some 10% of its activity over 3 days at ambient temperature.

Creatine phosphokinase (CPK or CK)

The highest concentrations of this enzyme are found in skeletal muscle, heart muscle and brain tissue. Modest increases follow hard exercise, but massive increases in the circulation are invariably associated with muscle damage (*rhabdomyolysis*). Serum CPK has good stability in transit.

Gamma glutamyl transferase (GGT or γGT)

This enzyme is found in the liver, renal tubules and pancreas of the horse. An increase in the circulating concentration is almost invariably associated with liver disease. Serum GGT has excellent stability in transit.

Glutamate dehydrogenase (GLDH)

GLDH is liver specific and increases in the circulating concentration reflect acute or ongoing hepatocyte damage. Unfortunately, its stability in transit is not good; serum GLDH will lose some 15% of its activity over 3 days at ambient temperature.

Glutathione peroxidase (GSH-Px)

GSH-Px is a red cell enzyme isolated from heparinized whole blood, but it is considered here under 'Serum enzymes' for convenience. It is a sensitive indicator of dietary selenium. GSH-Px activity will vary between stables (i.e. different feeding regimes), but should remain constant throughout the year.

Lactate dehydrogenase (LDH)

LDH is widely distributed in all tissues (including muscle, liver and intestine), and an increase in the circulating concentration is therefore of little diagnostic value. Subsequent estimation of the relative concentrations of its five iso-enzymes is more useful, since each of these is more organ specific. However, the more involved (and costly) analysis offers little advantage over other enzyme estimations. Serum LDH has good transit stability for up to 3 days.

Sorbitol dehydrogenase (SDH)

SDH is substantially liver specific and is used to detect acute or ongoing liver damage. It has a short half-life and therefore declines to a normal range once the hepatic insult ceases to be progressive. Unfortunately, it is not stable in blood and the assay must be undertaken as soon as possible after sampling and certainly within 24 hours. Serum SDH will lose well over 50% of its activity within 3 days at ambient temperature.

Blood urea and creatinine

An increase in the circulating concentrations of urea and creatinine (azotaemia) is consistent with a state of renal failure. However, some 75% of glomerular function is lost before azotaemia becomes apparent and it is therefore an insensitive indicator of the onset of failure. Nevertheless, once raised, urea and creatinine concentrations reflect improvements or deteriorations in the glomerular filtration rate and become useful monitors of disease progress.

Small increases in blood urea concentration alone (i.e. up to two-fold, with creatinine remaining within its normal range), frequently accompany dehydration and/or wasting diseases associated with increased tissue catabolism. Feeds which are high in protein may also raise blood urea slightly.

Blood glucose

An increase in blood glucose above the normal range is often transient and as such is relatively common. Causes include insulin resistance (stress, pregnancy and/or obesity) and corticosteroid or α_2 agonist administration. Persistent hyperglycaemia is uncommon in the horse and is most usually the result of hyperadrenocorticism (see 'Hyper-glycaemia' in Chapter 5: 'Endocrine diseases'). Hypoglycaemia is very uncommon in horses, but can be associated with anorexia or liver failure.

Serum bilirubin

An increase in total bilirubin may be sufficient to cause jaundiced membranes and is seen in a variety of equine diseases which include liver disease, haemolysis, impaction colic, and any condition associated with a chronic reduction in food intake. However, it is not usual for serum bilirubin to be elevated in equine liver disease; an increase may be diagnostically useful, but normal values do not discount liver disease. In fasting (or inappetance) there is a physiological decrease in the removal of bilirubin by hepatocellular transport. *Anorexia, for whatever reason, is probably the commonest cause of hyperbilirubinaemia and jaundiced membranes in the horse.*

Electrolytes

Sodium, potassium, chloride, calcium, magnesium and phosphorus can be measured in either serum or plasma. However, whole blood samples should be separated soon after collection because any tendency to haemolysis will alter electrolyte concentrations in both serum and plasma.

Sodium

Sodium is the major cation within the extracellular fluid and is largely responsible for maintaining the osmotic forces which regulate the compartment's fluid volume. However, the laboratory estimation of serum or plasma sodium should not be interpreted in absolute terms as a blood deficit or excess. This is because its concentration at any one time depends upon the exchangeable body stores of water, sodium and potassium, which are able move in and out of the circulation and produce changes in the serum or plasma sodium concentration.

Hyponatraemic states (<135 mmol/l) usually occur in diarrhoeic diseases where massive losses of fluid and electrolyte are followed by the oral intake of water and partial replacement of lost fluid. Hyponatraemia therefore indicates a relative water excess. Hypernatraemic states (>145 mmol/l) are rare but may be associated with acute dehydration in which water loss exceeds that of electrolytes. Excess sodium replacement during fluid therapy will also cause hypernatraemia.

Potassium

Potassium is the major cation of the intracellular fluid and estimations of its serum or plasma concentration are of very limited value in inferring total body potassium.

Hypokalaemia (<3.3 mmol/l) is often associated with increased intestinal loss (diarrhoea) or, importantly, a decreased food intake. *Large amounts of potassium are excreted by the normal equine kidney, so that deficits soon occur when the horse's feed intake is reduced.* Marked hypokalaemia is usually indicative of alkalosis because in alkalotic states cells take up potassium and release hydrogen.

Hyperkalaemia (>5 mmol/l) is unusual in the horse unless associated with haemolysis, impaired renal function, muscle necrosis, or severe acidosis. In acidotic conditions potassium leaves cells in exchange for hydrogen ions, so that the circulating potassium concentration increases. Spurious hyperkalaemia may follow blood sample spoilage by haemolysis or leakage of potassium out of red cells. If possible, hyperkalaemia should be confirmed by a second blood sample. For obvious reasons, whole blood samples are unsatisfactory if laboratory processing is delayed.

Chloride

Chloride is largely located in the extracellular fluid, so that changes in its serum or plasma concentration tend to reflect changes in its whole body status.

Hypochloraemia (<93 mmol/l) is usually the result of increased loss to the gastrointestinal tract (diarrhoea or high obstruction) or, alternatively, prolonged heavy sweating. In the extracellular fluid, chloride concentrations are inversely related to bicarbonate concentrations, so that hypochloraemia is usually accompanied by metabolic alkalosis.

Hyperchloraemia (>103 mmol/l) may be associated with acute dehydration (when water is lost in excess of electrolytes), or metabolic acidosis.

Calcium

Calcium exists in the blood in three states: ionized; chelated and protein-bound. In the laboratory, calcium estimation in serum or plasma measures the total of all three, but only the ionized portion is biologically active.

Hypocalcaemia (<2.86 mmol/l) is most usually associated with a reduced feed intake. Clinical hypocalcaemia develops only when the circulating concentration of ionized calcium falls below the homeostatic requirement. In these circumstances the patient may show a low total serum or plasma calcium concentration, but this is not a reliable measure of the biologically available (ionized) calcium.

Persistent hypercalcaemia is a rare disorder of horses which usually reflects a regulatory problem (see 'Hypercalcaemia' in Chapter 5: 'Endocrine diseases').

Blood calcium concentrations may be influenced by renal disease, but the effect is not consistent in horses. Acute or chronic renal disease may be accompanied by low, normal or high blood calcium levels.

Magnesium

Magnesium estimation in serum or plasma has little diagnostic value. Low concentrations occasionally accompany hypocalcaemia and as such may be associated with neuromuscular irritability and muscle stiffness ('tetany').

Inorganic phosphorus

Like calcium and magnesium, the estimation of phosphorus in serum or plasma may be of little diagnostic value. With the exception of acute conditions, such as clinical hypocalcaemia, the circulatory concentrations of these minerals are often within normal ranges, despite whole body abnormalities. This is because complex homeostatic mechanisms act to sustain their blood concentrations.

If renal function is believed to be normal, the investigation of whole body electrolyte status (including phosphorus) is best addressed by evaluating the urinary fractional excretion of electrolytes (see 'Rhabdomyolysis and the fractional excretion of electrolytes' in Chapter 13: 'Musculoskeletal diseases').

Triglycerides

In healthy animals under adequate conditions of nutrition, the serum triglyceride concentration is usually less than 1 mmol/l. Short-term fasting may produce a physiological lipaemia which is reversible and without clinical sequel. In hyperlipaemic states the value exceeds 5 mmol/l and the serum or plasma develops a visible opacity. In extreme cases a cloudy, milk-like appearance develops, which renders the sample unfit for any biochemical or haematological analyses.

Serum biochemistry profiles

Most clinical pathology laboratories offer an equine biochemistry profile at a cost advantage over the individual tests. The clinician should always aim to select laboratory investigations which are complementary to a thorough history and clinical examination, rather than 'trawling' a profile. However, when the clinical examination is inconclusive, such profiles can be useful in identifying further routes of investigation. A typical profile is shown in Table 1.5, together with a tentative interpretation of abnormalities and suggestions for further investigations.

Table 1.5. Tentative interpretation of a serum biochemistry profile with suggestions for further investigations.

Test	Result	Possible cause & investigation
Urea	Uraemia	Dehydration: check PCV Tissue catabolism: check indicators of inflammation High protein diet Renal failure: compare serum creatinine concentration
Total protein	High	Dehydration: check PCV High globulin: check SPE: 　　　　Raised alpha: acute inflammation 　　　　Raised beta: parasitism 　　　　Raised gamma: chronic inflammation
Albumin	Low	Protein-losing enteropathy: If diarrhoeic: check salmonellosis; faecal larvae and SPE (cyathostomiasis); rectal biopsy No diarrhoea: check strongylosis (FEC & SPE); SAP (or IAP) activity; oral glucose tolerance test Liver failure: check liver enzymes; function tests Renal disease: check urea and creatinine; urinalysis Loss to inflammatory effusion: check paracentesis
Globulin	High	Parasitism: check SPE Chronic inflammation: check SPE Liver failure: check liver enzymes; function tests
AST	High	Soft tissue damage: check indicators of inflammation Acute or progressive liver disease: check liver-specific enzymes; function tests Myopathy: check CPK activity
γGT	High	Liver disease: check other liver enzymes; function tests
SAP	High	Hepatobiliary disease: check liver-specific enzymes; function tests Gut damage: check SAP (or IAP) activity; serum albumin concentration Bone damage

Abbreviations: PCV = packed cell volume; SPE = serum protein electrophoresis; FEC = faecal egg count; SAP = serum alkaline phosphatase; IAP = intestinal alkaline phosphatase; CPK = creatine phosphokinase; AST = aspartate aminotransferase; γGT = gamma glutamyltransferase.

Further reading

Blackmore DJ and Brobst D (1981) *Biochemical Values in Equine Medicine.* Newmarket: Animal Health Trust.

Jain NC (1986) The horse: Normal hematology with comments on the response to disease. In: *Schalm's Veterinary Hematology*, 4th edn, pp 140–177. Philadelphia: Lea & Febiger.

2 Alimentary diseases

I. Practical techniques

Examination of the mouth

The usual indications for examination of the mouth are headshaking or refractory behaviour while being ridden, excessive salivation, and difficulty in chewing and/or swallowing (dysphagia). In addition, any horse suffering reduced food intake and/or weight loss should have its mouth examined.

Restraint

The horse should be reversed diagonally into a corner to prevent backward movement and a competent handler should stand close to the side of the head, facing forwards. A strong headcollar should be used, but the nose and jowl pieces should be sufficiently slack to allow the mouth to open wide. Some horses resent manipulation within the mouth to the extent that sedation may be necessary if clinical circumstances permit. The clinician should always be aware that he/she will be examining directly in front of the animal and will therefore be vulnerable to rearing and striking. Where appropriate, some protection is afforded by securing a horse blanket to the patient's neck and draping it in front of the forelegs.

External examination

An external examination of the mouth is made by standing to the side of the animal, facing forwards, and separating the lips with both hands to reveal the labial mucosa and incisor teeth. The colour of the mucous membranes is noted together with the presence of abnormal features such as petechial or ecchymotic haemorrhages. Inspection of the incisors may reveal abnormalities in bite (e.g. parrot mouth), deciduous teeth, supernumerary teeth, or undue wear owing to crib-biting or poor grazing (chronic close cropping at the soil surface). Sharp edges to the upper cheek teeth can be palpated through the cheeks, where associated regional pain may also be found.

Internal examination

The mouth may be held open for more detailed examination by using the patient's tongue as a gag or, alternatively, using a gag manufactured for the purpose.

Use of the tongue

Standing to one side or other of the horse, the clinician introduces his/her hand into the interdental space to grasp the free end of the tongue. This is brought out through the interdental space and gently lifted to a position between the cheek teeth to hold the mouth open (Fig. 2.1). Care should be taken not to injure the ventral frenulum by pulling the tongue too hard. The clinician should also beware of impaling the tongue on a canine tooth during manipulation. The hold is more assured if the little finger of the hand grasping the tongue is hooked around the halter or head collar.

The clinician's free hand may now direct a pen torch to view the teeth and soft structures on the opposite side of the mouth. The teeth on this side may also be palpated by careful insertion of the fingers inside the cheek. Providing the tongue is held between the horse's teeth on the opposite side, it will not attempt to bite the examiner's hand for fear of biting its own tongue.

The other half of the mouth may then be examined by releasing the tongue, taking hold of it again through the opposite interdental space, and repeating the procedure. The tongue itself should not be overlooked during examination, lack of normal tone during manipulation suggests paralysis.

Use of the Swale gag

The Swale gag, and allied designs, act by holding apart the cheek teeth on one side of the mouth, allowing the clinician to examine the opposite side. It is available in a range of sizes and is simple and safe in use (Fig. 2.2).

The clinician opens the mouth by moving the tongue to one side as described above and inserting the gag between the teeth of the opposite side (Fig. 2.3). The handle of the gag may be held by the assistant standing at that side or fastened to a ring on the headcollar by

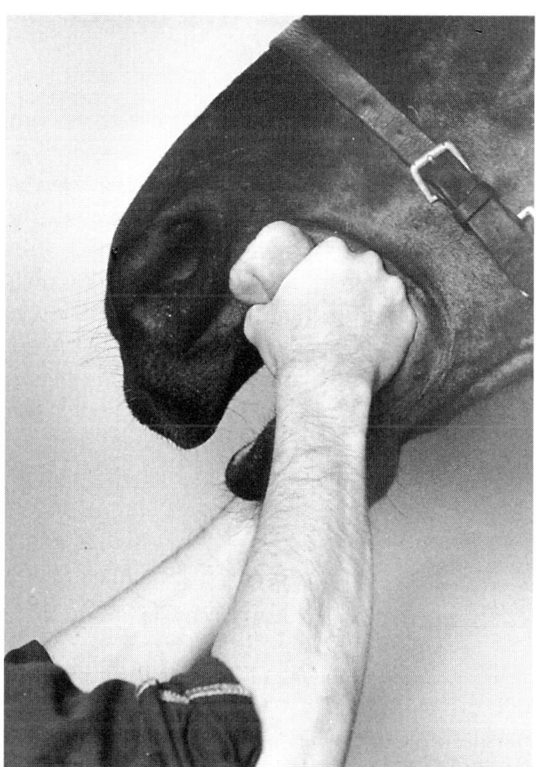

Figure 2.1 Examination of the mouth using the tongue as a gag.

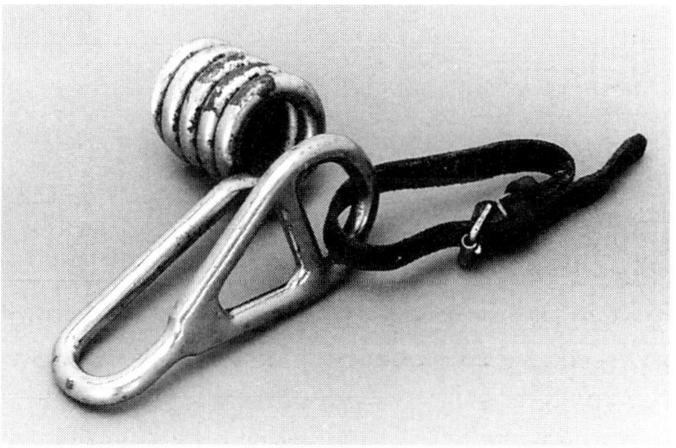

Figure 2.2 The Swale gag.

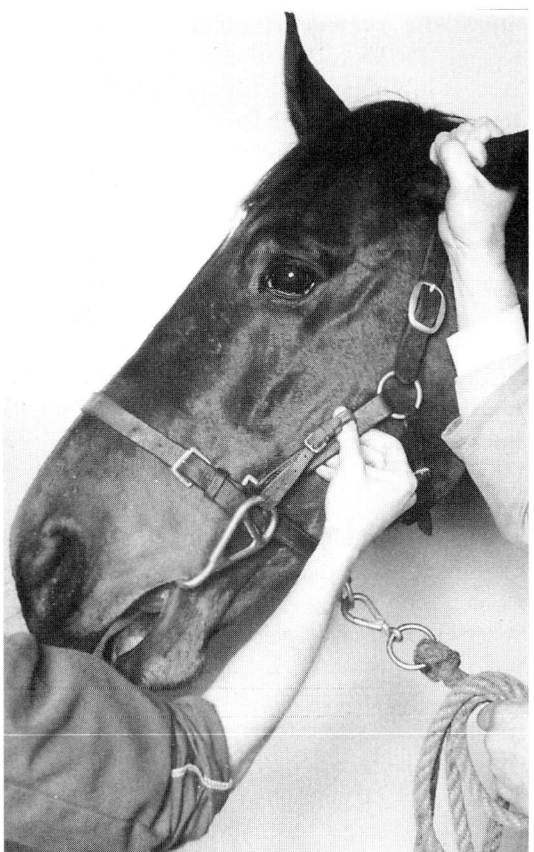

Figure 2.3   The Swale gag in position.

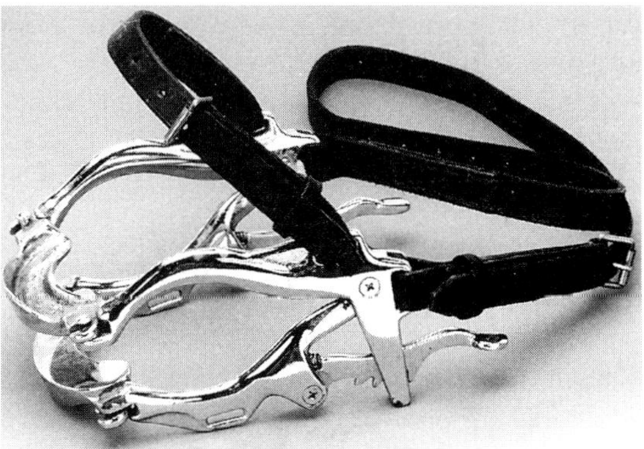

Figure 2.4   The Haussman gag.

a small strap supplied by the manufacturer for that purpose.

Use of the Haussman gag

This is a more sophisticated gag which is applied over the headcollar (Fig. 2.4). Two plates rest on the incisor tables and are moved apart by a ratchet system which prises the jaws to the required distance and then locks the position (Fig. 2.5).

This gag allows the maximum amount of room for examination and/or manipulation within the mouth and can be released instantly. Its disadvantage is the danger to personnel if the horse becomes fractious during adjustment or when the gag is in place.

Comments

● Examination should include an assessment of mouth odour — a distinct carious smell suggests entrapped food, caries or bone necrosis.

● On occasion a satisfactory examination of the mouth is only possible under short-term general anaesthesia.

Radiography of the upper alimentary tract

Comprehensive radiography and fluoroscopy of the upper alimentary tract are restricted to centres with specialized equipment. However, good quality diagnostic radiographs of the teeth, pharynx and oesophagus of adult horses are possible using portable units with settings ranging from 60 kV and 30 mA, to 90 kV and 15 mA. *This of course presumes that stringent safety precautions are possible in line with current ionizing radiation regulations.* The use of fast rare earth screen/film combinations and, where appropriate, positive contrast media, produces diagnostic films at lower exposures.

Radiography of the teeth

Radiographs are useful in determining the extent to which dental disease involves periodontal tissues. Diagnostic radiographs are best obtained under short-term general anaesthesia which also facilitates detailed inspection. Lateral and oblique views are

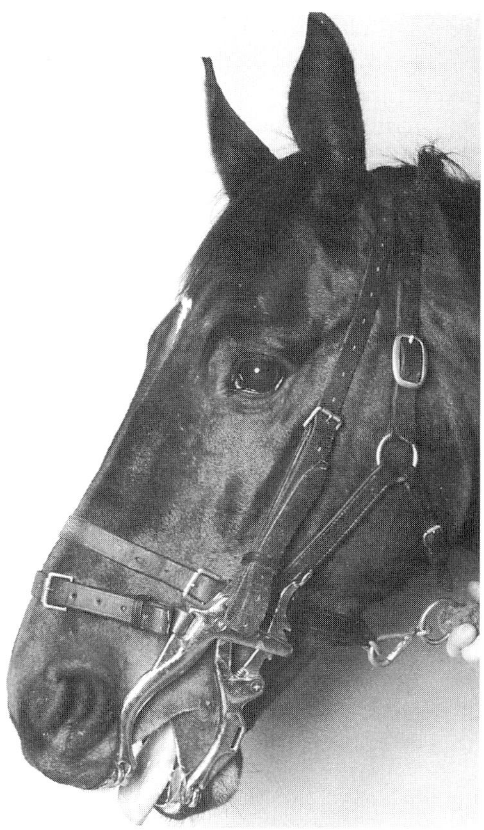

Figure 2.5 The Haussman gag applied.

obtained with the jaws held apart by an incisor gag and the horse positioned with the diseased side next to the cassette. An isolated image of the diseased root is best obtained using a 45° beam, which prevents superimposition of the images formed by the diseased and normal arcades. The X-ray beam should be directed from the nasal side for the maxillary cheek teeth, and from the mandibular side for the mandibular cheek teeth.

Radiography of the oropharynx

Plain lateral radiographic views of the pharynx reveal gross lesions, such as a retropharyngeal mass or guttural pouch enlargements (blood, pus or gas), which can compress the pharynx. On rare occasions fracture of the hyoid bone is diagnosed in this way.

Technique

Lateral radiographs of the pharynx are usually obtained in the conscious, standing animal. Sedation may be needed in fractious animals, but can also be useful in others to keep the head and neck in a lowered position.

The horse should be held in a rope halter with no metal attachments. The handler should stand directly in front of the horse and it may be useful for the horse's head to be supported under the chin by a lead-gloved hand. This also allows the height of the horse's head to be controlled and positioned within the primary beam. No part of the handler's body should encroach on the primary beam, even if shielded.

The cassette should be placed in a mechanical support and not held manually. A practical support can be contrived from a bag, into which the cassette is inserted, suspended from a drip stand. The cassette is then positioned against the side of the horse's head and aligned with the tube which is centred on the area of interest. Standard radiographs of the oropharynx are obtained by centering on the caudal edge of the vertical ramus of the mandible immediately dorsal to the larynx.

The presence of air in the nasopharynx, larynx, trachea and guttural pouches provides good contrast with the adjacent soft tissues. A short focus to film distance (1.0–1.3 m) allows a short exposure time to be used and thereby minimizes any movement blur on the radiograph. kV/mA settings will vary with the size of the horse.

Although gross lesions are identifiable using plain films, the more subtle soft tissue problems require contrast radiography. Barium sulphate suspension given orally by catheter syringe (60 ml) will outline the oropharynx, lateral food channels and cranial oesophagus. Obstructions such as a subepiglottic mass or oesophageal diverticulum/stricture may then be identified easily. In cases of dysphagia (e.g. pharyngeal paralysis), attempts at swallowing usually disperse barium sulphate into the nasopharynx, larynx and trachea. In cases of complete pharyngeal stasis no contrast medium is seen to reach the oesophagus.

Radiography of the oesophagus

The radiographic appearance of the normal, empty oesophagus is indistinct owing to its collapsed state. An outline is only apparent when air, fluid, food material or a radiopaque foreign body are present. Oesophageal radiography may therefore be of diagnostic use in the dysphagic patient.

Radiographs of the cervical oesophagus are possible in most adults using portable equipment, but investigations at the level of the thoracic inlet and shoulders require the use of more high powered equipment. However, views of the thoracic oesophagus behind the shoulder are also possible with portable equipment.

Technique

Radiographs of the oesophagus can be obtained in the conscious standing animal. Sedation may be used if necessary. The cassette is suspended against the side of the horse as described above for oropharyngeal radiography.

Multiple exposures are needed to cover the length of the oesophagus. The exposure factors will also vary along the length of the oesophagus according to the amount of soft tissue present at the various levels. For each exposure the beam is centred on the known path of the oesophagus down the neck and through the thorax. As a rough guide the oesophagus would be included in standard views of the cervical vertebral column and the dorsal lung fields.

The normal oesophagus is a collapsed soft tissue tube and as such is not visible on plain radiographs. However, the lumen may be delineated in pathological conditions or by the use of contrast agents. Impacted ingesta will be visible along a length of oesophagus in cases of choke and air will be visible in cases of megoesophagus.

Greater clarification of oesophageal anomalies is obtained using contrast radiography. This is achieved by giving 60–180 ml barium sulphate suspension *per os* by catheter syringe or via a nasogastric tube which is passed as far as the upper cervical oesophagus. In either case the suspension may

be given neat or in warm water. Investigation of the mid- to lower cervical oesophagus requires the larger volume given by a nasogastric tube.

Using contrast medium, the normal oesophagus appears collapsed and its longitudinal mucosal folds may be outlined. Any obstruction will disrupt the flow of medium, thus producing a radiolucent outline of the foreign body. Oesophagitis, e.g. following the relief of an obstruction, may be associated with thickening of the longitudinal folds and the pooling of contrast medium owing to a motility disturbance. Oesophageal diverticuli are also demonstrable using contrast radiography.

The narrowing of a column of contrast is consistent with either stricture, neoplasia or external compression by a perioesophageal mass, whereas an 'hour glass' shape indicates pre- and post-stenotic dilatation. NB A normal peristaltic contraction 'caught' at exposure may be confused with stenosis. This possibility can be investigated by taking a second radiograph of the same area.

Extensive dilatation and pooling of contrast media suggests megoesophagus which often accompanies the intestinal stasis and gastric distension of grass sickness — but it should not be regarded as a pathognomonic sign.

Oesophageal transit time

An assessment of oesophageal transit time can be achieved by serial radiography of the passage of contrast suspension. This must be given by catheter syringe, not a nasogastric tube. Alternatively, the passage of a food bolus, such as mash mixed with contrast agent, can be followed in the same manner.

In normal horses the passage of a fluid bolus from the cricopharynx to the stomach is rapid, occupying some 5–10 seconds, and solid boli are only a few seconds slower. Liquid contrast does not pool in the normal oesophagus and little contrast residue is left after the passage of a treated food bolus. In contrast, most oesophageal lesions are associated with significantly longer clearance times; minutes to hours. Post-obstructional oesophagitis, stricture, and all motility disorders are associated with impaired transit times, so that serial radiographs reveal minimal movement of a bolus.

Comments

- Normal oesophageal peristalsis will give the appearance of a 'false' stricture or dilatation when caught at exposure. In contrast studies it should be remembered that swallowing (of medium) is the trigger for a peristaltic wave. If the interpretation is in doubt, repeat the exposure.

- Dynamic studies using image intensification are more reliable and informative in assessing the swallow reflex and the speed of passage of a bolus through the oesophagus to the stomach. However, these techniques are only available at specialist centres.

- In dyspnoeic animals free gas may be seen in the oesophagus. This is usually secondary to an increased respiratory effort.

Endoscopy of the upper alimentary tract

Endoscopy should be used routinely to examine the nasal, pharyngeal, laryngeal and upper oesophageal regions in cases of dysphagia. Direct observation of swallowing enables assessment of pharyngeal function. In addition, foreign bodies, inflamed tissues, defects of the palate and pharyngeal cysts are easily identified.

Endoscopy of the nasopharynx

Most young horses show a dense aggregation of lymphoid tissue in the dorsal pharyngeal recess (lymphoid hyperplasia). On occasion plaques of lymphoid tissue extend down to the nasopharyngeal roof. In horses above six years of age the nasopharyngeal mucosa is relatively smooth (see also 'Endoscopy' in Chapter 12: 'Respiratory diseases').

Defects of the soft palate are readily recognised. The most common is a midline cleft extending through the soft palate. Touching the nasopharynx of a healthy horse with a catheter or forceps wire (protruded through the biopsy channel) usually stimulates a swallow in which the elevation of the soft palate is seen, together with the opening of both guttural pouch flaps. In cases of pharyngeal hemiplegia, one side of the pharynx may be seen to be immobile during the swallow. *In complete paralysis there are no pharyngeal movements and the soft palate remains permanently displaced above the epiglottis* (Fig.2.6). In such cases food material is often seen on the soft palate and within, and around, the larynx.

Comment

- In some healthy horses there may be a reluctance to swallow. In addition, the soft palate may be displaced above the epiglottis during endoscopic examination of a normal animal. A diagnosis of pharyngeal paralysis must therefore be made with care, after repeated attempts to stimulate swallowing.

Endoscopy of the oesophagus

The endoscope may be directed towards the oesophageal entrance and introduced into the oesophagus in the same way as a stomach tube. This can be achieved in the conscious horse with minimal restraint. Oesophagoscopy may complement oesophageal radiography but it is of unique value for inspection of the mucosal lining — especially after the relief of an obstruction. Transendoscopic procedures such as biopsy, foreign body retrieval and laser surgery are restricted to specialist centres.

Examination of the entire oesophagus of an adult horse requires an endoscope of at least 2 m length. Ideally, gastroscopic examination should accompany oesophagoscopy as gastric lesions are often associated with oesophageal disorders. However, the common endoscope lengths preclude this, allowing examination of the proximal oesophagus only.

Because normal oesophageal tone causes the wall to collapse on the endoscope, it is necessary to use inflation with air (insufflation)

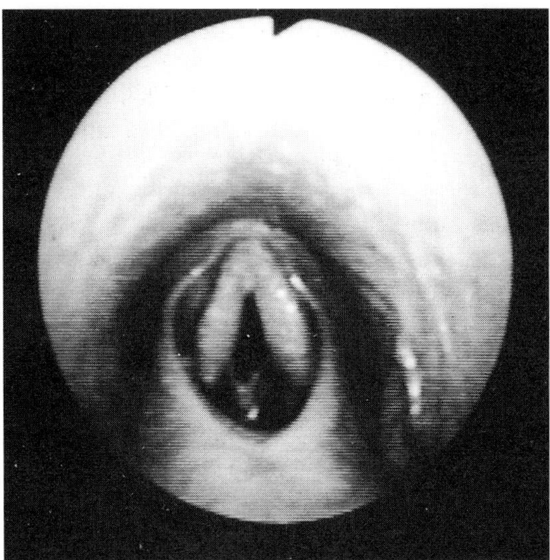

Figure 2.6 Endoscopic view of displacement of the soft palate above the epiglottis in a case of pharyngeal paralysis.

during examination. Observations are best made by starting with the endoscope fully inserted and then examining the mucosa during withdrawal under insufflation.

Normal appearance

The mucosal surface is pink and thrown into longitudinal folds which become more prominent in the distal oesophagus. There is a natural narrowing of the lumen in the postpharyngeal area, the thoracic inlet, the heart base and the terminal oesophagus.

Anomalies of appearance

Inflammation (oesophagitis) is readily apparent, with or without ulceration or perforation of the luminal wall. An inability to dilate the lumen at some point suggests a stricture or external compression of the oesophagus. The appearance of transverse mucosal folds under insufflation is pathognomonic of a mural lesion, but these must be distinguished from the folds that are inevitably produced by the forward passage of the endoscope in a collapsed oesophagus. Linear mucosal ulcers in the distal oesophagus which are progressively more abundant

towards the cardia are consistent with reflux oesophagitis and are typically associated with grass sickness. In some of these cases a retrograde movement of gastric fluid may be seen.

Comments

- The cranial cervical oesophagus is difficult to examine adequately by endoscope because repeated stimulation of the swallow reflex causes the tip of the endoscope to be directed dorsally. Structural anomalies in this region may be outlined on a radiograph following oral administration of a barium suspension by catheter syringe.

- In obstructive lesions of the oesophagus, food material may be packed down above the lesion so that endoscopy cannot identify the underlying cause of the problem. In these cases food deprivation for 24 hours may allow identification of a partial obstruction, such as a twig. If not, radiography may be more helpful.

- Oesophageal disorders are often best assessed by radiography or endoscopy and in many instances both techniques are required for a complete examination.

Gastroscopy

This is precluded in practice since commercial gastroscopes are insufficiently long for adult horses. An alternative is to pass the endoscope via a presternal oesophagotomy. However, oesophagotomy and its attendant complications can be justified only in cases of extreme urgency and the technique is best left to specialized surgical units.

Abdominal auscultation

Gut sounds reflect gut activity and the greatest value of abdominal auscultation is in the assessment of colic. As a routine, at least four sites are auscultated: both paralumbar fossae and both sides of the lower abdomen.

Normal sounds

Abdominal sounds are for the most part generated by the caecum and large colon. There are two components: weak sounds associated with localized bowel contractions (mixing the ingesta), and louder fluid sounds or borborygmi associated with peristalsis (propelling the ingesta onwards). One or both of these sounds should be audible during a minute's auscultation at each site.

Sounds heard in the right paralumbar fossa reflect ileocaecal (and possibly caecocolic) valve activity and differ from the other sites. Here, a period of silence is broken once or twice a minute by a sudden rush of fluid rumbling as secretions from one compartment pass through the valve and hit the gas/fluid interface of the next.

Anomalies of sound

A simple obstruction in an otherwise healthy gut provokes hyperperistalsis in adjacent gut segments. The best example is spasmodic colic in which continuous sounds, of greater than usual intensity, are heard at all sites.

In contrast, reflex movement is reduced by inflammation and ischaemia. An absence of sound, or infrequent sounds of reduced intensity, may therefore be associated with peritonitis or the development of gut hypoperfusion. A deteriorating colic with progressively diminishing gut sounds suggests the development of a crisis in which the blood supply to the gut is compromised. An absence of sound is also associated with alimentary paralysis as in post-operative ileus and grass sickness. A reduction in the intensity and frequency of ileocaecal sounds sometimes accompanies ileocaecal intus-susception.

The presence of entrapped gas (tympany) is denoted by low-pitched tinkling sounds which may be superimposed on other alimentary sounds — as, for example, in tympany associated with spasmodic colic. The localization of entrapped gas in a segment of the large bowel may be appreciated by simultaneous percussion and auscultation over the abdominal wall. A distinctive 'hollow' sound is audible where a volume of gas is trapped against the body wall. This area may be 'mapped out' on the side of the animal to determine its extent.

It is particularly useful to monitor gut sounds in assessing the progress of a colic, or the post-operative recovery from a colic. The re-establishment of a normal frequency and intensity of sound is a good prognostic sign. The authors find it useful to record these sounds at each site using a simple scale of intensity: 0; +–; + or ++ equivalent to absent, reduced, normal or increased.

Comment

- In assessing the colic patient, the significance of gut sounds must be evaluated within the context of all other clinical signs. In the case of a return to normal sound the prognosis is probably favourable, whereas the outcome for a reduction or absence of sound is more difficult to predict.

Examination of the alimentary tract per rectum

Contributed by Professor GB Edwards

Rectal examination is the single most important part of the clinical work up of a horse with colic. It should be carried out after reviewing the relevant aspects of the history and physical examination. In this way an attempt can be made to predict what should be felt and to compare the actual findings with the preconceived ideas.

While rectal examination is of considerable value in the diagnosis of benign problems (such as primary impaction and tympany of the large intestine, and the intestinal hyperactivity of spasmodic colic), it is of greater importance in recognizing those cases which require surgical intervention. Many of these can be diagnosed by rectal palpation before the animal deteriorates, or changes in the peritoneal fluid become apparent. *The early diagnosis and referral of these cases significantly improves the prognosis and reduces the occurrence of post-*

operative complications. Rectal examination should therefore be performed in all colic cases whenever possible, but it must be approached with a respect for its value and the risks involved.

Restraint

Adequate restraint is essential to prevent damage to the horse or examiner. When rectal examination is carried out in a stable or barn, restraints may include the use of a twitch, sedation (e.g. xylazine) or raising a foreleg. For right-handed examination, the horse is positioned with its right flank against the wall and the handler restrains the animal to the left of the head, which should be drawn into the corner. In this way, forward and right-sided movement are restricted. If the clinician uses the left hand for rectal examination, the horse should be positioned with the left flank against the wall and the head should be restrained on the right side. Stocks provide a safeguard against being kicked, but the examiner must always be wary of the horse going down suddenly.

Technique

The examiner should stand to the side of the tail base, close to the horse's quarters, with his/her back to to the animal's head. This minimizes injury in the event of a sudden kick. The tail is raised with the free hand and a well-lubricated rectal sleeve is introduced into the rectum. In doing this the fingers and thumb should be brought together to form a cone for slow introduction through the anal sphincter. Any resistance on the patient's part usually relates to the width of the knuckles passing through the sphincter. Care should be taken to ensure no tail hairs are carried into the rectum and all faeces within reach must be removed prior to any attempt to palpate structures. Thereafter, forward movement of the hand should always be performed slowly with the fingers and thumb brought together in a cone shape. Exploratory palpation should not be undertaken with a wide spread of fingers and

thumb since this can predispose rectal trauma. If confronted with a strong peristaltic wave the cone shape should be resumed and the examiner should be prepared to withdraw the hand.

Assuming patient compliance by the time the forearm has been introduced, the examiner can move to a position behind and in line with the horse in order to allow the full reach of his/her arm during examination. Once the arm has been introduced to its full length it is advisable to hold it still for 30 seconds, during which time the colon usually relaxes. In particularly difficult cases, injecting 60 ml of xylocaine into the rectum or applying xylocaine gel to the rectal sleeve may be helpful.

The abdominal and pelvic contents should be palpated by running the hand along the surfaces rather than by grasping any structures through the gut wall. At the end of any examination the hand should be checked for any bloodstained faeces or frank blood. If there is concern that a rectal tear has occurred, greater sensitivity in exploring the lesion is achieved by wearing a plastic sleeve, with the fingers cut off, under a surgical glove.

A systematic examination can now begin bearing in mind that it is limited to the caudal 40% of the abdomen even in small horses and ponies.

Normal structures

The normal structures palpable in the left dorsal quadrant include the spleen, the caudal pole of the left kidney and, linking the two, the nephrosplenic ligament (Fig. 2.7). Moving to the right and extending forwards in the midline below the spine, the root of the mesentery can be palpated — although in large horses the reach may be difficult. Specific arterial identification may be impossible and it is frequently easier to identify the caecocolic artery at the base of the caecum rather than the cranial mesenteric artery.

In the right dorsal quadrant the base of the caecum is identified. Normally the caecum is not full and the caudal and medial taeniae

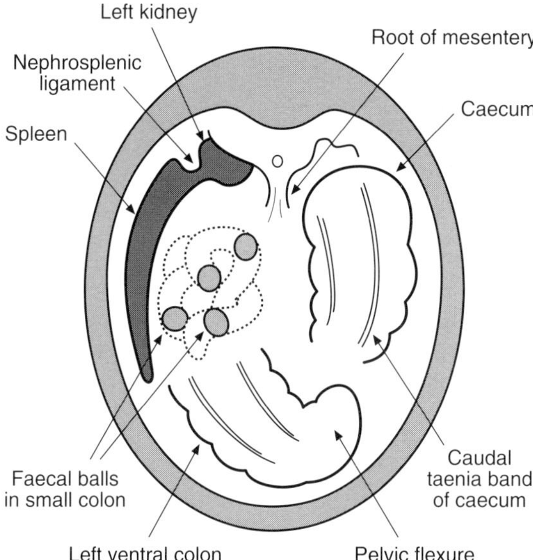

Figure 2.7   Normal disposition of structures which are palpable per rectum.

bands, running from dorsal to ventral, are fairly relaxed and allow the fingers to be hooked around one or other of them so that painless traction can be applied to the caecum.

Moving ventrally to the pelvic brim and somewhat to the left, the pelvic flexure of the large colon containing soft ingesta can usually be detected. Extending cranially from the pelvic flexure are the left ventral colon, with its large diameter and clearly recognizable longitudinal bands, and the narrower, smooth left dorsal colon.

The space above this and to the left of the caecum is usually occupied by the small intestine and small colon. The normal small intestine is usually not palpable unless it happens to contract when touched, but the small colon is easily recognized by the formed faecal balls it contains.

The inguinal canals can be felt in the stallion to either side of the pelvic opening at the pubic brim. The bladder, when distended, can limit palpation of organs cranial to it. This problem can be alleviated by catheterization, or stimulating the animal to urinate by putting it in a box with clean bedding.

In general, easy entry, the presence of normal faeces and a relaxed abdomen with ample room for movement of the arm, tend to rule out a serious lesion. However, tense painful loops of intestine distended with gas and fluid which are displaced back towards the pelvic inlet and upwards towards the roof of the abdomen, indicate a severe obstruction.

Abnormal structures

Although specific diagnoses can be made on the basis of rectal findings, more often the examiner can only determine distension in a specific segment of bowel, or a particular position which identifies an obstruction.

Abnormalities of the stomach and small intestine

Diseases of the stomach are rarely identifiable on rectal examination. The spleen may give the impression of being pushed caudally by gastric distension but splenic enlargement is common and will mimic this finding. The author has, on two occasions, palpated a massively impacted stomach which was found at laparotomy to extend almost to the umbilicus.

Obstructions of the small intestine or adynamic ileus produce distension recognizable as one or more distended loops containing gas and fluid. Strangulating lesions usually lead to tighter distension. The number of loops palpable depends on the nature, duration and location of the lesion. In the early stages of obstruction, careful and patient palpation over a period of several minutes may be necessary before a distended loop is recognized. As the small intestine continues to distend it folds onto itself forming accordion-like loops (Fig. 2.8). These may be positioned vertically or horizontally and can occupy any quadrant of the abdomen, but eventually the tightly distended loops push back into the pelvic inlet making examination difficult. *The presence of distended small intestine almost always indicates a problem requiring surgical correction.* Early identification greatly enhances the chances of recovery.

In *anterior enteritis* (proximal duodeno-

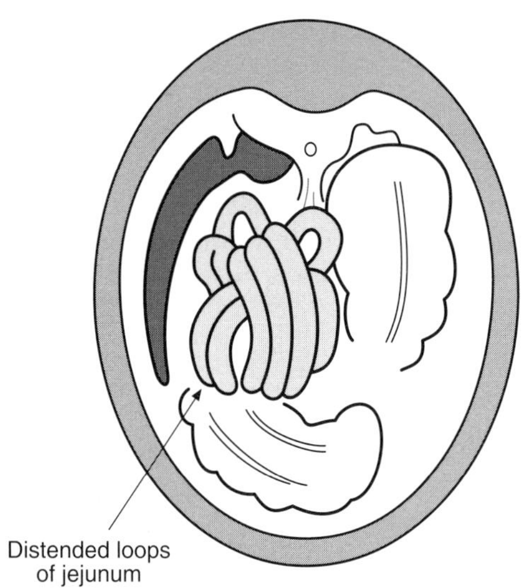

Figure 2.8 Well-established obstruction of the small intestine.

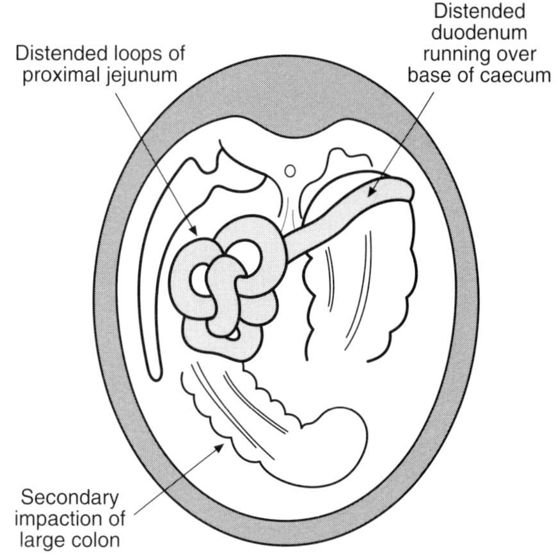

Figure 2.9 Palpable anomalies associated with anterior enteritis.

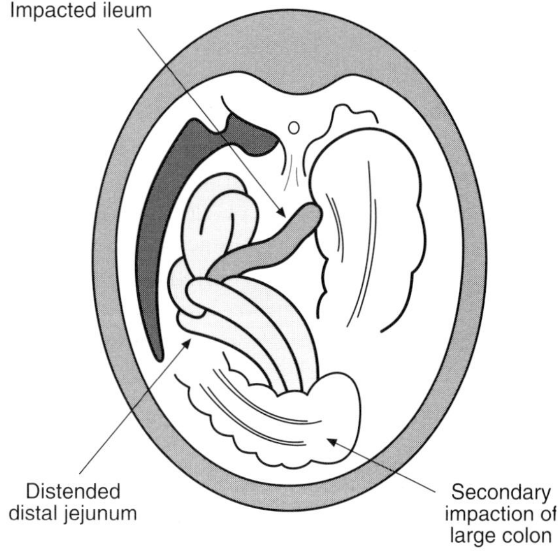

Figure 2.10 Palpable anomalies associated with impaction of the ileum.

jejunitis) the duodenum is distended and can readily be felt as a tubular structure over the base of the caecum in the right dorsal quadrant (Fig. 2.9). Some distension of the proximal jejunum may also be present, but the gut is not so tightly distended as in obstructions.

Impaction of the ileum can be identified in the early stages as a firm tubular structure 12–16 cm in diameter, medial to the base of the caecum (Fig. 2.10). Later on, distension of much of the jejunum, if not all, will prevent palpation of the ileum.

Ileocaecal intussusception can be recognized as a firm, enlarged, tubular or coiled structure (depending on the length invaginated) within the base of the caecum in the right dorsal quadrant (Fig. 2.11).

In stallions, palpation of the inguinal rings, either side of the midline at the pubic brim, should always be perfomed. In *strangulated inguinal hernia*, distended painful small intestine can be felt at the ring on the same side as the scrotal enlargement resulting from the engorged testis (Fig. 2.12).

Chronic obstruction causing intermittent bouts of colic, and often weight loss, may be due to a partial obstruction of the small intestinal lumen by intussusception, muscular hypertrophy or intramural neoplasia. As a result of the increased workload necessary to propel ingesta through the constricted segment, marked secondary muscular hypertrophy occurs in the intestine proximal to the obstruction. As a result, several metres of intestine may dilate to a diameter of 10 cm or

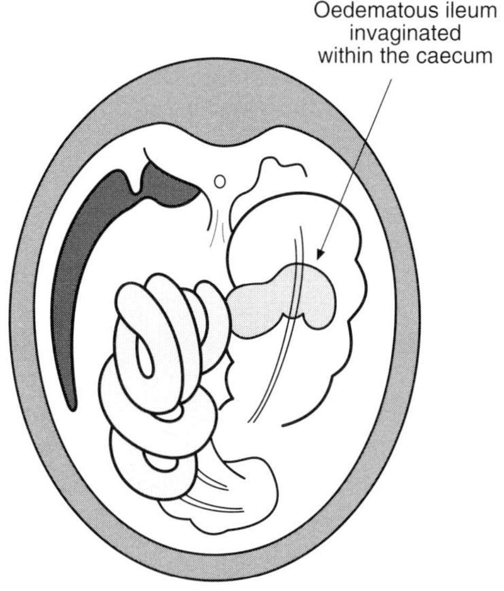

Figure 2.11 Ileocaecal intussusception: high obstruction with a palpable caecal anomaly.

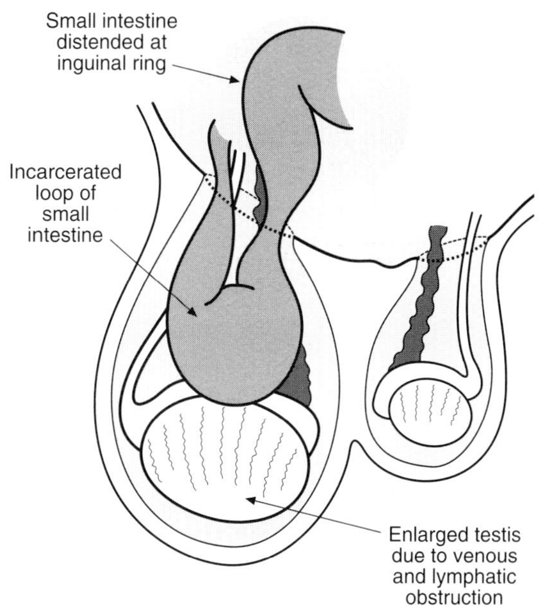

Figure 2.12 Strangulating inguinal hernia.

more and have a wall 1 cm thick (Fig. 2.13). A single loop can be mistaken for pelvic flexure but the presence of other identical loops and the fact that they become 'solid' when they contract, helps to distinguish between them.

Although the precise cause of small intestine obstruction can be identified only infrequently, some indication of the level of obstruction is usually possible. The absence of palpable distension of the small intestine in the presence of gastric reflux indicates a gastric problem, pyloric stricture or a high small intestinal obstruction. Distended small intestine with no gastric reflux often indicates a distal small

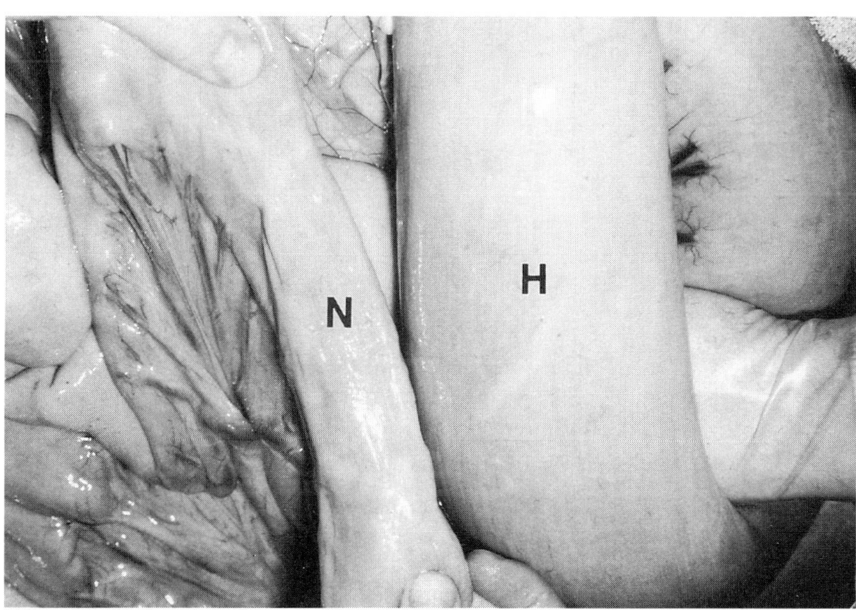

Figure 2.13
Chronic obstruction of small intestine: H = hypertrophied jejunum proximal to partial obstruction; N = normal jejunum.

intestinal obstruction, but this conclusion can only be reached with reference to the length of time that the obstruction has been in existence. Further evidence of a distal obstruction may be obtained by applying gentle traction to the medial caecal band. A pain response is often elicited in horses which have epiploic foramen incarceration or some other ileal obstruction.

Abnormalities of the caecum

A number of caecal obstructions can be identified per rectum. Located in the right caudal abdomen, the caudal aspect of the caecal base and the ventral aspect of the caecal body are within reach even in large horses. In the normal horse the ventral taenia, which is vertical in position, is readily identified as a flaccid narrow band which is without covering by mesocolon or vessels. In small horses the medial taenia is also palpable. The tension within the ventral band and its direction will vary with the contents and the degree of distension of the caecum. Because of the normal dorsal mesenteric attachment, the examiner's hand cannot pass dorsal to the caecum.

Rectal examination allows differentiation of gaseous distension from accumulation of solid or fluid ingesta. Tympany pushes the caecum back to the pelvic inlet and the tense ventral taenia can be felt running diagonally from the right dorsal to the left ventral quadrant (Fig. 2.14).

Care must be taken to differentiate *caecal impaction* from impaction of the colon, right dorsal colonic displacement and caecal intussusception. Caecal impaction usually presents as a firm to hard digesta-filled viscus with a distinct ventral band. A hand can be passed to the right of, but not dorsal to, the viscus. Typically, the caecal base fills before the body and little or no gaseous distension is evident. Repeated rectal examinations over a period of 12 hours or more may be necessary before the impaction is palpable. Palpation of the overhanging part of the caecal base may be impossible in large horses. The mass of ingesta tends to be oval and can be moved from side to side like a pendulum (Fig. 2.15). Difficulty in recognizing the relatively empty large colon is another significant feature of caecal impaction.

A type of caecal dysfunction has been described in which the immobile caecum is grossly distended with feed and fluid. Pain is often severe and the rectal findings are more akin to tympany, except that the caecum

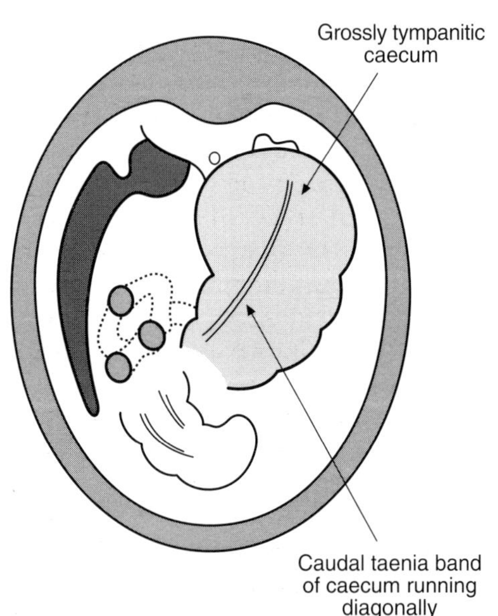

Figure 2.14 Caecal tympany.

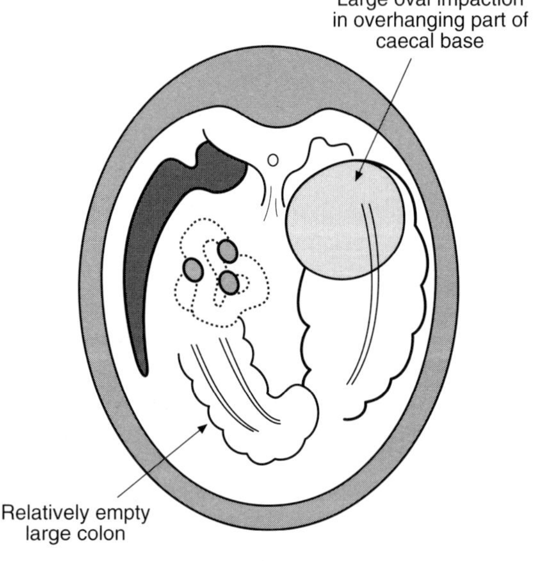

Figure 2.15 Caecal impaction.

is pulled cranially by the weight of the contents.

Caecal intussusceptions take one of two forms. Following the initial invagination of the apex, intussusception of the body of the caecum into the base (caeco–caecal intussusception) may occur or the invagination process may continue until most of the caecum has passed through the caeco–colic opening into the right ventral colon (caeco–colic intussusception). On rectal examination the firm, oedematous body of the invaginated caecum can be palpated in the right dorsal quadrant either within its base (Fig. 2.16) or within the right ventral colon.

Rectal examination is generally unhelpful in diagnosing non-strangulating infarction of the caecum. Infarctive changes commence at the apex, which is out of reach, but in some cases oedema of the caecal body and pain on palpation are evident. Caecal torsion and typhlitis (owing to enteric clostridiosis) also result in mural oedema which is palpable on rectal examination. However, it is rare for either to be a primary disease process and usually there is concurrent involvement of the large colon.

Abnormalities of the large colon

Rectal examination is particularly helpful in diagnosing large colon problems. Primary *impaction of the pelvic flexure* is characterized by an enlarged, firm, evenly-filled viscus which is often located on the pelvic floor or, alternatively, is palpated in the right ventral quadrant. In severe cases it is palpable within a few centimetres of the anal sphincter. Typically, as the hand and arm are moved cranially there is an obvious mass on the pelvic floor which displaces the rectum in a dorsal direction. The doughy mass can be indented by manual pressure with the indentation remaining for 5–10 seconds. The gut wall around the impaction is smooth, taeniae bands can be felt on the more cranial portions of the left colon and the impaction often extends beyond arm's reach. Occasionally there may be some gaseous caecal distension.

Evaluation of the firmness and extent of the impaction will give an indication of the severity

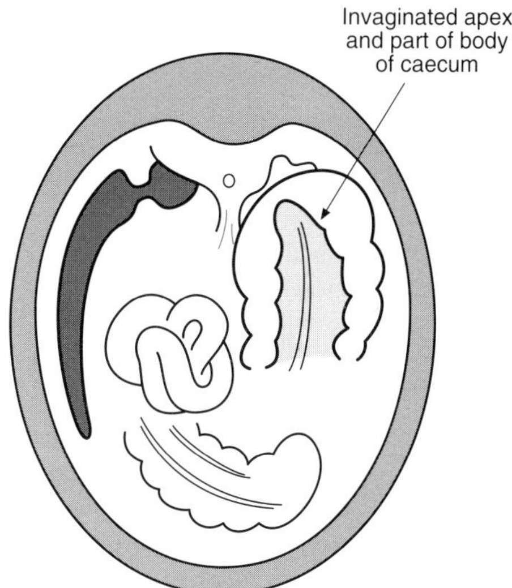

Figure 2.16   Caeco–caecal intussusception.

of the problem and will allow the effectiveness of treatment to be assessed at subsequent examinations. The thickness of the colon wall should also be assessed. In the majority of cases it will feel normal, but oedema indicates a degree of vascular obstruction, usually owing to torsion. This can occur (rarely) when the impaction is beginning to clear. In contrast to impaction, gaseous distension of the colon presents as a taut viscus which resists indentation.

A common error is to mistake a secondary impaction for a primary impaction. Secondary impactions are encountered in horses with grass sickness, anterior enteritis and ileal impaction; conditions in which gastric and small intestinal fluid distension lead to hypovolaemia. As a result of the body's attempt to conserve as much fluid as possible, the contents of the colon become very dry and shrink. The large colon contracts onto the firm ingesta and the constrictions and sacculations give it a characteristic corrugated feel (Fig. 2.9), in contrast to the smoothly distended colon of the horse with a primary impaction. Recognition of a secondary impaction will avoid the mistake of giving large volumes of mineral oil by nasogastric tube with the risk of rupturing an already distended stomach.

In *left dorsal displacement* (nephrosplenic entrapment), varying lengths of left colon are draped over the nephrosplenic ligament. If the displaced portion is large the bands hang down in a diagonal direction and the pelvic flexure cannot be palpated (Fig. 2.17). Considerable tympany of the left ventral portion may obscure the spleen. An impaction is often palpable in the left dorsal colon just caudal to the nephrosplenic ligament. If only a short length of colon lies caudal to the spleen, the impacted pelvic flexure is easily recognized (Fig. 2.18). Deviation of the spleen away from the left abdominal wall suggests incomplete entrapment. Oedema of the colon wall indicates marked constriction in the nephrosplenic space or a degree of torsion.

In *right dorsal displacement* a slight to moderately distended large colon lies horizontally in front of the pelvic canal, caudal to a tympanitic caecum. The mesocolon containing fat and large vessels can be recognized and traced to the right where it can be felt passing between the caecum and the abdominal wall (Fig. 2.19). Oedematous thickening of the mesocolon indicates a degree of torsion.

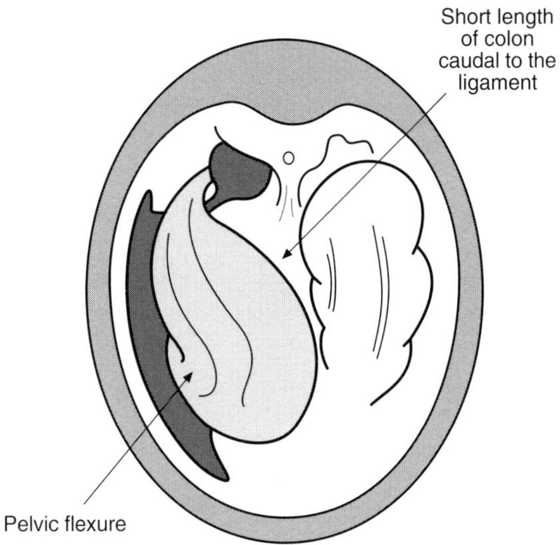

Figure 2.18   Nephrosplenic entrapment associated with a short length of palpable colon.

Severe *torsion of the large colon* produces such great distension that it is often impossible to explore beyond the pelvic inlet. The characteristic features are a horizontal colon with palpable thickening of its wall and mesocolon as a result of oedema (Fig. 2.20). Severe pain and a marked abdominal distension causing respiratory distress are other characteristic signs.

In obstruction of the large colon by an *enterolith*, the stone can occasionally be palpated, but in the majority of cases the only detectable abnormality is severe tympany (Fig. 2.21).

Abnormalities of the small colon

Obstructions of the small colon are characterized by tympany proximal to the obstruction. *Impactions* present as a solid tube of ingesta without formed faecal balls. The antimesenteric band can be felt and helps to distinguish small colon from distended small intestine. Occlusion of the lumen by a submucosal haematoma may be identified if the lesion is located far enough distally. In cases where the overlying mucosa has split, frank blood will be present in the lumen. Abrupt deviation of the small colon to left or right may be felt in mares in which it has become hooked

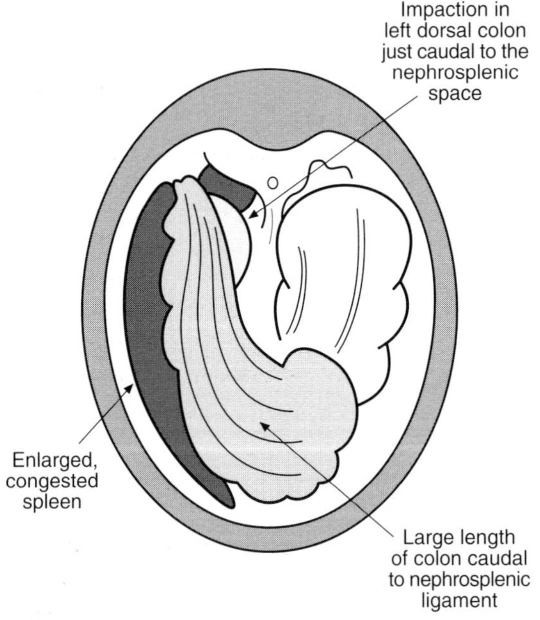

Figure 2.17   Nephrosplenic entrapment of the large colon.

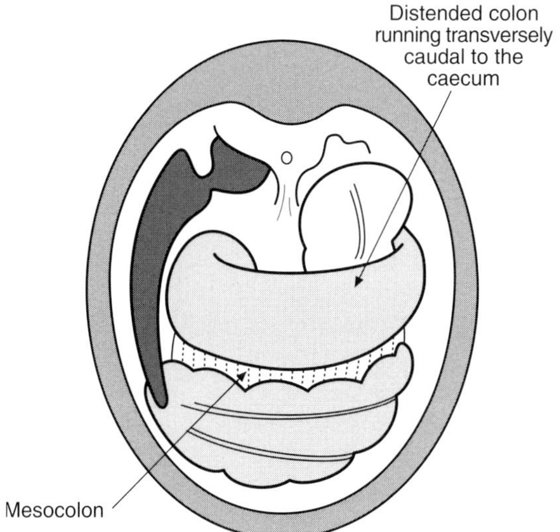

Figure 2.19 Right dorsal displacement of the large colon.

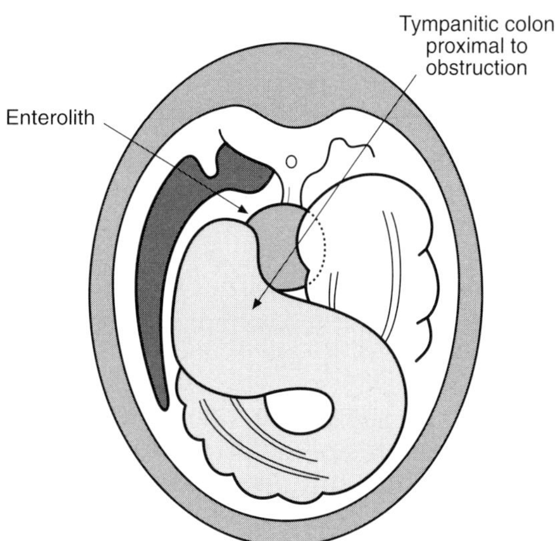

Figure 2.21 Obstruction of the large colon by an enterolith.

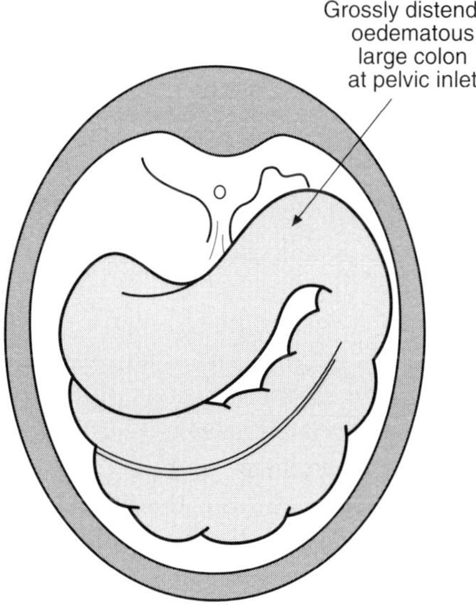

Figure 2.20 360° torsion of the large colon.

around an ovarian pedicle. Submucosal oedema, possibly associated with salmonella infection, can lead to small colon impaction. Passage of a well-lubricated hand along the oedematous section is difficult due to partial occlusion of its lumen and roughening of the mucosa. Sand colic can be suspected on the basis of gritty rectal contents, and can be confirmed by floating faeces in water and allowing any sand to settle to the bottom.

Other abnormal masses

Occasionally, mesenteric abscesses or tumours are felt on rectal examination. Mesenteric abscesses, which usually develop secondary to upper respiratory infections several months previously, present as large firm masses in the midline. The closer their location to the root of the mesentery, the less mobile they are. Distended loops of adherent small intestine may also be palpable. Splenic abscesses or tumours cause splenic enlargement with medial and caudal deviation. The enlarged spleen feels irregular or nodular.

Gut rupture

Rupture of the stomach or intestine can be diagnosed on the basis of the roughened granular feel to the surface of the gut owing to adherent particles of food. Emphysema of the bowel wall or gaseous distension of the abdominal wall may also be detected. Gas and fluid within the peritoneal cavity separate the loops of bowel, and movement of the arm is less restricted than would be expected when multiple loops of intestine are present.

Comments

- Rectal examination should be carried out routinely in all colic cases if possible — only rarely does the examination fail to provide significant information.

- Negative findings may indicate the absence of any serious problem, but on the other hand may simply mean that any affected bowel is out of reach.

- The examination should be repeated every 1–2 hours if the case is presented close to the onset of colic and/or other clinical findings indicate obstruction or strangulation of the bowel.

- Identification of the precise cause of the obstruction is more likely when it involves the large intestine. Few causes of small intestinal obstruction can be recognized per rectum, but the presence of distended fluid and gas-filled loops is sufficient indication in the vast majority of cases for surgical intervention.

Abdominal paracentesis (peritoneal tap)

Changes in the composition of peritoneal fluid reflect changes occurring at the peritoneal surfaces of organs within the abdominal cavity. The analysis of peritoneal fluid is most useful in monitoring the progression of persistent, intractable colics and identifying peritonitis. It is also indicative of much rarer conditions such as pancreatitis, rupture of the bladder and chyloabdomen. Abdominal tumours may occasionally be revealed by paracentesis if they are sufficiently exfoliative. However, the commonest abdominal tumour of the horse, lymphosarcoma, is not usually exfoliative.

Technique

Peritoneal fluid may be collected using a sterile needle or, alternatively, using a sterile bovine teat cannula.

Needle technique

The horse is restrained with its head in a corner and the right side of its body against the side of a wall. Additional physical restraints such as twitching are usually unnecessary. Sedation may be used in fractious animals providing the clinical circumstances permit.

The clinician stands close to the left foreleg facing towards the animal's back. From this position of relative safety the operator can work in full view of the hindlegs and avoid injury if a foot strikes forward during the procedure.

The hair is clipped 5 cm either side of the linea alba from the xiphisternum to the umbilicus. The xiphisternum is recognized as the point at which the costal arches meet in a 'V' shape at the midline. The clipped area is then prepared as for surgical intervention.

Ideally, paracentesis is performed at the lowermost point of the belly since this forms a natural basin in which peritoneal fluid accumulates. In all cases the point of insertion should be approximately a handsbreadth behind the xiphisternum to avoid damage to its cartilage. It is also important to place the needle in the midline through the linea alba, since this is relatively avascular and free of sensory nerve endings. In most cases the linea alba is readily seen in the midline and is palpable at the finger tips as a shallow channel, roughly the width of a pencil.

A 1.5 inch x 18G (40 x 1.2 mm) sterile needle is held by its hub between the forefinger and thumb of a surgically gloved hand. The site of insertion is visualized and the channel of the linea alba is located by the remaining fingers. If the needle is held at 90 degrees to the linea alba and in line with the fingers as they are located in the channel (Fig. 2.22), then it is possible for the operator to withdraw his/her head to safety before placing the needle in the skin, knowing

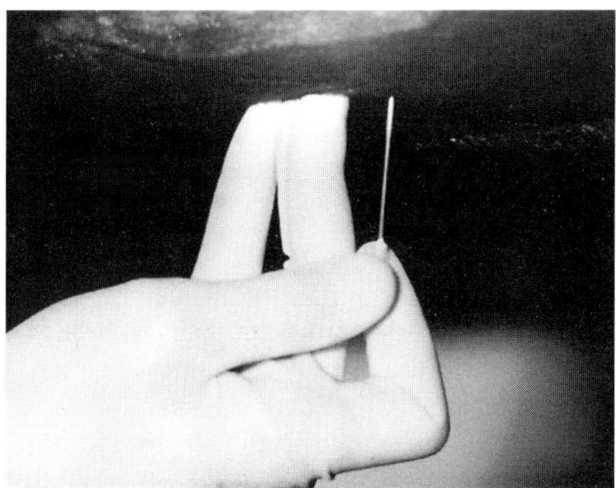

Figure 2.22   Position of the needle for abdominocentesis.

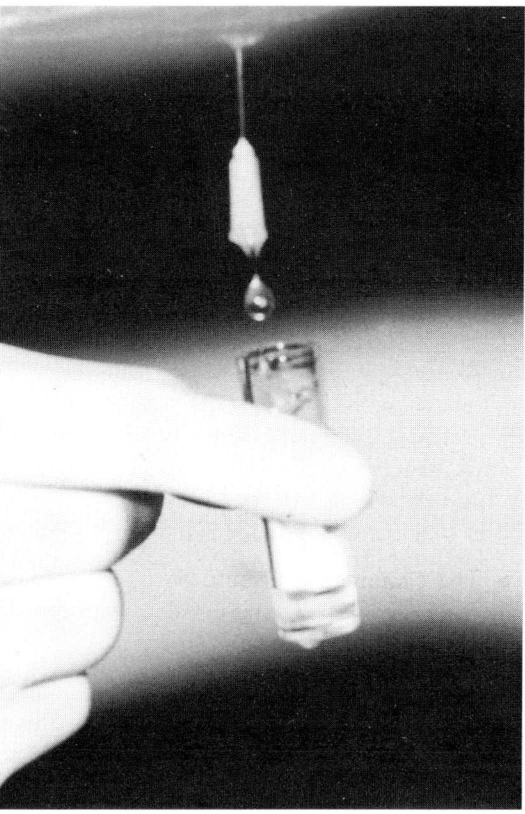

Figure 2.23   Dropwise collection of peritoneal fluid into EDTA for cytology.

that it is positioned accurately. The needle is pushed through the skin and into the linea alba, gently but firmly, to a depth of no more than 5 mm. This should allow the needle to be self-retaining when released. As the point of the needle penetrates the peritoneum there may be a pain response, but this is not always apparent.

Having placed the needle, the operator must exercise patience in manipulating it to obtain fluid. Unless the production of fluid is enhanced by some pathological process, it is usual to obtain occasional drips at the needle hub. This dropwise collection occurs intermittently as the viscera move to and fro with respiratory movements over the site of paracentesis. In trying to obtain a sample the operator must therefore spend up to 10 seconds watching the hub, at a safe distance from the hindlegs, before attempting to manipulate the needle further. If no fluid is forthcoming, the hub should first be rotated between finger and thumb to free the point from any potential blockage. If there is still no fluid drip, the needle is advanced 2–3 mm only and the process is repeated. When the point of the needle comes into contact with the serosa of some part of the alimentary tract, the hub is seen to move or 'course' with respiratory excursions. At this stage the needle should be withdrawn slightly and redirected.

Once fluid appears it should be collected into EDTA and plain sample tubes for cytology and biochemistry/microbiology respectively (Fig. 2.23). One ml of fluid is sufficient for each purpose.

NB When attempting to obtain peritoneal fluid from the donkey it is essential to use a long needle (e.g. a disposable spinal needle, minimum 3.5 inch/90 mm), since there are usually deep deposits of retroperitoneal fat. This will be the case even when the animal is in poor condition.

Sampling failure. The accidental contamination of a sample with blood is recognized by a swirling of blood into the sample, possibly after a short period of clear fluid collection. Overt haemorrhage is recognized as fresh and accidental if it clots in a plain tube. On the other hand, blood which has collected in the abdomen as a result of some pathological process is defibrinated and will not clot.

Very dark blood that clots rapidly is likely to be the result of tapping an enlarged spleen. With splenic enlargement it may be impossible to obtain a fluid sample from the midline. In these cases ultrasound may be used to determine a 'window' to the side of the midline through which fluid may be reached.

A green-brown sample suggests accidental gut penetration (enterocentesis) or, alternatively, gut rupture. The fluid is likely to smell of ingesta and is obvious at microscopy. Accidental gut taps are rarely attended by complications (see later).

Occasionally, no fluid is obtained; even after the needle is inserted to the hub. In such cases, if the hub shows no coursing movement the point may be resting in fat and a longer 2 inch x 19G (50 x 1.0 mm) sterile needle should be used. In fat horses and ponies it is advisable to start with the longer needle.

In any of these instances the procedure may be repeated with a fresh needle 3–4 cm caudal to the original point of insertion. Up to three attempts to obtain a sample may be made at different sites along the midline.

Cannula technique

Although needle collection is quick and relatively simple, it suffers the disadvantage of occasional accidental contamination of the sample by blood or gut contents. An alternative technique is to collect fluid using a blunt bovine teat cannula. This technique is preferable where intestinal distension against the belly wall is suspected, or where organs are repeatedly felt at a needle tip despite manipulation. The major disadvantages are its more invasive nature and the greater number of procedures to be undertaken under direct vision at a difficult location. In general, it requires greater patient cooperation.

The site is prepared as previously described and 1–2 ml of local anaesthetic are infiltrated below the skin at the site of proposed insertion using a 25G needle. A short stab incision is then made with a scalpel through the skin and a sterile 3.8 cm or 7.0 cm teat cannula is pushed through the linea alba using steady pressure. Once again, a pain response may be noticed as the blunt end of the cannula pierces the parietal peritoneum. A sterile swab wrapped around the hub should prevent blood contamination from the wound entering the sample. The cannula is manipulated, several mms at a time, until an adequate flow of fluid is obtained.

Gross appearance of peritoneal fluid

Useful empiric information may be obtained from the gross appearance of the sample as it is produced.

Volume

It is usual to obtain 5–10 ml of peritoneal fluid in dropwise fashion over 4–5 minutes. A copious flow of fluid under pressure is unusual and suggests that its production is enhanced by some pathological condition, but laboratory confirmation of pathology is required. An absence of fluid ('dry tap') may be experienced in dehydrated patients, but fluid is unobtainable from normal horses on occasion.

Colour and turbidity

Normal fluid is straw-coloured to deep yellow (depending on the bilirubin concentration) and is visually clear because of its low cell content. The yellow intensity increases with the bilirubin concentration during periods of reduced feed intake.

In colic patients an amber colour and slight turbidity suggests a vascular compromise of the gut (hypoxia) which is associated with diapedesis of red and white cells from serosal capillaries. Subsequent necrotic change causes a dark red-brown discolouration and an increase in fluid turbidity as the leucocyte count escalates. Visual assessment of sequential samples during the course of a colic is therefore valuable in confirming the need for laparotomy.

Dark sanguinous fluid should be run into a plain container to see if it clots. Clotting suggests accidental haemorrhage during the procedure. However, abdominal haemorrhage produces a reservoir of defibrinated blood which does not clot. In cases of colic this dark colour in a non-clotting sample could be indicative of gut necrosis; in which case the leucocyte count is also elevated.

A fawn colour in turbid solution is consistent with peritonitis and reflects a high leucocyte count. If the sample is left to settle for 10–20 minutes, the volume occupied by inflammatory cells is readily appreciated (Fig. 2.24). In healthy horses the cell deposit is scarcely visible.

A greenish brown colour in turbid solution is suggestive of gut contents. The sample usually has a distictive pungent smell of ingesta and in the laboratory a stained smear will reveal food debris, protozoa and bacteria in the presence of few leucocytes. This sample may well be the result of enterocentesis. In a case of gut rupture the sample will have a similar appearance, but in addition there will be a large leucocyte component and, more significantly, the clinical signs will be consistent with impending shock.

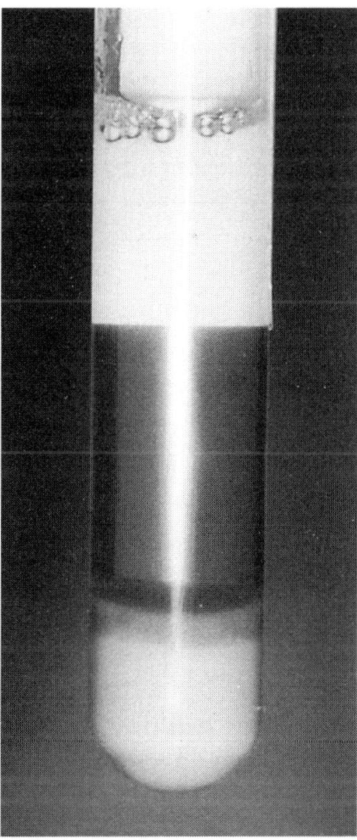

Figure 2.24   Huge volume of cellular deposit in the peritoneal fluid obtained from a patient with peritonitis.

Complications of abdominal paracentesis

Potential complications of abdominal paracentesis are: gut perforation or laceration; the introduction of infection at the site (resulting in cellulitis or peritonitis), and damage/infection at the xiphoid cartilage by sampling too far forward.

Gut perforation is a relatively common accident which is rarely attended by complications. The small puncture hole quickly seals over but a local peritonitis is evoked which increases the nucleated cell count of the peritoneal fluid within a few hours. The count then remains raised for 4–5 days.

Laceration of the bowel by needle point is an extremely rare complication, but it is a potential catastrophe. It is more likely to occur if the bowel is abnormally distended, or suffering vascular compromise, and the procedure is interrupted by sudden violent movement on the patient's part.

Cellulitis of the ventral abdominal wall or iatrogenic peritonitis are also extremely rare but could follow the introduction of infection by careless technique. It is also possible that a needle contaminated by enterocentesis could infect the abdominal wall as it is withdrawn.

Comments

- When peritonitis is suspected the fluid in the plain sample container should be submitted for bacteriology. Ideally, fresh paracentesis samples should be drawn by syringe and transferred to aerobic and anaerobic blood culture bottles for immediate dispatch to a microbiology laboratory. However, it is not unusual to obtain a negative culture, even when the clinical signs and peritoneal fluid smears indicate sepsis.

- Turbid exudates may occasionally clot if the associated peritonitis is severe enough to allow fibrinogen to enter the peritoneal fluid.

- During the treatment of peritonitis, the composition of sequential peritoneal fluid samples may fluctuate considerably. Having established that a state of peritonitis exists, it is easier to assess progress by measuring plasma fibrinogen concentration. This is a sensitive and reliable monitor of septic inflammation which simply requires a blood sample (in EDTA).

● Following castration or abdominal surgery, the cell counts and protein concentration of peritoneal fluid are usually raised, even in the absence of complications, and return to normal limits within 7–14 days. The use of abdominal paracentesis to distinguish between post-operative tissue reactions and post-operative infection is therefore limited. Equally, increases in the leucocyte count and protein concentration in peritoneal fluid after castration or abdominal surgery are not necessarily indicative of clinically significant peritonitis. Clear exceptions are where these parameters are greatly elevated and/or accompanied by the presence of bacteria. Where doubt exists, it is advisable to use sequential plasma fibrinogen concentrations as a monitor of post-operative septic inflammation.

Interpretation of peritoneal fluid analysis

Cytology

Cytological analysis is highly specialized and requires the services of a veterinary pathologist. The interpretation of the laboratory report is discussed here.

Normal fluid has a PCV of less than 1% with a total leucocyte count well under 10 x 10^9/l and frequently below 5 x 10^9/l. In differential count the predominant cell types are neutrophils, followed by mononuclear cells and a few lymphocytes.

Neutrophils. In cases of peritonitis, the cell count greatly exceeds 10 x 10^9/l and the neutrophil predominates. Neutrophils are often reported as either non-degenerate or degenerate. The presence of degenerate neutrophils in a sample indicates the activity of bacterial toxins — i.e. sepsis. These injured neutrophils may be seen in the absence of demonstrable bacteria, but the supernatants of such samples should nevertheless be submitted for culture. Occasionally degenerate cells are reported in association with intracellular or extracellular bacteria.

Mononuclear cells. Two types are recognized. Mesothelial cells form the peritoneal lining and are present in normal samples, where mitotic forms are occasionally seen. In acute inflammation they become pleomorphic and may be difficult to differentiate from neoplastic cells. In chronic inflammation they may be reported as phagocytic. Macrophages are present in low numbers during acute inflammation but their numbers increase as the condition resolves and they may be reported to contain degenerate neutrophils and aged erythrocytes.

Lymphocytes. Very low numbers are present in normal fluid. High numbers of lymphoblasts in a sample suggest abdominal lymphosarcoma, but exfoliation of abdominal tumours in the horse is rarely sufficient to enable diagnostic cytology in peritoneal fluid.

Other cells. Scant eosinophils are occasionally seen. Increased numbers within a slightly raised leucocyte count suggest strongyle parasite migration or hypersensitivity reactions. A few erythrocytes are usually present as a contaminant of collection or as a result of inflammation associated with abdominal pathology. Large numbers in a non-clotting sample indicate intra-abdominal haemorrhage. In these samples there is a lack of platelets and erythrophagocytosis may be reported. Although neoplastic cells are not commonly seen in cases of equine abdominal neoplasia, the total leucocyte count may increase according to the extent of any associated inflammation.

Biochemistry

The most useful biochemical parameter in peritoneal fluid is total protein, which is usually <20 g/l in health. Increases in the concentration of protein reflect the severity of inflammatory effusion.

Peritoneal alkaline phosphatase activity (ALP) is increased in conditions of bowel ischaemia owing to the release of the intestinal isoenzyme with which the intestinal mucosa is richly endowed. An elevation in conditions of colic is therefore consistent with the need for laparotomy. However, the colour of the fluid sample and the associated clinical signs would be of more immediate value in electing laparotomy.

Peritoneal amylase activity is elevated in acute necrotizing pancreatitis. However, acute pancreatitis is extremely rare in horses although the presenting signs, acute intractable colic, are relatively common. Because the indications for choosing to estimate amylase are not specific, the condition is usually diagnosed as a post-mortem finding.

When rupture of the bladder is suspected, the urea concentration of peritoneal fluid may be very similar to that of the blood, because it dialyses freely. However, creatinine is less freely diffusible and its peritoneal concentration will usually be more than double that of blood, despite the presence of azotaemia.

Significance of effusions

The leucocyte count and total protein concentration of peritoneal fluid can be used to identify effusions as transudates, modified transudates or exudates. The type of effusion may reflect the mechanism of its formation. However, it must be remembered that the nature of the effusion may change swiftly with the dynamics of the disease process.

Transudates are clear, colourless fluids of low cell count, normal cell differential and low protein concentration (<20 g/l). These fluid characteristics may be present in healthy horses, but large volumes of sample, pouring out under pressure, are abnormal and may be associated with hypoalbuminaemia or venous congestion.

Modified transudates are transudates featuring a modest increase in cell count and/or total protein (20–30 g/l). They therefore appear slightly turbid and are amber to red in colour. They reflect early or low grade abdominal disease or, alternatively, they accompany a systemic disease.

Exudates are turbid, amber to red fluids of high cell count (10 x 10^9/l). The predominant cells are neutrophils, and the protein concen-trations are high (>30 g/l). These fluids usually reflect inflammation of the peritoneal surface. Much more rarely, the predominant cell type may indicate a chylous effusion (small lymphocytes amongst numerous fat globules) or neoplasia (exfoliative cells).

Nasogastric intubation

Apart from therapeutic applications, a naso-gastric tube may be used to deliver glucose or xylose solutions in absorption tests, to assess fluid reflux and permit decompression in cases of high alimentary obstruction, or (with great care) to indicate the site of oesophageal obstruction.

Proprietary tubes are manufactured in foal, pony or horse sizes. Soft tubes which are easily folded or misdirected in the warmth of the oropharynx should be avoided. Tubes that are too narrow for the patient may also be folded or misdirected during attempted intubation. However, this is preferable to attempting to pass a tube that is too large, since the inevitable result is a traumatic nosebleed. Tubes with an additional hole set in the side of the leading end are recommended and transparent tubes are preferable because they allow the clinician to see the passage of fluid.

As tubes are not graduated along their length, it is extremely useful to make an indelible mark around their circumference at a point which indicates that the leading end is approaching the entrance to the larynx or oesophagus. This distance is approximately 30 cm for pony tubes and 35 cm for horse tubes. It is also useful to make an orientation mark indicating the 'top' of the tube — i.e. on its outer curvature.

In cold weather a rigid tube may be softened by passing warm tap water through it. This also reduces objection by the patient as it traverses the sensitive mucosa of the nasal cavity.

Restraint

The horse is stood diagonally in a corner with its quarters   against the wall to restrict backward and lateral movements. The handler should stand to the left of the horse's head with his/her back to the horse to minimize injury if rearing occurs. A sound headcollar is essential but additional restraints will depend upon the horse's temperament. A horse that struggles during intubation is more likely to suffer a nosebleed and such patients are best twitched. Where clinical circumstances permit, sedation is possible – but this will diminish the swallow reflex as the tube is passed and could affect the results of an absorption test if intubation is used for this purpose. In extreme circumstances the handler may apply an ear hold, but this must only be undertaken by a competent, experienced handler.

Passing the tube

A coiled tube is cumbersome to handle and an uncoiled tube will trail on the floor. The uncoiled tube is therefore draped around the clinician's neck, leaving the hands free to control its passage.

The first 10–12 cm of the leading end is liberally coated with a water-soluble lubricant and the tube is grasped just behind this point for controlled insertion. The clinician must avoid getting lubricant on the hands, otherwise the tube will constantly slip beneath the grasp.

The right-handed clinician will be most comfortable if stood to the right of the horse's head with his/her back to the horse. The handler should attempt to keep the head in a flexed position and the clinician rests his/her left hand on the bridge of the nose above the muzzle. Care should be taken not to occlude the opposite nostril inadvertently. The thumb is then used to elevate the alar cartilage of the right nostril, thus opening wide the entrance to the nasal cavity. The lubricated end of the tube is then placed on the floor of the open nostril, slightly inclined towards the nasal septum, with its curvature directed downwards (Fig. 2.25). It is then pushed gently forwards so that it follows the floor of the ventral meatus and the alar cartilage is released. Failure to place the tube on the floor of the nasal cavity may result in its passage along the middle

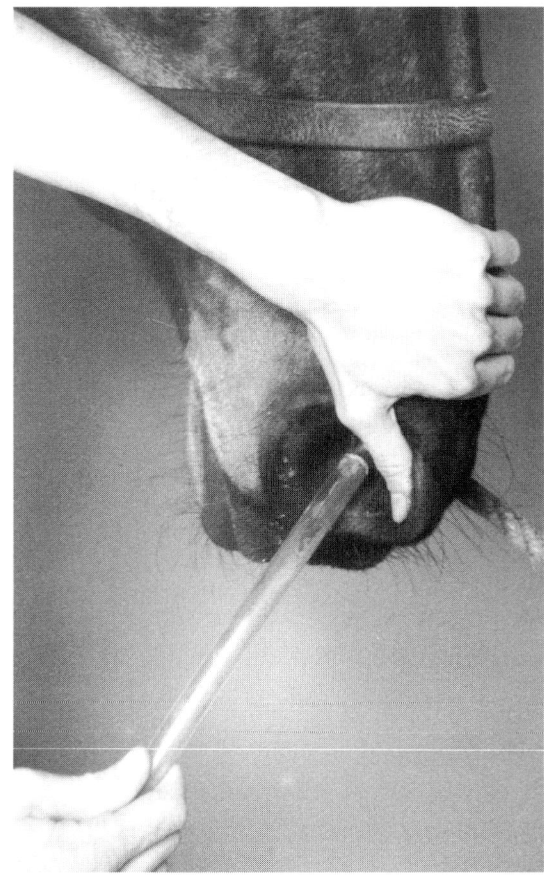

Figure 2.25   Placement of the stomach tube prior to passage along the ventral meatus.

meatus with consequent trauma to the ethmoturbinates. High placement may direct the tube into the nasal diverticulum ('false nostril').

Passage of the leading end of the tube through the nasal cavity is usually the part of the procedure which is most resented by the patient. The tube's advance is stopped once its preset mark arrives at the nostril, indicating that the leading end is approaching the larynx or oesophagus. In most cases, onward passage will result in entry into the larynx and trachea. To avoid this, the tube should be turned through 90 degrees before being advanced further. This has the effect of raising the level of the leading end with respect to the larynx, thereby bringing it closer to the opening of the oesophagus which is above the larynx. If successful, gentle pressure by advancing the leading end against the oesophageal opening will cause the tube to be admitted by a swallow.

If the tube is accidentally passed into the larynx, it should be withdrawn to the nostril mark, given an additional 90 degree turn to raise the leading end higher, and advanced again.

Alternatively, if gentle pressure meets total resistance the tube is withdrawn 2–3 cm and gently re-advanced in the hope of provoking a swallow. If this fails on 3–4 occasions, the operator should suspect that the end is pushing against the pharyngeal recess above both the larynx and the oesophagus. In this instance the leading end is lowered by turning the tube back through approximately 90 degrees before being advanced again. This trial and error manipulation of the tube to bring it adjacent to the oesophagus and provoke a swallow is the most difficult part of the procedure to master.

Checking the tube position

The commonest error is to pass the tube into the larynx. Tell-tale signs are as follows:

- Air can be blown or sucked through the tube without resistance.
- Shaking the larynx produces a palpable 'rattle' because of the tube within.

If the tube is clean, then untoward effects are unlikely — it is simply withdrawn and repositioned as described above. NB If the tube does enter the larynx, there may be no associated coughing. Equally, when coughing does occur it may coincide with swallowing of the tube and is not necessarily indicative of misplacement.

When the tube enters the oesophagus, there is often an accompanying swallow which may be repeated on the downward passage of the tube. Signs of successful intubation are as follows:

- There is some resistance to passage (oesophageal tone).

- A swelling may appear in the upper third of the left jugular groove and move down the neck as the leading end follows the line of the oesophagus along the left side of the trachea.
- There is resistance to air being sucked through the tube due to oesophageal collapse at the leading end.
- When the leading end is in the neck region, a short, sharp blow of air down the tube produces a momentary inflation of the oesophagus which is seen in the jugular groove. This is a useful test if a distinct swelling has not been seen to travel down the jugular groove. *Blowing should be repeated until the clinician is satisfied that the effect is truly inflation and not incidental swallowing.*

Once the tube is correctly placed, it is advanced to the stomach. On entry, there is usually an audible release of gas and listening at the open end reveals gaseous 'popping' sounds.

Aspiration of reflux

High intestinal obstruction causes fluid accumulation in the small intestine and stomach. The release of fluid and gas from the stomach at intubation is therefore indicative of high obstruction (Fig. 2.26). However, it is not always the case that fluid is released spontaneously and it is often necessary to create a siphon in the tube's dead space. This can be achieved by filling the tube with water, but the most consistent success is achieved by sucking on the open end of the tube — providing the operator ensures that the tube is dropped from his/her mouth as soon as fluid is seen to reflux!

It should always be borne in mind that the tube's leading end may not be immersed in gastric fluid and attempts to create a siphon should occupy at least 2 minutes of aspiration, moving the tube to and fro over 15–30 cm, before abandoning the procedure. In the absence of any fluid accumulation, gastric mucus is often seen in the leading end of the tube after withdrawal.

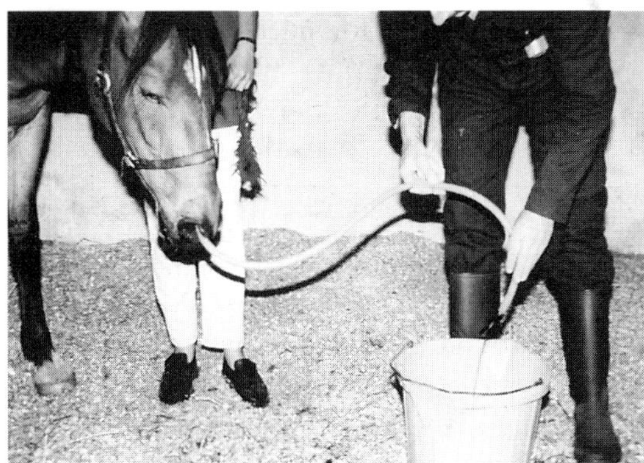

Figure 2.26   Reflux of fluid from the distended stomach of a pony with high intestinal obstruction.

Tube withdrawal

Any fluid medication which has been given by tube and is occupying its dead space should be blown through to the stomach before removal. Failure to do so may result in inhalation of spilt fluid as the tube is withdrawn over the larynx.

The tube should be withdrawn slowly and carefully. Particular care should be taken not to rush out the last 50 cm, otherwise trauma to the highly vascular turbinate mucosa will result in a nosebleed.

Potential problems

Nosebleeds look dramatic but are seldom a clinical problem. Raising the head may help to slow the bleed and promote clotting. Packing the nostril may reduce the external signs of haemorrhage, but it rarely hastens clotting time.

An unsuitably small or soft tube which folds over in the oropharynx may emerge from the opposite nostril, which is merely embarrassing, or may be swallowed with the leading end doubled on itself. In the latter instance, a swelling will probably be seen in the jugular groove, but inflation will not be possible due to a complete seal at the tube's end. If this is suspected, the tube should be passed into the stomach to release the kink rather than raking it back through the oesophagus.

There are rare but harrowing instances of

excess pressure being exerted to pass the tube when not engaged with the oesophageal opening. In these cases the tube has been pushed through the pharyngeal recess and onward progression has caused it to dissect down the neck towards the thoracic inlet. The result is invariably extensive sepsis. Attention to the technique outlined above should avoid this catastrophe.

Tubes should be kept in good condition and replaced as necessary. Frayed or chewed ends will traumatize mucosal surfaces. There are also infrequent reports of tube severance with retention of the leading end in the oesophagus, necessitating endoscopic or surgical removal.

Comment

- It is almost impossible to pass a stomach tube in an agitated patient without practice. Whilst acquiring the technique it is advisable to twitch the horse, irrespective of temperament.

Rectal biopsy in the horse

Lesions within the mucosa/submucosa of the hindgut are usually associated with chronic diarrhoea and can be characterized with surprising frequency in the histopathology of the rectal mucosa. Since rectal biopsy is easily undertaken in the standing horse it offers a clear advantage over intestinal biopsies which must be obtained under general anaesthesia. Bacterial colitis may be demonstrated by inflammatory changes in the specimen, while verminous colitis may be revealed by the presence of cyathostome larvae and/or eosinophil infiltration. Rarer causes of chronic diarrhoea that may be identified by biopsy are the malabsorption syndromes associated with cellular infiltrations such as lymphosarcoma, granulomatous enteritis and avian tuberculosis. Additionally, it may be possible to isolate salmonella from homogenized biopsy samples when faecal isolation has proved unsuccessful.

A variety of human rectal and cervical biopsy instruments are suitable for this purpose. The most suitable have a folding

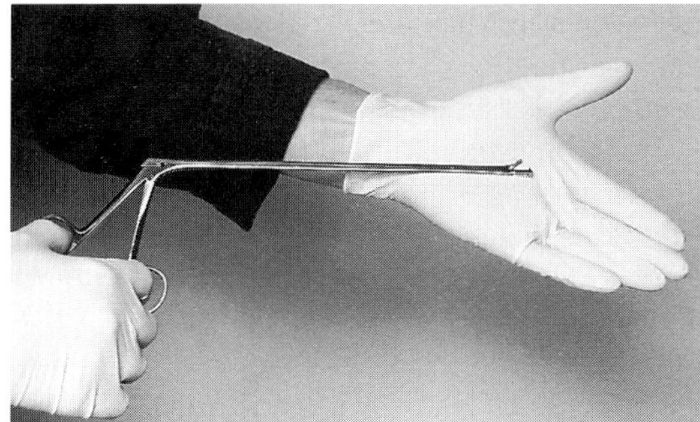

Figure 2.27 Rectal biopsy instrument.

upper jaw which cuts the specimen against a rigid lower jaw (Fig. 2.27).

Technique

The horse is restrained as for rectal palpation. Apart from passing the hand into the rectum, the procedure is usually without discomfort to the patient and the necessary restraints are minimal. A lightly lubricated gloved hand is introduced through the anal sphincter to wrist depth and the closed end of the sterilized instrument is passed into the cupped palm using the other hand (Fig. 28).

A mucosal fold in the roof of the rectum is palpated and held between finger and thumb and the instrument advanced with the jaws open to 'snag' the fold in an adjacent dorsolateral position. Taking biopsies from a dorsolateral position (at '1 or 11 o'clock') avoids damage to the dorsal vasculature. The jaws are closed and the sample is removed and transferred to fixative.

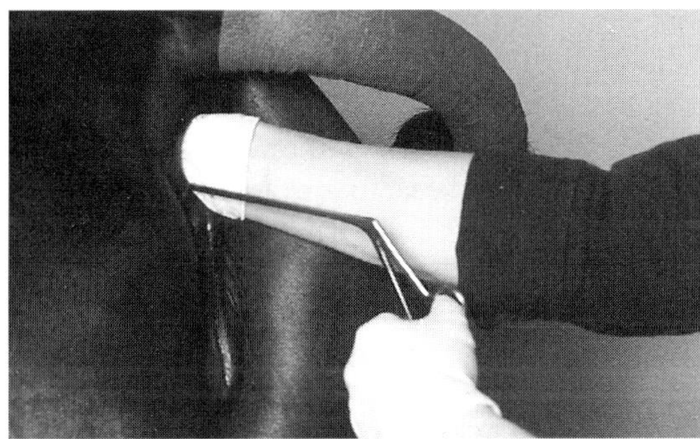

Figure 2.28 Passing the rectal biopsy instrument along the wrist and into the cupped palm.

A second biopsy for microbiology may be attempted in the opposite dorsolateral position. This specimen should be transferred to sterile saline.

Comments

- It is essential that the instrument is well maintained and cuts efficiently, otherwise the surrounding mucosa tears as the closed jaws are withdrawn.

- Whilst rectal biopsies can reflect pathology in the more cranial large bowel, normal (negative) specimens do not rule out the presence of colonic lesions.

Ultrasonography of the alimentary tract

Abdominal ultrasonography may occasionally be used to complement other investigations of the alimentary tract. However, a prerequisite for successful examination is a thorough knowledge of the normal topographical anatomy of the abdomen and the ultrasonographic appearance of organs. Both percutaneous and rectal approaches are possible, depending upon the area of interest.

Equipment

Adequate sound penetration is vital for a satisfactory examination. Low frequency transducers, in the range 2–3.5 MHz are preferred for the general examination. Linear array transducers allow a more rapid evaluation of a large area but sector scanners, with a smaller transducer/patient contact area, may be more useful where access is restricted, between ribs. A higher frequency transducer, in the range 5–8 MHz, is an advantage when a greater degree of resolution is required after initial scanning reveals a superficial area of interest. For percutaneous ultrasonography the hair must be clipped and the skin cleansed with povidone–iodine, before finally degreasing with spirit.

A rectal transducer is particularly useful for evaluation of the mid-caudal abdomen, especially where an abnormal structure can be palpated per rectum. In addition, a higher frequency transducer can be used per rectum as the depth of penetration required is not so great, and a corresponding increase in image quality may be achieved.

Appearance of organs

In the normal horse the greater curvature of the stomach can be imaged on the left side, in close apposition to the spleen. At this site the echogenic reflection of gas in the stomach allows the normally thin hypoechoic gastric wall to be identified. Thickening and abnormal echogenicity of the stomach wall suggests the development of a tumour. Although rare, the commonest gastric tumour in horses is the squamous cell carcinoma. Ascites is commonly found with these tumours and secondary spread may be recognized ultrasonographically as nodules associated with the liver, spleen, omentum, intestines or diaphragm.

Normal intestine is less easily identified and examined. Large intestine is usually seen as a thin-walled hypoechogenic structure around the echogenic reflection of gas in the lumen. Small intestine can be recognized as a tubular structure with a thin hypoechoic wall. Both are recognized by their heterogeneous contents and the movement associated with peristalsis.

Recognizable abnormalities in cases of obstruction include distended lengths of intestine containing fluid with little or no peristalsis. The appearance of double-walled areas of intestine (with a 'doughnut' appearance in transverse section) is suggestive of an intussusception.

In cases of intestinal neoplasia only the secondary effects may be detected and these can include changes to the volume or echogenicity of peritoneal fluid. The commonest intestinal tumour of horses is lymphosarcoma which may or not be associated with recognizable thickening of the bowel wall; this is also true of gross inspection at post-mortem examination.

When an abdominal mass is identified, the commonest differentials for neoplasia are abscessation or haematoma formation. The fluid-filled nature of an abscess or haematoma may be appreciated by the swirling motion of its contents as seen by real-time ultrasonography. This may be enhanced by external ballottement or moving the patient. However, it may be impossible to differentiate a primary abscess from an area of tumour necrosis and/or infection using ultrasonographic criteria alone.

II. Clinical evaluation of the colic patient

This section deals with the clinical assessment of colic and the indications for exploratory surgery (laparotomy) and summarizes a strategy for dealing with the colic patient.

Several of the practical techniques described in this chapter are of particular relevance to clinical evaluation of the colic patient. The vast majority of colics seen in practice are benign in nature, i.e. they are resolved by medical treatment alone and sometimes in the absence of any treatment at all. Most of these are 'spasmodic' colics.

In clinical examination it is rare to establish a precise diagnosis of the lesion causing colic, but it is essential to determine whether the situation is life-threatening or not. In the case of the spasmodic colic this conclusion can be achieved fairly quickly. However, in the case of the persistent colic continued monitoring of the clinical parameters is essential. In simple terms, the clinician must decide on the basis of these parameters whether the colic can be managed and resolved by medical treatment alone, or whether surgical intervention is necessary. The success of surgery is directly proportional to the speed at which a decision is made following the onset of colic.

Clinical parameters of colic

Once a history is obtained, the following observations should be made before handling the animal.

Behavioural signs

A state of colic is characterized by an abrupt change in normal behaviour in which various degrees of restlessness are seen. Mild colic produces behaviour such as: stretching of the abdomen; looking at the flanks; repeated yawning and/or teeth grinding. Geldings will occasionally prolapse the penis for protracted periods and even achieve erection. Signs of moderate colic include: persistent pacing of the box; pawing at the ground; kicking at the belly; adopting a crouching stance; occasional grunting; getting up and down frequently. Prolonged periods of lateral recumbency are possible. Severe colic signs include the above, but with profuse sweating, rolling and self-inflicted trauma.

Exceptions to these behaviour patterns occur in donkeys and heavy draught horses. These animals are often more stoical and less demonstrative of pain, even in a state of severe colic. Another consideration at this stage of observation is that the patient's behavioural signs may not reflect gut-associated pain, nor even abdominal pain. Table 2.1 indicates some differential diagnoses of colic behaviour.

Abdominal enlargement

Distension of the abdomen is often indicated by a convexity of the paralumbar fossae and suggests tympany or, in cases of severe pain and rapid deterioration, torsion of the large bowel. Rupture of the gut will also cause a gaseous distension of the abdomen, accompanied by signs of toxic shock.

Respiration

Rapid, shallow respiration can be a feature of pain and/or metabolic acidosis. Dyspnoea can accompany pressure exerted upon the diaphragm by severe gastric distension or hindgut tympany. Rupture of the diaphragm (rare) with prolapse of the gut into the thorax can also cause dyspnoea; particularly if the hindgut is prolapsed.

Muscle tremors

Occasionally, muscle fasciculation is seen over the flank and shoulders in moderate–severe colics. This is probably an autonomic response. Together with patchy sweating it is one of the characteristic features of grass sickness.

Table 2.1. Conditions presenting colic behaviour owing to discomfort that is not of gut origin.

Straining to urinate, e.g. urolithiasis and/or cystitis

Acute hepatitis, cholangitis or cholelithiasis — abdominal pain ± pyrexia

Peritonitis which is unassociated with a gut lesion

Rhabdomyolysis ('azoturia') — associated with exertion

Iliac thrombosis — usually associated with exercise

Laminitis — can be associated with prolonged recumbency

Acute pleuritis — anxiety; pain on movement + pyrexia

Complications following castration

Pregnancy
- — hypermotility of the foetus in late gestation
- — abortion
- — parturition or dystocia
- — postparturiant haemorrhage from the uterine artery
- — retained placenta
- — uterine contractions at involution

Pancreatitis — extremely rare in horses

Hypocalcaemia — muscle stiffness ± synchronous diaphragmatic flutter

Hepatic encephalopathy — behavioural disturbances

Pendulous ovarian tumours or haematomas

Splenomegaly (uncommon), e.g. abscessation; tumour; immune-mediated haemolysis

Cessation of defaecation

Defaecation ceases for the duration of any gut obstruction, although the faeces behind an obstruction may be passed initially. Small quantities passed irregularly suggest a partial obstruction. However, if faeces are passed regularly over 24 hours in a patient showing colic behaviour, the diagnosis of alimentary colic should be reviewed (see Table 2.1).

Having checked these observations, a 'hands on' clinical evaluation must include the following.

Heart and pulse rate

The heart and pulse rate are influenced to some extent by pain, but most particularly by haemoconcentration (dehydration), decreased venous return and toxaemia (as in gut devitalization). A heart/pulse rate increasing beyond 60 beats per minute in a patient with moderate–severe colic behaviour indicates a deterioration of the circulation and a need to scrutinize other parameters with a view to laparotomy. A persistent high pulse rate, the quality of which becomes weaker, suggests impending shock.

Rectal temperature

Slight increases can be associated with pain. However, temperatures in excess of 38.6° C (101° F) suggest a differential diagnosis of a systemic disease for which colic is an early incidental sign. The major differentials are salmonellosis and acute peritonitis. Anterior enteritis, an uncommon form of colic featuring ileus with thickening and haemorrhage of the anterior small intestine, is also associated with pyrexia.

A decreasing temperature, coupled with a rapid weak pulse, indicates the development of shock and carries a grave prognosis.

Mucous membrane colour and capillary refill time

The membrane colour and capillary refill time (CRT) reflect the circulatory status of the animal. The normal membrane appearance is moist and pink. Dry congested membranes suggest dehydration and circulatory disturbance. The CRT, observed by blanching out the gum adjacent to an incisor tooth and judging the time to colour restoration, indicates whether perfusion, hydration and vascular tone are impaired. In health, the normal CRT occupies less than two seconds. Increasing refill times indicate progressively inadequate perfusion and are usually accompanied by dryness and discolouration of the membranes.

Gut sounds

Gut sounds reflect gut motility (see above under: 'Abdominal auscultation'). In a healthy individual there should be sounds of movement at all sites. An absence of sound is abnormal and suggests gut stasis (ileus). An excess of sound suggests hyperperistalsis and is often a feature of spasmodic colics. Low-pitched tinkling suggests associated tympany.

Rectal examination

All cases of colic should be examined *per rectum* (see above under: 'Examination of the alimentary tract per rectum'). Essentially, the examination is a systematic search to reveal one or more of the following abnormalities:

- Distended loops of small intestine, indicating a high obstruction
- Impaction of the large bowel. This may variously be associated with nutritional impaction, large bowel displacement and/or entrapment, or reduced gut motility — as in peritonitis or grass sickness
- Taut distension of the large bowel, indicating tympany
- Taut bands of mesentery that are painful on manipulation, indicating a dependent lesion such as volvulus
- Solid masses. Possibilities include enlarged lymph nodes, tumours, enteroliths or adhesions.

Stomach intubation

The release of fluid and/or gas following stomach intubation is consistent with obstruction or stasis of the stomach and/or small intestine (see above under: 'Nasogastric intubation').

Abdominal paracentesis

Pathological change, in particular vascular compromise of the gut, is reflected in the colour changes seen in peritoneal fluid. This technique is particularly useful for monitoring persistent colics (see above under: 'Abdominal paracentesis').

Laboratory aids

In general, the most useful laboratory aids assess the extent of the physiological problems associated with a developing 'crisis', i.e. fluid and electrolyte losses and the development of metabolic acidosis. Of these, the most convenient in the field are assessments of dehydration by packed cell volume (PCV) and/or total plasma protein estimation. In most cases PCVs above 45% indicate haemoconcentration.

In summary, clinical evaluation of the colic patient should encompass all the above parameters. A trend to improvement or deterioration in the patient's condition is readily appreciated by monitoring these parameters over a period of time. The usual experience in practice is that the spasmodic colic resolves fairly quickly; however, it is important that the clinician identifies as soon as possible the 'acute abdomen' that requires exploratory surgery. For the best prognosis, surgery must be carried out within a few hours of an obstruction. Under 6 hours the prognosis is good; at 8–12 hours it becomes doubtful, and after 12 hours the prognosis for a successful recovery is progressively poorer.

Indications for surgical exploration (laparotomy)

Only on rare occasions is the precise cause of a 'surgical colic' diagnosed prior to laparotomy.

One such example is the umbilical hernia in which the intestine is incarcerated and strangulated. Most usually, the collective evaluation of clinical parameters indicates a deterioration in the patient's condition which requires surgical intervention. The collective indications for urgent laparotomy are as follows:

- Relentless pain despite analgesia*
- Pulse rate rising (> 60 bpm) and deteriorating in quality
- Congested mucous membranes and extended CRT
- Distension of the abdominal wall
- Gut sounds much reduced
- Fluid reflux on nasogastric intubation
- Positive findings on rectal examination*
- Abdominocentesis indicating gut devitalization

*NB Both intractable pain and positive rectal findings are justifications alone for surgical exploration.

In most instances the clinician will seek to refer the horse to a specialist centre. It must be emphasized that in these cases time is of the essence for a favourable prognosis. The delay in arranging transport and the distance to be travelled should therefore be borne in mind and the present condition of the patient must be carefully assessed. *It is inhumane to subject a mortally sick animal to a protracted and stressful journey.* In the client's interests the potential costs should be discussed with the centre when referral is requested.

A final indication for laparotomy is the undiagnosed chronic or recurrent colic which persists for days or weeks. In these cases laparotomy may provide the only remaining diagnostic step. However, the clinician should ensure that exhaustive clinical examinations have been undertaken and that both larvicidal and cesticidal anthelmintics have been administered before electing for exploratory surgery in these cases (see Table 2.2).

Table 2.2. Some causes of chronic or recurrent colic.

Possible cause	Aids to diagnosis
Gastric ulceration (probably rare in adults)	Gastroscopy at a specialist centre
Gastric squamous cell carcinoma (rare)	Gastroendoscopy and biopsy (specialist centre); ultrasonography; check abdominal paracentesis for exfoliation
Ileal obstruction: – intussusception – hypertrophy (uncommon) – tapeworm	Colic often follows soon after feeding See below Rectal examination Response to treatment
Intussusception (fairly common): – ileocaecal / caeco–caecal / caeco–colic	Rectal examination; ultrasonography
Hindgut impaction (common) – usually pelvic flexure – occasionally descending colon – rarely caecum	Rectal examination; response to liquid paraffin
Non-strangulating displacement of the large colon (fairly common)	Rectal examination
Sand colic (uncommon)	Relates to sandy top soil or muddy streams; rectal examination may indicate impaction; sand in diarrhoiec faeces
Enteroliths; faecoliths; foreign bodies in the colon (all rare)	Rectal examination
Recurrent ischaemia due to redworm migration	Recurrent 'spasmodic type' colics; check parasite parameters; response to larvicidal anthelmintics
Chronic grass sickness (fairly common in the UK)	Subtle signs of dysphagia; patchy sweating and muscle tremors; radiography to check megoesophagus and oesophageal transit time; ileal biopsy (specialist centres); histopathology of the coeliacomesenteric ganglion at post-mortem
Peritonitis (fairly common cause of chronic colic)	Abdominal paracentesis
Adhesions: – post-operative complications – chronic peritonitis – transabdominal parasite migration	Rectal examination; ultrasonography History or evidence of previous surgery Abdominal paracentesis Check β globulin; worming history
Progressive obstruction — tumour or abscess interfering with gut patency or peristalsis (uncommon)	Rectal examination; abdominal paracentesis

Table 2.2. Some causes of chronic or recurrent colic *(continued)*.

Possible cause	Aids to diagnosis
Infiltrative bowel diseases (uncommon)	Not usually associated with appreciable colic; investigate chronic wasting / malabsorption
Differentials of colic pain	See Table 2.1

A strategy of approach to the colic case

If the behaviour suggests mild–moderate pain and there are no systemic complications (i.e. no evidence of high obstruction or circulatory collapse), and a positive response follows the administration of a spasmolytic/analgesic drug, the prognosis is fair–good. A state of affairs is established; the colic can be treated medically for the present, but should continue to be monitored. NB The use of non-steroidal anti-inflammatory drugs with anti-endotoxic effects (e.g. flunixin, ketoprofen, phenylbutazone) should be avoided in the first instance since these analgesics can mask the clinical signs of a developing crisis, and valuable time can be lost in diagnosing an acute abdomen. Table 2.3 lists acute colics that are usually responsive to medical treatment.

If the pain is severe and difficult to control using various analgesics, the prognosis is much poorer. If the collective clinical parameters indicate deterioration, there are only two choices: surgery or euthanasia. In all cases where surgery is elected there will be one of three conclusions which the owner should understand in advance:

(1) The lesion is operable, but the procedure constitutes major surgery, which is necessarily expensive and carries a guarded prognosis in the first instance.

Table 2.3. Acute colics that are usually responsive to medical treatment.

Type	Aids to diagnosis
Spasmodic colic (very common)	Response to spasmolytic treatment; good prognosis
Tympanitic colic (fairly common) — often accompanies other types	Gut auscultation; rectal examination; response to treatment of underlying colic; good prognosis NB Extreme distension is a surgical emergency
Hindgut impaction (common)	Rectal examination; responsive to treatment with liquid paraffin; good prognosis
Gastric colic — grain overload or impaction (both uncommon)	Response to decompression by stomach intubation; prognosis guarded
Acute peritonitis (uncommon)	Abdominal paracentesis; response to antibiotics; guarded prognosis since aetiology unknown
Heat exhaustion/exercise dehydration	Immediate history; PCV and electrolyte estimations; blood gas estimations; usually fair–good prognosis

(2) The lesion is inoperable and the situation demands euthanasia while the horse is under general anaesthesia.

(3) Nothing of significance is found because the lesion is functional or inaccessible. This is rarely the case in the acute abdomen, but can arise at surgical exploration of the chronic or recurrent colic. The inevitable dilemma is then between reviving the animal or destroying it under general anaesthesia. To avoid this predicament, the course of action to be taken must be agreed by prior consultation with the owners before surgery. It is for this reason that elective laparotomy for the chronic or recurrent colic must only follow exhaustive clinical examinations (see Table 2.2).

III. **Clinical pathology**

Serum biochemistry

Total protein

Sequential total protein estimations may be used to monitor dehydration in cases of colic. However, in the severely compromised gut there may be a concurrent and progressive loss of protein into the peritoneal cavity or bowel lumen, thus rendering the technique inferior to sequential determinations of packed cell volume (PCV) in whole blood. Similarly, mucosal lesions associated with enteropathies such as malabsorption, parasitism or diarrhoea are usually accompanied by protein loss (hypoalbuminaemia) and in these cases progressive dehydration must also be judged by changes in the PCV.

Albumin

In horses hypoalbuminaemia is almost invariably associated with a protein losing enteropathy as a result of some lesion of the intestinal mucosa. Much rarer causes are glomerulonephropathy, liver failure or massive exudative effusion. In all these lesions albumin is lost preferentially because it has the smallest molecular weight of the plasma proteins. The exception is end stage liver failure, in which case the synthesis of albumin declines.

Globulins

Apart from dehydration, total globulin concentrations may also be increased by acute and chronic inflammatory processes (caused by increases in acute phase protein and immunoglobulin concentrations respectively), strongyle parasitism (caused by increases in $IgG_{(T)}$), or liver failure (caused by decreased catabolism of globulins). Some commercial laboratories offer an assay of serum $IgG_{(T)}$ concentration. If raised above the normal range, it is good evidence of active strongyle migration.

Albumin/globulin (A/G) ratios

In health, the A/G ratio approximates to 1.0. Shifts in the ratio may occur in a number of pathological states. However, the information is seldom useful since it lacks specificity. It follows from the preceding paragraphs that a fall in this ratio, due to a decrease in albumin and/or an increase in globulin, may be a feature of either inflammatory intestinal disease, strongyle parasitism or liver failure.

Serum protein electrophoresis

Routine serum protein electrophoresis may help the clinician to identify certain categories of disease, some of which will be alimentary in nature. Agarose gel electrophoresis separates equine serum proteins into four fundamental bands, characterized in order of their electrophoretic mobility. These bands are stained and identified as albumin with subdivisions of alpha, beta and gamma globulins. Once the total protein concentration is known, the individual protein concentration within each band may be determined in the laboratory by densitometer. However, the results of electrophoretic analysis of horse serum are not always comparable between laboratories because of differences in the separative technique. As a result there are conflicting data regarding the 'normal' concentrations and ranges of the various protein fractions. It is therefore advised that clinicians interpret protein shifts as empirical increases or decreases rather than absolute values. Table 2.4 shows an empiric interpretation of protein shifts.

Comment

- In diarrhoeic horses, the identification of high beta globulin levels is suggestive of cyathostomiasis. However, the presence of normal beta globulin levels cannot be regarded as a reliable indicator of the absence of significant parasitism.

Serum alkaline phosphatase (SAP or ALP)

The brush border of the intestinal epithelium is richly endowed with alkaline phosphatase and cellular damage increases the circulating SAP concentration. However, alkaline phosphatase is not organ specific and damage to bone or the biliary tract of the liver will also cause an increase in the circulating SAP concentration. Many laboratories will assay the isoenzyme intestinal alkaline phosphatase (IAP). However, in the authors' experience the accurate quantitation of this enzyme on a reproducible basis is technically difficult and it is arguably preferable to consider the total SAP. Thus an increased SAP concentration, in the absence of either bone disease or clinicopathological evidence of liver disease (Chapter 4), is indicative of gut pathology.

Pancreatic enzymes

Pancreatitis is extremely rare in horses and the indication for pursuing its clinicopathological diagnosis only follows the exclusion of other causes of moderate to severe abdominal pain.

Albeit on the basis of limited experience, useful indicators of acute necrosing pancreatitis seem to be estimations of amylase and lipase activity in both serum and peritoneal fluid. In health, amylase and lipase estimations are

Table 2.4. Empiric interpretation of serum protein shifts as revealed by electrophoresis.

Disease	Albumin	Alpha	Beta	Gamma
Acute infection	Normal	++ (APPs)	Normal	Normal
Chronic infection	Normal	+ (APPs)	+ (IgG$_{(T)}$)	++ (Igs)
Viral infection	Normal	Normal	+ (IgG$_{(T)}$)	++ (Igs)
Intestinal parasitism	Low (PLE)	++ (APPs)	++ (IgG$_{(T)}$)	Normal
Hepatic failure	Low	Normal	Normal	+++ (Igs)

Notes: PLE = protein losing enteropathy; APPs = acute phase proteins; Igs = Immunoglobulins; IgG$_{(T)}$ = Immunoglobulin G (subclass T).

usually very low in horses, but normal ranges vary between laboratories reflecting different assay techniques. In horses that have had demonstrable pancreatitis, the concentration of these enzymes has been greatly elevated. However, these enzymes are not organ specific and relatively modest amounts may be released following injury to the intestinal mucosa or renal tubules. Modest increases could also occur following ischaemic change to the pancreas (secondary pancreatitis), as may be associated with an intercurrent disease such as distension of the adjacent bowel.

Fluid, electrolyte and acid–base balance

Fluid, electrolyte and acid–base disturbances are associated with those acute colics in which fluid is sequestered in the gut lumen and/or there is associated strangulation. Examples include all forms of high obstruction, and displacement with torsion of the large intestine. In diarrhoea, the extent of fluid and electrolyte losses and the development of acidosis depends upon the severity of the enteric lesion and whether or not the patient continues to drink during the illness. The diagnostic assessment of fluid, electrolyte and acid–base balance in various disease states is considered in depth in Chapter 11: 'Fluid, electrolyte and acid–base balance'. Brief details of clinical pathology are given below.

Fluid balance

Simple blood parameters such as packed cell volume (PCV) and total plasma protein can be used to indicate the severity of dehydration. However, where facilities are available they are best used in a serial manner to follow the course of dehydration over a critical period.

Packed cell volume

In general terms, a PCV >45% indicates a reduction in extracellular fluid volume and a loss of sodium. Colic patients with a PCV >60% usually have a poor prognosis, but this is not invariably so.

Total plasma protein (TPP)

TPP estimation can be undertaken in the field using a refractometer. However, a patient suffering a concurrent protein loss (e.g. protein-losing enteropathy), as well as dehydration, may show a total plasma protein which is within the normal range.

Urea and creatinine concentrations

Most serum or plasma biochemistry parameters, including urea, are raised by acute dehydration. However, increases in both urea and creatinine beyond their normal ranges reflect prerenal failure associated with hypovolaemia (i.e. renal hypofusion).

Electrolyte balance

The interpretation of serum or plasma electrolytes in alimentary disease should be undertaken with caution. Increases in sodium, potassium and chloride concentrations are consistent with dehydration, but there may be a concurrent loss of electrolytes to the gastrointestinal tract. High obstructive colic is associated with a loss of water, sodium and chloride from the plasma. In cases of lower bowel pathology, relatively more potassium and bicarbonate ions are lost. A meaningful interpretation of electrolyte shifts can only be undertaken with a knowledge of the concurrent acid–base status.

Acid–base balance

Metabolic acidosis is the most common acid–base disorder in horses. It occurs most frequently in association with obstructive gastrointestinal disease and diarrhoea. The underlying causes of acidosis in these situations are either increased base loss and/or reduced peripheral perfusion causing a switch from aerobic to predominantly anaerobic metabolism in tissues, with a consequent build up of lactate.

Although blood gas and pH measurements provide the only accurate guide to acid–base status, plasma bicarbonate estimations are acceptable for most clinical situations. Even so, this requires venous blood samples to be collected anaerobically into syringes treated with lithium heparin and processed as soon as possible using sophisticated equipment which is not usually available in practice. In practical terms, however, the need to correct a metabolic acidosis by specific bicarbonate therapy is rare if fluid and electrolyte requirements are met (see Chapter 11: 'Fluid, electrolyte and acid–base balance).

Haematology

Useful aspects of haematology in the evaluation of alimentary disease are the PCV, indicators of anaemia and the white cell count. In chronic conditions the plasma fibrinogen concentration should also be requested. Although strictly a biochemical parameter, fibrinogen is often estimated by the haematologist and must be submitted in anticoagulant (either EDTA or sodium citrate depending upon laboratory requirements).

Erythrocyte parameters

As indicated above, the PCV is a useful monitor of dehydration and hypovolaemia if used on a sequential basis.

Chronic anaemia in the horse is often nonregenerative and associated with chronic inflammatory processes, but a chronic regenerative anaemia could reflect chronic haemorrhage into the gut or abdomen. Techniques for investigating anaemia are detailed in Chapter 8: 'Blood disorders'.

Acute haemorrhage is only reflected in the haematology profile after 12–24 hours, by which time there is a compensatory influx of tissue fluid to expand the plasma volume. The effect is to reduce the PCV, RBC and Hb concentration, and dilute plasma protein concentrations.

Leucocyte parameters

Leucopenia

Leucopenia (white cell count less than 6.0 x 10^9/l) is a feature of peracute/acute diseases of the gastrointestinal tract, e.g. gut ischaemia (as in surgical colics), gut perforations or salmonellosis. In these situations the count may fall to 2–3 x 10^9/l. It is attributed to localization of cells at the site of injury and is most pronounced in the presence of endotoxin. A number of morphological changes to the border and cytoplasm of neutrophils may be reported as toxic changes. These reflect the production of chemicals by neutrophils which are toxic to bacteria. The magnitude of these changes is proportional to the severity of sepsis, and persistence over several days in sequential samples is consistent with a poor prognosis.

Leucocytosis

Leucocytosis may accompany acute, progressive or more chronic inflammation of the gastrointestinal tract. This 'reactive leucocytosis' usually features neutrophilia and may be accompanied by immature band forms in acute conditions (left shift) and a monocytosis in chronic conditions.

Eosinophilia

Eosinophilia is popularly associated with parasitism, but high burdens of mature worms do not seem to affect the eosinophil count. In many instances eosinophilia probably reflects some form of hypersensitivity response.

Plasma fibrinogen concentration

The fibrinogen concentration is raised by inflammation, most particularly septic inflammation, and its level indicates the severity of disease. Concentrations increase within 1 or 2 days of an infection, but peaks are not attained until 3 or 4 days. A modest increase may therefore reflect early disease or alternatively, a chronic low-grade inflam-mation. High concentrations indicate advanced and serious disease with a poorer prognosis.

Comments

- In horses, plasma fibrinogen concentration is usually a more sensitive and reliable monitor of recovery from inflammation, or efficacy of treatment, than the peripheral white cell count.

- The normal range of fibrinogen concentration varies markedly between laboratories depending upon the technique used for its quantitation. *The clinician should always refer to the normal range given by the laboratory.*

Tests of intestinal malabsorption

These tests are indicated where weight loss is occurring in the absence of an obvious cause, despite an adequate food intake. The tests assess the functional integrity of the small intestine by measuring the efficiency of sugar absorption from the intestinal lumen. Pathological changes that interfere with cellular transport mechanisms reduce uptake into the bloodstream.

The oral glucose tolerance test (OGTT)

This test is inexpensive, simple to perform using readily available reagents, and offers good empiric information on the efficiency of small intestinal absorption.

Technique

- The horse's weight is estimated as accurately as possible (e.g. girth weighband) and it is fasted overnight on an inedible bedding. Access to water can be allowed until 2 hours before the test begins.

- One g/kg bodyweight of anhydrous or monohydrate D-glucose is weighed out and a fresh solution is prepared as 20% w/v in warm water. The quantity and concentration of glucose are important since stomach emptying is delayed by excessive concentrations of glucose, and the test depends

upon the rapid entry of the administered solution into the lumen of the small intestine.

- A 'fasting' sample of blood is taken immediately before the test and designated 'time zero'. *All samples must be collected into potassium oxalate–sodium fluoride anticoagulant.*

- A nasogastric tube is passed and the entire solution is delivered as a bolus into the stomach.

- Further blood samples are taken at 30, 60, 90, 120, 180 and 240 minutes and submitted to the laboratory for glucose estimation. These samples will be sufficiently stable in oxalate–fluoride to send in the post.

NB If the patient is insufficiently fasted, residual food in the stomach will mix with the incoming glucose solution and reduce its rate of delivery to the small intestine, thus producing a spurious result.

Interpretation

The tolerance curve is plotted arithmetically and in conditions of normal absorption has two phases (Fig. 2.29a). In the first 2 hours glucose is continuously absorbed from the small intestine and the plasma glucose concentration doubles. Quite apart from mucosal cell integrity, this absorption phase is influenced by the rate of gastric emptying, intestinal transit time and previous dietary history. A recent dietary history of a high energy intake will be associated with the production of reduced peaks. The second phase is insulin-dependent and shows a progressive fall to a resting level which is achieved by 6 hours. The sampling times suggested above should reveal these features in cases where absorption is not compromised.

A flat line indicates a state of total malabsorption (Fig. 2.29c) and usually constitutes a grave prognosis because the principal causes are progressive inflammatory cellular infiltrations of the gut wall. These include lymphosarcoma, granulomatous enteritis, eosinophilic gastroenteritis and avian tuberculosis. Diagnosis is defined by histo-

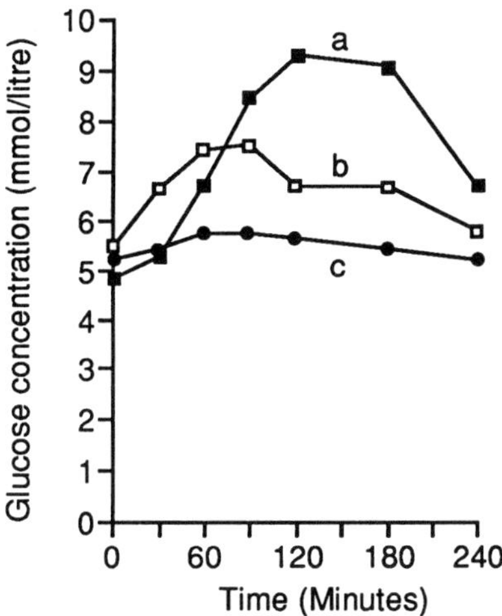

Figure 2.29   Oral glucose tolerance curves for three horses: (a) normal absorption; (b) partial malabsorption; (c) total malabsorption.

pathology of the small intestine; gross lesions are usually not visible or palpable at laparotomy or post-mortem examination.

An intermediate curve between normal absorption and total malabsorption suggests a state of partial malabsorption (Fig. 2.29b) which is more difficult to interpret. Causes are likely to be variable and could include, for example, circulatory disturbances, villous atrophy or reversible inflammatory changes associated with parasitism. In some cases the associated histology may be normal, suggesting other causal factors such as protracted stomach emptying, rapid intestinal transit time, inherent anomalies of cellular uptake and metabolism of glucose, or an overgrowth of intestinal bacteria which metabolize the test sugar. Without knowing the precise nature of the lesion or functional disturbance, it is not possible to be certain that such cases will not revert to normal given time and supportive treatment. However, the test can easily be repeated at a later date to monitor the patient's progress. Repeated 'partial malabsorption' results require bowel wall biopsy for further diagnosis. Alternatively, subsequent deterio-ration to a state of 'total malabsorption' suggests the end stage of a severe infiltrative lesion in the small intestinal wall.

Comment

- Lesions causing malabsorption in the small intestine may also infiltrate the hindgut, where malabsorption causes chronic diarrhoea. Lesions causing malabsorption may therefore affect the small intestine alone, the large intestine alone, or the whole intestinal tract. In patients with chronic diarrhoea of unknown cause, an OGTT will indicate whether or not there is associated small intestinal malabsorption.

The D-xylose absorption test

The principle of this test is essentially the same as the OGTT, but the shape of the xylose absorption curve is unaffected by the endogenous metabolic events which can influence the blood glucose concentration. In addition, it is not a normal constituent of the plasma. Because of this, it is said to provide a more accurate assessment of absorption. It is also believed to be a more sensitive indicator of malabsorption, registering decreases in absorptive function before the glucose uptake curve. This may be because xylose is passively absorbed from the intestine whereas glucose is actively absorbed. However, the shape of the curve is influenced by a number of factors which can also cause anomalies in the glucose absorption curve, i.e. the rate of gastric emptying, the intestinal transit time, intraluminal bacterial overgrowth, and the immediate dietary history. In addition, the costs of xylose and its assay are considerably more than those of glucose and at present commercial laboratories do not process the samples routinely. On balance, the practitioner is advised to use the OGTT.

Technique

- The horse is weighed and prepared as for the OGTT (above).
- The xylose solution is prepared as 0.5 g/kg bodyweight in 10% solution.
- A 'fasting' sample of blood ('time zero') is taken into potassium oxalate–sodium fluoride anticoagulant immediately before the test.

- A nasogastric tube is passed and the solution is delivered as a bolus to the stomach.
- Further blood samples are taken at 30-minute intervals for 2 hours.

Interpretation

In conditions of normal absorption, blood xylose concentrations rise from zero to a peak concentration of 1.33–1.67 mmol/l within 60–90 minutes of administration.

As with interpretation of the oral glucose tolerance curve (above), normal absorption and total malabsorption are easily appreciated. A flattened, intermediate curve suggests partial malabsorption and requires re-evaluation.

Faecal analysis

Intestinal parasites

The faeces should be examined grossly for large parasites and tapeworm proglottids.

Faecal egg count (FEC)

Parasite eggs are separated from the faecal mass by a floatation technique using solutions of high specific gravity. The results are calculated as eggs per gram (epg) of faeces. Faecal samples should be fresh and taken from the rectum if possible. A half universal volume (approximately 10 ml) is sufficient. Samples may be stored in a refrigerator for a short time before submission if necessary.

Strongyle eggs are readily identified in the laboratory, but it is difficult to distinguish between large and small species. However, small strongyle (cyathostome) eggs usually comprise the vast majority of the count (> 90%).

Interpretation

It is impossible to determine the number of parasites present in the gut on the basis of a faecal egg count. Egg production varies greatly between, and possibly within, species of worms and also varies with individual host factors such as age and immune status. Most importantly, intermediate larval stages do not produce eggs — thus parasitic infection may be a significant problem without a significant faecal egg count. However, some positive counts do reflect the severity of strongyle burdens: 500 epg suggests a mild burden; 800–1000 moderate, and >1500 severe. In general, counts greater than 500 epg indicate the need for control measures to be implemented.

Faecal egg reduction and anthelmintic resistance

Resistance amongst cyathostome species to several benzimidazole anthelmintics is well known. When evaluating the efficacy of a parasite control programme, particularly where drug resistance is suspected, it is useful to monitor the faecal egg count prior to worming and again 10–14 days after the routine anthelmintic treatment.

Following effective anthelmintic treatment, the faecal egg count reduction (FECR) at 10–14 days should be at least 90% and preferably close to 100%. If not, resistance should be suspected and the test repeated following a change of anthelmintic from one chemical group to another. The FECR is calculated as follows:

$$\text{FECR}\% = 1 - \left(\frac{\text{epg after 10–14 days}}{\text{epg at worming}} \right) \times 100\%$$

Within a group of horses, the FECR will vary between individuals (because of shifts in the individual host–parasite relationship), and as many horses as possible should be monitored to give an overview of the efficacy of control. In the case of a large group it is ideal to divide the horses in order to compare a subgroup, treated with the usual anthelmintic, with a positive control group which has been treated with an anthelmintic against which there is no known resistance (currently pyrantel and ivermectin).

Presence of faecal larvae

Unlike parasite eggs, faecal larvae are separated from a sample by sedimentation using the Baermann apparatus. Alternatively, a wet faecal smear may be examined under the microscope. Samples should be taken freshly for rapid analysis and not subject to refrigeration.

Presence of tapeworms

The laboratory test for diagnosing an *Anoplocephala* burden is unsatisfactory. Eggs are rarely floated out of faecal solution and are found primarily in gravid proglottids from which they are released after the segments have been passed in the faeces. Gravid segments or even whole tapeworms may be seen intermittently in the faeces, but usually there is no conclusive evidence of infection.

When investigating the possibility of tapeworm infection it may be more cost-effective to treat prophylactically, with a double dose of oral pyrantel embonate (38 mg/kg), than to attempt laboratory diagnosis. In positive cases, tapeworms may appear in the faeces 24 hours after treatment.

Presence of *Oxyuris equi*

Oxyuris (pinworm) eggs may be identified on the anal sphincter by pressing a strip of transparent adhesive tape onto the mucosal folds of the external sphincter and attaching it, adhesive side down, over a water droplet on the surface of a clean microscope slide. The operculated eggs show at 100x magnification.

Bacterial culture of faeces

Faecal samples inevitably contain a great many organisms with differing requirements for culture *in vitro*. When submitting samples it is therefore necessary to define the organism(s) of interest to enable selective culture.

Salmonella

In patients suffering salmonellosis the numbers of salmonellae shed may be very low, even during the acute stage of disease. In consequence, a minimum of 3 and preferably 5 faecal samples should be collected from the rectum at 24 hour intervals to increase the possibility of detection. An adequate sample should occupy half a universal tube (approx. 10 ml) — swabs are unsatisfactory.

At the laboratory the sample is inoculated into direct medium and an enrichment broth. A positive culture in the direct medium can be reported within 24 hours, but this does not always grow sufficiently well. The enriched culture needs to be subcultured to a selective medium for a further 12–24 hours. Suspect cultures are then subcultured again for biochemical test. The turn around time for samples is thus a minimum of 48 hours and may be as much as 72 hours.

Comments

- There appear to be no host-adapted salmonellae that affect horses, but horses are known to excrete salmonellae asymptomatically and they may act as carriers or reservoirs of infection. This occasionally calls into question the significance of some isolates of salmonella in horses with chronic diarrhoea. Whereas a positive isolate always carries the suspicion of being the primary aetiological agent in patients with colitis, excretion may accompany concurrent bowel diseases such as verminous colitis or lymphosarcoma.

- Despite the fact that salmonella may not be isolated in the faeces of a patient during life, it may be detected at fresh post-mortem in homogenates of the large intestinal mucosa and/or mesenteric lymph nodes.

- The concurrent submission of rectal mucosal biopsy specimens for culture improves the likelihood of detecting invasive salmonellae.

Clostridia

Clostridiosis (usually *Clostridia perfringens*) is uncommon in horses but is certainly a differential diagnosis to salmonellosis in cases of peracute/acute toxaemic colitis. Whilst faecal samples should always be cultured for salmonella, clinical circumstances may also dictate examination for clostridia. In some cases this may be an investigation of intestinal contents post-mortem. A half universal of faeces taken from the rectum is submitted for anaerobic culture as soon after collection as possible — swabs are unsatisfactory. A positive result is indicated by a high faecal count (>100 colony forming units per gram of faeces).

In the acute case it is possible to submit blood in anaerobic blood culture bottles (see 'Blood culture' in Chapter 8: 'Blood disorders'). Up to three samples should be taken during a 24-hour period. The isolation of clostridia from the blood is obviously significant.

Faecal leucocytes

The presence of leucocytes and occasionally epithelial cells in faecal samples suggests inflammatory injury to the distal intestinal mucosa. Consequently, they are a feature of severe diarrhoea (fluid faeces), particularly in the acute stage. High numbers suggest the presence of an intestinal pathogen such as salmonella or clostridia.

Technique

- Fresh faeces should be taken from the rectum and strained through a thin medical gauze to remove fibrous matter.
- If necessary, the sample is diluted to a watery consistency with saline (0.9%). A drop is smeared on a 1 x 3 inch microscope slide.
- The smear is air dried, stained with modified Wright's stain and mounted with a coverslip.
- The feathered (trailing) edge of the sample is viewed under low power (10x) to assess the presence or otherwise of leucocytes.

Interpretation

Large numbers, often in the presence of epithelial cells, are significant and suggest salmonellosis, but their presence is not pathognomonic for salmonellosis. Equally, the absence of faecal leucocytes does not rule out salmonellosis.

Faecal blood

When blood is clearly visible in the faeces, a red discolouration suggests a recent, distal source such as the small colon or rectum. A dark to black discolouration (melaena) suggests a

source in the proximal gastrointestinal tract or large colon. Chronic gastrointestinal loss is usually occult and may be associated with a state of chronic regenerative anaemia.

Occult blood may be detected qualitatively using a commercial kit. A small amount of specimen from deep within a faecal mass is smeared on a reagent impregnated paper slide. Two smears are made from different parts of the mass to increase the chances of detection. In the laboratory, the presence of haemoglobin is detected in the smear by reagents that produce a dye. Specimen preparations are stable if kept dry and may be sent through the post for development.

Comment

- Occult bleeding may be intermittent and ideally three faecal samples should be checked on separate occasions. Chemical tests for the determination of blood in faeces are highly sensitive but not specific. Potential sources are neoplastic infiltration of the bowel, parasitism or mucosal ulceration. A positive finding must be interpreted with great care, taking into consideration all the presenting clinical signs and the associated clinical pathology.

Faecal sand

Sand ingestion from topsoil or water courses may be associated with colonic impaction and, following abrasion of the intestinal mucosa, severe diarrhoea. If this is suspected, faeces should be tested for the presence of sand.

One volume of faeces is mixed vigorously with two volumes of water in a clear container and allowed to settle. Sand sediments to the base of the mixture.

Comment

- Minimal amounts of sand are often present in the faeces of grazing horses but amounts vary with the regional differences in soil type. A clearly defined layer of sand in a small faecal sample is abnormal, but if there is doubt as to its significance, the faeces of a healthy individual from the same region should be tested for comparison.

Chapter appendices

The appendices suggest applications of some of the diagnostic techniques covered in this chapter for the investigation of two common problems of the equine alimentary tract: dysphagia (Appendix 2.1) and diarrhoea (Appendix 2.2).

Further reading

Edwards GB (1992) Rectal examination. In: *Proceedings of the 14th Bain-Fallon Memorial Lectures, July 2nd–5th, Sydney, Australia*, pp. 93–101.

Greet T (1989) Dysphagia in the horse. *In Practice* (supplement to the Veterinary Record) **11**: 256--262.

Hunt JM (1987) Rectal examination of the equine gastrointestinal tract. *In Practice* (supplement to the Veterinary Record) **9**: 171–177.

Kopf N (1982) Rectal findings in horses with intestinal obstructions. In: *Proceedings of the 1st. Equine Colic Research Symposium, Georgia, U.S.A*, pp. 236–260.

Mair TS, Hillyer MH, Taylor FGR and Pearson GR (1991) Small intestinal malabsorption in the horse: an assessment of the specificity of the oral glucose tolerance test. *Equine Veterinary Journal* **23**: 344–346.

Schramme M (1995) Investigation and management of recurrent colic in the horse. *In Practice* (supplement to the Veterinary Record) **17**: 303–314.

Appendix 2.1. Some applications of diagnostic techniques for the investigation of dysphagia.

Possible cause	*Aids to diagnosis*
Choke/oesophageal foreign body	Stomach intubation to determine the level of obstruction (care!); endoscopy of the oesophagus; radiography of the oesophagus
Foreign body lodged in the mouth/oropharynx	Examination of the mouth; endoscopy of the upper alimentary tract
Oesophageal stricture	Endoscopy; contrast radiography
Oesophageal ulceration	Endoscopy
Squamous cell carcinoma involving the oesophagus	Endoscopy and biopsy (specialist centre); thoracic radiography
Teeth problems	Mouth examination; radiography
Pharyngitis, e.g. acute 'strangles' or viral infection	Endoscopy; nasopharyngeal swab (see Chapter 12)
Obstruction of the oropharynx or oesophagus, e.g. 'strangles' abscessation	Radiography of the oropharynx/oesophagus
Pharyngeal paralysis: – guttural pouch infection – trauma of the head or neck – lead poisoning – botulism	Endoscopy of the nasopharynx Endoscopy of the guttural pouches Neurological examination (see Chapter 14) Lead estimation in: blood (check lab's preferred anticoagulant); liver or kidney, and top soil Check clinical signs and feedstuff (see Chapter 14)
Hyoid abnormalities	Radiography of the oropharynx
Hepatic encephalopathy	Check blood ammonia (specialist centre); serum enzymes; liver function (see Chapter 4)
Tetanus	Check clinical signs
Grass sickness	Check clinical signs; radiography of the oesophagus (megoesophagus and pooling of contrast medium); endoscopy of the oesophagus ('reflux oesophagitis'); ileal biopsy (specialist centres); post-mortem histopathology of the coeliacomesenteric ganglion
Myopathies	Estimation of serum muscle enzymes (see Chapter 13)
Hypocalcaemia	Estimation of serum calcium, magnesium and phosphorus; response to treatment (see Chapter 5)

Appendix 2.2. Some applications of diagnostic techniques for the investigation of diarrhoea.

Possible cause	Aids to diagnosis
Acute diarrhoea	
Dietary changes	Dietary history
Salmonellosis (fairly common)*	Check clinical signs (colic, pyrexia, toxaemia and leucopenia suspicious); sequential culture of faeces; faecal leucocytes; rectal biopsy for histopathology and culture of homogenized specimen; post-mortem examination of fresh carcase (haemorrhagic inflammation of the caecum and colon/culture of tissues)
Intestinal clostridiosis (rare) **Colitis X (uncommon)**	Clinical signs and investigation as above for acute salmonellosis; the major differential between all three is the ability to isolate a causative organism; Clostridiosis: high faecal bacterial counts on anaerobic culture (>100 cfu/g faeces); Colitis X: no organisms isolated
Iatrogenic causes, e.g. antibiotics	History of drug treatment
Poisons, e.g. mycotoxins in feed, acorns, etc. in grazing	Check spoilage/adulteration of feedstuffs; grazing history
Endotoxaemia, e.g. acute peritonitis	Clinical signs; check WBC and plasma fibrinogen concentration
Sand colitis	Sandy grazing or muddy streams; sand in faeces
Hyperlipaemia (ponies and donkeys)	Milky opacity to plasma; a metabolic consequence of some other problem (see Chapter 16)
Chronic diarrhoea	
Salmonellosis (fairly common)*	Repeated faecal culture (at least five occasions)
Cyathostomiasis (common)	Faecal redworm egg and larvae counts; serum albumin, globulin and β-globulin estimations; rectal biopsy for histopathology
Malabsorption syndromes associated with various cellular infiltrations (uncommon)	Check serum albumin and ALP (or IAP); oral glucose tolerance test (to assess small intestinal involvement); rectal biopsy; full thickness colonic biopsies under general anaesthesia

*The clinician should *always* investigate the possibility of salmonellosis in a diarrhoeic horse.

3 Chronic wasting

The purpose of this chapter is to consider a strategy for the investigation of chronic wasting that occurs in the absence of an obvious predisposing cause. A horse that is losing weight for no obvious reason usually falls into one of two categories. It is either healthy, but suffering from some imposed stress or deprivation; or it is unhealthy, but not displaying any obvious signs of disease. A further possibility is that it is geriatric.

Wasting and the healthy horse

Problems of management which result in an imposed stress should become apparent during a careful consideration of the history. The clinician should consider the following possibilities:

- Inadequate parasite control
- Dental problems; especially sharp points on the cheek teeth
- Insufficient food; especially when supplementation is required owing to poor grazing or a high stocking density. Increasing work loads, cold weather, pregnancy and lactation will also increase nutrient demands. Infre-

quent feeding of a stabled animal may be associated with insufficiency
- Bullying of the individual within a group of horses, preventing adequate access to food
- Poor quality or unpalatable food owing to spoilage
- Inappropriate or unsuitable food
- Insufficient water. This is a particular danger where ad-lib supplies are not possible. The healthy adult horse requires 20–30 litres per day, the demand fluctuates with the level of work and changes in the ambient temperature
- Excessive work or irregular hard work in an unfit horse

Wasting and obscure disease

When disease is suspected but the associated clinical signs are obscure, the patient requires careful observation over a protracted period. Too often a visit by the clinician is associated with aroused interest and the patient is distracted to the extent that subtle signs disappear temporarily. In such circumstances it is preferable to hospitalize the animal for several days so that distractions cease and behavioural signs can be properly assessed.

Careful observations of behaviour, locomotion, eating and drinking are essential. These observations are complemented by a thorough and systematic clinical examination. Depending upon the findings, a logical strategy of clinicopathological investigation is then required. However, clinical pathology is no substitute for painstaking examination and the clinician should beware of heavy (and expensive) reliance on laboratory diagnosis.

Potential causes of obscure chronic wasting disease include:

- Persistent low grade pain
- Conditions interfering with feeding and drinking
- Conditions interfering with digestion and intestinal absorption
- Chronic liver diseases
- Chronic heart diseases
- Chronic kidney diseases
- Chronic low grade infection
- Neoplasia

These conditions will now be considered in more detail, together with pointers to diagnosis. At appropriate points the reader is referred elsewhere in the text for details of the relevant practical techniques.

Persistent low grade pain

Persistent low grade pain compromises the animal's welfare and can reduce its appetite or willingness to move about and graze. Examples are:

- *Chronic colic.* Causes of low-grade colic may be associated with subtle signs of discomfort such as persistent yawning, stretching of the abdomen (often misinterpreted as a desire to urinate), grinding of the teeth, or protracted prolapse of the penis in geldings (often with intermittent erections). Typical causes are chronic low grade peritonitis, chronic grass sickness, or progressive cellular infiltrations of the gut wall associated with a chronic inflammatory or neoplastic process. These conditions also

interfere with intestinal absorption (see below).
  Diagnostic aids. Colic assessment (see 'Clinical evaluation of the colic patient' in Chapter 2: 'Alimentary diseases'). Abdominal paracentesis will demonstrate peritonitis, but rarely discloses alimentary neoplasia. A serum biochemistry profile may reveal hypoalbuminaemia consistent with a protein-losing enteropathy. If so, an oral glucose tolerance test is indicated to check whether intestinal absorption is compromised. If low grade chronic grass sickness is suspected, the clinician should check carefully for signs of dysphagia. Other signs could include intermittent muscle fasciculation, patchy sweating and the development of a 'tucked up' abdomen.
- *Bilateral lameness;* most usually of the forelimbs. Examples include laminitis, navicular disease, 'splints', bruised soles, or chronic bilateral joint disease. However, they arc unlikely to be a cause of significant weight loss without being clinically obvious.
  Diagnostic aid. If the length of stride is shortened or pain is suspected in both forelimbs, a unilateral nerve block will reveal obvious lameness in the contralateral limb (see under: 'Musculoskeletal diseases').

Conditions interfering with feeding and drinking

Most obviously the teeth should be inspected for evidence of uneven wear or disease. The ability of the horse to flex its neck and eat/drink from the ground should also be checked. Otherwise, the clinician should look for subtle signs of difficulty in chewing and/or swallowing (dysphagia). These include: protracted time to eat a feed; dropping of food while eating ('quidding'); food and/or water returning down the nose; gulping water but swallowing little; dipping and splashing the muzzle in water. Dysphagia can be associated with the following conditions:

- Chronic grass sickness
- Pharyngeal paralysis (e.g. guttural pouch disease; neck trauma; lead poisoning)

- Pharyngitis
- Ulceration of the oropharynx/oesophagus
- Myopathy
- Low-grade botulism
- Hypocalcaemia
- Hyoid abnormalities
- Neoplasia of the upper alimentary tract

Diagnostic aids. Mouth examination. Endoscopy of the oropharynx to assess the swallow reflex (see 'Endoscopy of the upper alimentary tract' in chapter 2: 'Alimentary diseases'). Rare associations with myopathy or hypocalcaemia can be demonstrated by estimation of serum muscle enzyme and electrolyte concentrations respectively.

Conditions interfering with digestion and intestinal absorption

Conditions causing maldigestion in the horse are hardly described and poorly understood. In the absence of suitable laboratory tests for the horse, maldigestion is either rare or under-diagnosed. That said, maldigestion may accompany problems of intestinal absorption, which are much better defined in the horse.

In general, those enteropathies which affect the hindgut, or both the fore- and hindgut, are associated with diarrhoea. In such cases diarrhoea is an obvious clinical sign and a diagnosis is pursued by investigating the cause of diarrhoea (see Chapter 2: 'Alimentary diseases'). In the absence of diarrhoea, enteropathies that interfere with intestinal absorption are usually confined to the foregut. Lesions responsible for these *malabsorption syndromes* include:

- *Diffuse cellular infiltrations of the intestinal wall* by chronic inflammatory or neoplastic cells. These conditions present as chronic weight loss despite an apparently adequate food intake, but are relatively uncommon. A definitive diagnosis is obtained only by histopathological examination of an intestinal biopsy — it is important to realize that in such cases no visible or palpable lesion is likely to appear at laparotomy or gross post-mortem examination. Diseases defined by histopathology include: granulomatous enteritis; eosinophilic enteritis; avian tuberculosis and diffuse alimentary lymphosarcoma. In the authors' experience alimentary lymphosarcoma is the commonest of these diseases in the UK (see Chapter 10: 'Lymphatic diseases').

Diagnostic aids. Hypoalbuminaemia in the wasting horse is strongly indicative of a protein-losing enteropathy; only on rare occasions is it associated with liver or renal failure. Enteropathies may also be associated with raised concentrations of alkaline phosphatase, in particular intestinal alkaline phosphatase, but this is not an invariable finding. Evidence of a protein-losing enteropathy should always prompt an evaluation of intestinal absorption using the oral glucose tolerance test (see 'Tests of intestinal malabsorption' in chapter 2: 'Alimentary diseases'). Definitive diagnosis requires full thickness biopsy under general anaesthesia, but several are necessary as one may miss an affected region. However, since the prognosis for treatment in all cases is so poor the procedure is rarely justified.

- *Chronic diffuse peritonitis* can be associated with malabsorption.
  Diagnostic aids. Abdominal paracentesis; oral glucose tolerance test.
- *Heavy parasitism*. Large numbers of migrating and adult alimentary parasites can be associated with nutritional deprivation. However, most horses tolerate large parasite burdens without wasting — unless there is an associated enteropathy.
  Diagnostic aids. Faecal egg count; beta-globulin estimation by serum protein electrophoresis.

Chronic liver diseases

Chronic liver diseases such as ragwort poisoning or progressive cirrhosis can be associated with chronic wasting in the absence of obvious clinical signs.
Diagnostic aids. Estimation of serum liver enzyme concentrations. Liver function tests (see Chapter 4: 'Liver diseases').

Chronic heart diseases

Heart disease is not usually synonymous with wasting, but occasionally the investigation of a wasting horse reveals chronic conditions such as congestive heart failure, endocarditis or atrial fibrillation.

Diagnostic aids. Heart auscultation and evaluation of associated parameters; ECG; echocardiography (see Chapter 9: 'Cardio-vascular diseases').

Chronic kidney diseases

Intrinsic kidney diseases are rare in horses. However, chronic renal failure, for whatever reason, is invariably associated with weight loss and few tangible clinical signs.

Diagnostic aids. Estimation of serum urea and creatinine concentrations. A state of azotaemia indicates the need for further investigation of renal function (see Chapter 6: 'Urinary diseases').

Chronic low grade infection

Chronic internal abscessation, as in lymph nodes or other tissues, can pass undiagnosed in the wasting animal if no associated signs are present. On rare occasions systemic diseases such as leptospirosis, brucellosis or avian tuberculosis can be associated with depression and loss of weight in the absence of specific signs.

Diagnostic aids. Frequent monitoring of the rectal temperature by competent owners may reveal recurrent pyrexia. Haematology and plasma fibrinogen estimation may indicate a chronic septic inflammatory process. Abdominocentesis should be used to investigate the possibility of an abdominal location. Specific serology is required to implicate leptospirosis or brucellosis. Demonstration of a tubercular mycobacterium requires acid-fast staining of a suitable biopsy specimen. Unfortunately, tissue lesions become obvious only at an advanced state of disease. Tuberculin testing in horses is unreliable.

Neoplasia

Internal neoplasia often develops to an advanced state before significant clinical signs are apparent. In the meantime, obscure chronic wasting may be all that is apparent. In general terms, developing tumours can produce a variety of interrelated effects which are consistent with wasting:

- Reduced, variable or occasionally capricious appetite
- Low grade pain
- Physical obstruction, e.g. causing dysphagia or recurrent low grade colics
- Malabsorption (see above)
- Competition for absorbed nutrients owing to increasing metabolic demands
- Secondary anaemia

The commonest internal tumour of clinical significance in horses is lymphosarcoma, which most usually takes an abdominal form; either as a diffuse cellular infiltration of the intestine associated with malabsorption, or as a discrete mass acting as a space occupying lesion — both forms may occur together. Thoracic forms are less common. Leukaemias associated with lymphosarcoma are extremely rare in horses, so that haematology is often unhelpful.

Diagnostic aids. See 'Lymphosarcoma in horses' in Chapter 10: 'Lymphatic diseases'.

Clinical pathology and obscure wasting disease

When clinical signs are vague there is a natural tendency to place greater reliance on laboratory diagnosis. This can be expensive and unrewarding. Bearing in mind the conditions associated with wasting listed above, it is possible to unify the various clinicopathological investigations into a strategic approach to diagnosis using simple haematology and a routine serum biochemistry profile. The initial biochemistry profile should include: urea; acute and chronic liver enzymes; protein estimation (albumin and globulin), and muscle enzymes. Some interpretations of potential findings in wasting horses are summarized below.

Haematology

Anaemia most usually suggests dyserythropoiesis associated with chronic infection or, less commonly, neoplasia. Dyserythropoiesis can be confirmed by bone marrow aspirate or biopsy (see Chapter 8: 'Blood disorders').

Leucocytosis featuring a neutrophilia with a monocytosis is indicative of a chronic inflammatory process associated with infection or, less commonly, neoplasia.

A raised *fibrinogen* concentration is a sensitive indicator of septic inflammation. This is usually associated with bacterial infection, but could reflect necrosis within a tumour.

Serum biochemistry

Urea. Raised concentrations, say two-fold, simply indicate a high protein diet or, more likely, an increased tissue catabolism and protein turn-over associated with disease. Dehydration is also a possible cause. Higher concentrations suggest renal failure and should be corroborated by estimation of serum creatinine. Subsequent urinalysis can be helpful (see 'Analysis of urine' in Chapter 6: 'Urinary diseases').

Increases in the concentrations of acute and chronic *liver enzymes*, e.g. SDH and γGT respectively, suggest an active (ongoing) liver problem. When the insult ceases the chronic enzyme remains raised for a variable period of weeks to months, depending upon resolution of the lesion. When liver enzymes are raised, the total serum bile acid concentration should be requested in order to assess liver function. Percutaneous ultrasonography and biopsy may be helpful (see Chapter 4: 'Liver diseases').

The *serum globulin concentration* is raised by: inflammatory processes; infections; parasitism; liver failure and often, but not always, by lymphosarcoma. Serum protein electrophoresis may subsequently distinguish between parasitism and these other conditions; the beta-globulin concentration is often raised in response to migrating redworm (see 'Interpretation of blood biochemistry' in Chapter 1: 'Submission of samples and interpretation of results').

Hypoalbuminaemia is most usually the result of a protein-losing enteropathy. This is often associated with parasites or a malabsorption syndrome. Occasionally, hypoalbuminaemia is the result of chronic liver failure or a substantial inflammatory effusion such as chronic peritonitis. Only rarely is it associated with kidney disease (protein-losing nephropathy). In cases of hypoalbuminaemia, if parasites have been ruled out (serum globulin analysis, faecal egg count and/or larvicidal treatment) and liver or kidney diseases are not indicated, then an oral glucose tolerance test is necessary to assess absorption in the small intestine (for technique and interpretation see Chapter 2: 'Alimentary diseases').

Muscle enzyme concentrations (AST and CPK) are raised in all forms of myopathy. NB CPK is muscle specific, but an increase in AST alone is unlikely to be the result of muscle damage and could reflect active liver disease (see 'Interpretation of blood biochemistry' in Chapter 1: 'Submission of samples and interpretation of results'). However, there should be no confusion if other liver enzymes are requested in the profile.

Additional tests

A *faecal egg count* reflects the presence of adult redworm in the colon but not the burden of migrating parasites.

Abdominal paracentesis will provide evidence of abdominal inflammatory disease but rarely discloses exfoliative neoplastic cells.

Oral glucose tolerance test. A horse that is eating well but wasting in the absence of associated clinical signs should undergo an oral glucose tolerance test, even if hypoalbuminaemia is not identified (see above).

Serology can be used to detect occult infections such as leptospirosis (see Chapter 8: 'Blood disorders') and brucellosis (see Chapter 13: 'Musculoskeletal diseases').

Comment

- In the absence of any defined clinical abnormality, normal clinicopathological profiles should prompt a reconsideration of the history, i.e. the horse may be healthy but suffering from a management stress.

Further reading

Brown, CM (1989) Chronic weight loss. In: C.M. Brown (ed) *Problems in Equine Medicine,* pp. 6–22. Philadelphia: Lea & Febiger.

4 Liver diseases

I. Clinical pathology

Liver disease is relatively common in the horse but often occurs in the absence of specific clinical signs. It is usually diagnosed on the basis of a serum biochemistry profile and for this reason clinicopathological techniques are considered first in this chapter. Any horse with an obscure, non-specific history of malaise, lethargy, inappetance and/or weight loss should be screened for the possibility of liver disease.

The liver has great powers of regeneration and the more overt clinical signs associated with its failure do not appear until some 70–80% of the functional capacity is lost. *Obscure signs of liver disease are therefore much more common than overt signs of liver failure.* Signs of failure include central disturbances and are usually acute, even if the underlying liver disease has developed over a protracted period. This 'hepatic encephalopathy' is associated with toxic blood levels of ammonia and intestinal amines, which would normally be detoxified by the liver.

Acute liver disease can present as a mild, reversible condition of non-specific malaise with depression. In acute disease with liver failure a severe encephalopathy develops rapidly. There is defective vision, head-pressing, ataxia, compulsive walking and at the extreme, hyperexcitability with mania.

Chronic liver disease often features an obscure subclinical malaise with mild anaemia and weight loss over many months. This may be punctuated by acute episodes of more obvious depression and mild encephalopathy. Eventually the condition can terminate in a

Blood glucose

Hypoglycaemia develops in conditions of liver failure and therefore indicates a state of affairs requiring therapeutic support. The situation is aggravated by inappetance and a loss of efficient gluconeogenesis by the liver. Hypoglycaemia contributes to hepatic encephalopathy, the central disturbance associated with liver failure.

Blood ammonia

Because detoxification is impaired as a consequence of liver failure, there is an increase in the circulating concentrations of intestinal amines and ammonia (the products of protein degradation in the gut). These are associated with the development of encephalopathy.

Blood ammonia is the most convenient for routine laboratory estimation, but unfortunately it is labile and requires collection into anticoagulant (EDTA) for rapid plasma separation followed by prompt laboratory analysis (within two hours). Where facilities are available, serial estimations of blood ammonia can indicate an impending encephalopathy and also provide a sensitive monitor of the response to treatment.

Comment

- In conditions of liver failure the impaired detoxification of intestinal amines and ammonia is accompanied by a decrease in the circulating concentration of BUN (blood urea nitrogen) — the form in which they are normally detoxified. An increase in blood ammonia in the presence of a low BUN or urea is therefore consistent with liver failure.

Hyperlipaemia

Hyperlipaemia is a metabolic disease in which there is an abnormal mobilization of fat deposits caused by some form of stress or nutritional deprivation. It is most often seen in ponies and donkeys and is frequently associated with inadequate nutrition during late pregnancy. It also occurs secondary to any disease process which induces anorexia. The increased circulatory concentration of lipid induces fatty liver disease in which the serum liver enzymes are raised.

Evidence of hepatopathy associated with any disease process, or with advanced pregnancy in ponies and donkeys, should raise the suspicion of intercurrent hyperlipaemia. The condition is diagnosed by an abnormal increase in serum triglyceride concentration (>5 mmol/l), which in the extreme produces a milky discolouration of the plasma. The latter is readily apparent to the naked eye if a heparinized blood sample is allowed to stand and settle. See 'Hyperlipaemia' in Chapter 16: 'Fat diseases'.

Haematology

Haematology provides no specific information in cases of liver disease. Anaemia may accompany chronic disease and patients suffering bacterial infection, as in cholangitis or abscessation, will show leucocyte shifts and an increase in the plasma fibrinogen concentration.

In advanced liver failure there is a decrease in the production of coagulation factors and a consequent increase in clotting time (see 'Coagulation tests' in Chapter 8: 'Blood disorders'). In practical terms, the clinician is more likely to appreciate significant clotting defects as petechiation of the mucosae, or haematoma formation following venepuncture, rather than by pursuing elaborate coagulation tests.

Liver function tests

Bromosulphthalein (BSP) clearance

When BSP is introduced into the bloodstream it binds to albumin and accumulates in liver cells. Here it dissociates from albumin, conjugates with glutathione, and is excreted in the bile. Its clearance from the bloodstream can be used as a measure of the liver's functional capacity.

The clearance of BSP is defined as the time taken to reduce a given concentration in the circulation by half ($T_{1/2}$ BSP). Essentially, BSP is injected into the circulation and sequential blood samples are taken at recorded time intervals to calculate its speed of removal.

Prepared BSP solution can be obtained from the commercial laboratory which undertakes the assay and BSP plasma samples are sufficiently stable to be sent in the post. The technique is as follows:

- Before injecting BSP, a heparinized blood sample is taken from the jugular vein.
- 1 g of BSP is given intravenously and a stopwatch started *on completion of the injection.*
- Using heparinized 'Vacutainers' (Becton-Dickinson, UK) samples are collected from the opposite vein at 2, 4, 6 and 8 minutes after injection. Three sampling times will suffice, but the exact time of sampling must be recorded when the tube is approximately half full. Heparinized syringes may be used to draw a sample more promptly, but this necessitates an indwelling catheter.
- A portion of the BSP used for injection (e.g. 1 ml) should accompany the samples when submitted for analysis — this enables the laboratory to prepare a standard solution of known concentration against which the samples will be compared by colorimetry.
- From the assay results, the concentration of BSP in each sample is plotted on semi-logarithmic paper against a linear time scale. The result should be a linear plot, from which the time taken for a given circulating concentration to fall to half its value can be measured (Fig. 4.1).

The accepted clearance time ($T_{1/2}$) for a healthy horse is 2–3.5 minutes. Clearance times in excess of 4 minutes suggest a functional disturbance of the liver.

Comments

- In healthy horses BSP clearance occurs in two distinct exponential phases. The first and steepest part of the curve is associated with BSP uptake by liver cells and lasts roughly 7–10 minutes. This is followed by a well-defined convexity of the curve and a second exponential begins some 20–30 minutes later. This second phase is associated with the excretion of BSP into the bile by liver cells. The practical consequence is that samples taken after 10 minutes may produce results that lie on the curve between the two exponentials, thus confounding the calculation of a linear slope which is essential to $T_{1/2}$ measurement. It is therefore advisable to restrict samples to within the 10-minute period so that a linear clearance slope is obtained (Fig. 4.1).
- In healthy horses a period of fasting is associated with a delay in the hepatocellular transport time of all metabolites. In any disease process associated with inappetance the same physiological effect will occur and may result in a prolonged $T_{1/2}$ despite normal liver function.
- The test is contraindicated in any situation where the circulating concentration of total bilirubin is elevated — i.e. in all cases of jaundice. Bilirubin competes with

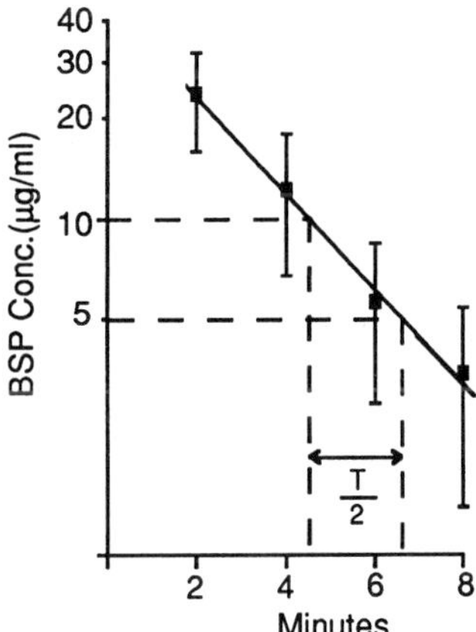

Figure 4.1   BSP clearance in five healthy ponies following the intravenous injection of 1 g of BSP (mean plots ± SD). The clearance time ($T_{1/2}$) is derived by selecting a blood concentration (10 μg/ml in the above example) and measuring the time scale required to reduce its value by half. Mean $T_{1/2}$ = 2.2 minutes (range 1.8–2.5).

BSP for clearance and will produce a spurious $T_{1/2}$.

- Since BSP binds to albumin and then dissociates in hepatocytes prior to conjugation and excretion, any condition causing hypoalbuminaemia has the potential to shorten $T_{1/2}$ values.

- Poor circulation through the liver (e.g. cardiac insufficiency) will be associated with poor clearance of BSP.

Total serum bile acids (TSBA)

Bile acids are synthesized and conjugated with amino acids in the liver and excreted in the bile. Assuming a similar function to that in man, they are important for the digestion of dietary fats and the absorption of fat-soluble vitamins. Following excretion they are largely reabsorbed from the gut and re-excreted in the bile, thus undergoing an 'enterohepatic cycle' (Fig. 4.2). A small portion enters the peripheral circulation after reabsorption and can be measured as the total serum bile acid concentration.

In cases of liver malfunction the re-excretion of bile acids is reduced, resulting in higher circulating levels of TSBAs. The estimation of TSBAs from a single blood sample therefore provides a liver function test without the need for more invasive (and expensive) procedures. It also allows liver function to be monitored routinely during disease and treatment.

Many commercial laboratories now undertake TSBA estimation and require only a clotted blood sample (serum). Interpretation should always be based on the normal range for horses as supplied by the individual laboratory.

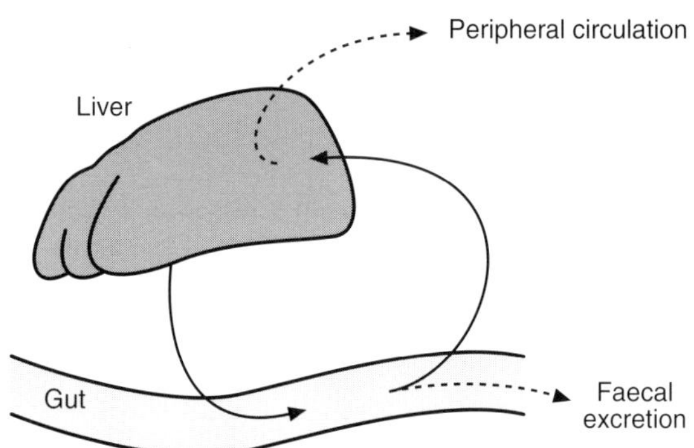

Figure 4.2   The enterohepatic cyle of bile acids. In liver malfunction the circulating concentration of bile acids is increased.

Comments
- TSBAs will be raised (but not grossly elevated) by fasting or inappetance.
- Poor liver circulation will increase TSBAs.

Liver fascioliasis

Horses are known to be parasitized by the sheep/cattle fluke *Fasciola hepatica*. The longevity of the adult fluke could mean that infected horses suffer low-grade hepatitis and associated poor performance for several months after removal from the source of infected grazing. However, in an abnormal host the parasite does not develop to full patency and few (if any) eggs are produced in the faeces.

As proof of infection, the conventional faecal analysis requires adaptation to detect a low number of eggs in a large amount of faeces. In most instances this is not practical. Where there is circumstantial evidence in the history of access to fluke pastures it is advisable to treat the horse for fascioliasis (e.g. oxyclozanide: 10 mg/kg *per os*) and assess the clinical/clinicopathological response.

II. **Practical techniques**

Clinical examination and, in particular, clinical pathology can conclude that a state of hepatopathy exists, but in most instances the cause is inapparent. Ultrasonography and liver biopsy may help to provide aetiological information — but not invariably. However, they will provide information concerning the severity and prognosis of the lesion. They also establish a comparison for future examinations.

Ultrasonography of the liver

In normal adult horses the bulk of the liver is situated on the right side of the cranial abdomen but it may be 'scanned' beneath the ribs of both sides by percutaneous ultrasonography. A low frequency transducer, in the range 2–3.5 MHz, is suitable for liver ultrasonography and a sector scanner, with a small transducer/patient contact area, is preferred because of the restricted access between ribs.

On the left side, the liver is found ventral to the lung margin extending from the diaphragm in a caudal direction over several rib spaces to where it lies adjacent to the spleen (7th–11th intercostal spaces). On the right side, the liver is found ventral to the lung margin extending from the diaphragm to the level of the right kidney (7th–15th intercostal spaces). The exact position is variable and alters with age, bodily condition and breed. Careful skin preparation is essential for percutaneous ultrasonography and in most cases this involves clipping the hair, cleansing the skin with povidone–iodine and then degreasing with spirit.

Ultrasonography of the liver should include an assessment of the following:

- *The volume and nature of the surrounding peritoneal fluid.* Increases in peritoneal fluid cause displacement of the liver away from its normal close contact with the body wall. The echogenicity of the fluid increases with its turbidity and cellularity.

- *The overall size of the liver.* Liver size is very variable in horses. However, a subjective assessment of overall size can be made by considering the area of surface contact between the liver and body wall relative to the animal's size, and the depth of tissue which is present over this area.

- *The capsular surface of the liver and the angle of its ventral margin.* The healthy liver has a capsule which provides a smooth and sharply defined border, with an acute angle at its ventral limit.

- *The texture of the hepatic parenchyma.* Healthy hepatic parenchyma has a uniform echogenicity. Variations in overall echogenicity may result from changes in transducer/patient contact, transducer frequency and control settings, or hepatic disease. Experience with a standard examination protocol will allow a subjective assessment of hepatic echogenicity to be made. Diffuse increases in echogenicity may result from fibrosis or cellular infiltration. Focal changes in echogenicity are more readily appreciated and may result from liver abscessation, hydatid cysts, cholelithiasis, or neoplasia. The appearance of these abnormal areas may suggest an aetiology and usually enable a 'targeted' biopsy to be obtained.

- *The appearance of the hepatic vasculature.* Images of hepatic veins and hepatic portal veins can be identified. The latter tend to have more echogenic borders. Alterations in the size or shape of these vessels can be appreciated readily and usually reflect other (e.g. cardiovascular) disorders.

Liver biopsy

Most lesions which afflict the horse liver are diffuse so that a biopsy usually provides a representative sample for histopathology. The severity of the lesion is usually apparent, which may help in terms of prognosis, but the precise cause is not always revealed. Exceptions are cases where the pathology is characteristic, e.g. the hepatomegalocytosis of ragwort poisoning. Contraindications for biopsy are evidence of concurrent coagulopathy, or suspicion of liver abscessation.

Instruments

Several medical biopsy instruments are suitable for the purpose. The 14 gauge disposable 'Tru-cut' needle (Baxter Healthcare Corporation, California) retrieves good specimens with practice. A 6 inch (153 mm) length is suitable for most horses. When a biopsy is obtained using ultrasound guidance, the use of a single-handed automated biopsy system is a considerable advantage.

Site of biopsy

If ultrasound is available, the optimal site for biopsy will be shown by the liver image. In the absence of ultrasound the approach is the same for all instruments. A site is selected in the 13th intercostal space on the right hand side, just in front of the 14th rib, midway between a wedge whose upper and lower limits are delineated respectively by imaginary lines drawn from the point of the hip to the point of the shoulder, and from the point of the hip to the point of the elbow (Fig. 4.3). The 14th rib is located by

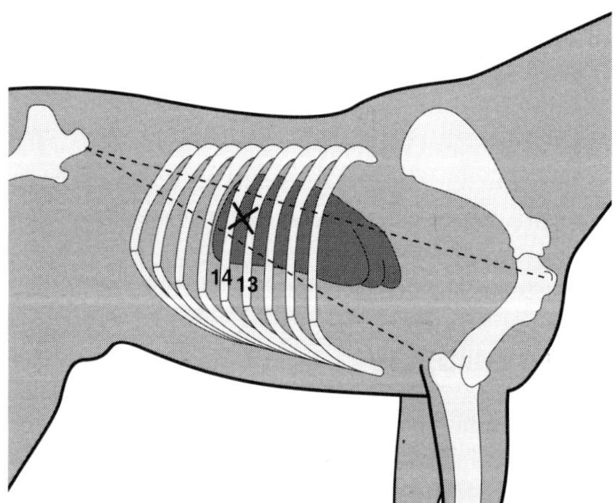

Figure 4.3 Landmarks indicating a suitable site for liver biopsy in the absence of ultrasound guidance.

counting back from the 18th rib, ignoring 'floating ribs'.

Procedure

- An area 4 x 4 inches (10 x 10 cm) is clipped and surgically prepared at the chosen site.
- Depending upon temperament, the horse may require sedating.
- Using sterile precautions the skin and intercostal muscle beneath are infiltrated down to the parietal pleura with 4–5 ml of 2% lignocaine using a 1.5 inch x 21G (39 x 0.8 mm) needle.
- A 5 mm skin incision is made just in front of the 14th rib. *It is important to avoid the intercostal vessels and nerves which run caudal to the border of the adjacent rib.*
- The biopsy needle is introduced through the incision, into intercostal muscle and then directed some ten degrees backwards to pass through the lung and diaphragm. If inserted at the point of full expiration, the amount of lung involved is minimized. It is possible to feel the diaphragm 'pick up' on the instrument as it passes through. If released from the operator's grip, the instrument will now be seen to move with the respiratory excursions of the diaphragm.
- The biopsy needle is advanced 5 cm or so into the liver, which has a 'solid' feel, and at this point the instrument is operated. At withdrawal the core of tissue should be dark in colour and sink in fixative. If the first attempt yields nothing (or a pale tissue which does not readily sink), two further attempts may be made through the same incision, redirecting the needle slightly and maintaining sterile precautions. If there is clinical/clinicopathological evidence of liver infection, a sample (or part of a sample), should be submitted for culture in a sterile container.
- A single interrupted suture is placed in the wound, although a dab of wound powder is often sufficient for such a small incision. The horse is rested at least one hour to permit clotting within the biopsy tract.
- If unsuccessful, it is possible to repeat the procedure at a different site, preferably after

24 hours. Using a 'blind' procedure it is advisable to try one intercostal space farther back, but in older horses atrophy may cause the liver to be drawn forward. The advantages of ultrasound-guided biopsy are obvious.

- The patient's tetanus status should be assessed and the appropriate action taken.

Complications of liver biopsy

These are rare. Tissues other than liver (e.g. diaphragm, lung, colon) may be inadvertently sampled without undue effect. However, if the core of tissue obtained does not have the 'feel', colour or texture of liver, it is advisable to give a short course of antibiotics in case of bowel penetration.

Haemorrhage may occur into the abdomen or thorax. Serious haemorrhage is a rare complication of liver biopsy, even in advanced disease. Where there is evidence of extended clotting time, such as haematoma formation following venepuncture, an estimation of bleeding time may be helpful (see 'Coagulation tests' in Chapter 8: 'Blood disorders').

Comments

- On occasion normal tissue will be obtained at biopsy. Depending upon the clinical and clinicopathological circumstances, this may suggest a discrete liver lesion such as abscessation, fascioliasis or (rarely) neoplasia.

- The ultrasound-guided technique offers the opportunity to biopsy the liver from the left side of the horse. Blind biopsy of the left side is not recommended.

Further reading

Divers, TJ (1991) Hepatic disease. In: N.E. Robinson (Ed). *Current Therapy in Equine Medicine*, 3rd edn, pp. 253–259. Philadelphia: W.B. Saunders.

5 Endocrine diseases

This chapter covers the diagnosis of those disease states which are known or thought to have a basis in endocrinopathy. Clinical endocrinopathies of the horse are less well defined than in other companion animals. However, this situation is likely to change as more equine hormone assays and dynamic tests are developed. In recent years the diagnosis of equine hyperadrenocorticism (Cushing's disease) has received a lot of attention and it now seems that many more cases are recognized than formerly.

Hyperadrenocorticism

In horses hyperadrenocorticism (HAC) is caused primarily by an adenoma of the intermediate lobe of the pituitary gland. The tumour is functional, producing an excess of secretions including adrenocorticotrophic hormone (ACTH). This in turn can cause adrenocortical hypertrophy accompanied by an increase in circulating cortisol. The increased blood cortisol concentration has a number of potential effects. It may inhibit insulin (resulting in hyperglycaemia), antagonize antidiuretic hormone activity (contributing to polyuria/polydipsia), promote immunosuppression, and mediate the development of laminitis. In addition, the tumour mass itself can exert pressure locally, producing a variety of bizarre clinical signs. Dorsal expansion will put pressure on the posterior lobe of the pituitary, the hypothalamus or the optic chiasma. Compression of the posterior lobe can interfere with antidiuretic hormone (ADH) secretion and further contribute to polyuria/polydipsia. Pressure on the hypothalamic thermoregulatory centre may be responsible for excess hair growth (hirsutism) and excess sweating. In the extreme, expansion can produce central effects including visual impairment, but this is uncommon.

Unlike other species, adrenal tumours are almost unknown as a cause of HAC in horses and diagnostic techniques are therefore directed to demonstrating the presence and effects of a pituitary adenoma.

HAC is usually suspected on the basis of a number of appropriate clinical signs which lead to an investigation of clinical pathology and thence to the use of a dynamic function test. However, definitive diagnosis is usually only possible at post-mortem examination when a pituitary adenoma and adrenocortical hypertrophy are confirmed. Although HAC is not curable, there are a number of promising treatments which serve to alleviate the condition and improve the horse's quality of life. Consequently, the pursuit of an ante-mortem diagnosis is well justified.

Presentation and clinical signs

The condition occurs in older animals (usually >12 years) of either sex and the prevalence is greater in ponies. There is a wide variation in the clinical signs exhibited by an individual case, but such signs commonly include one or more of the following:

- A long, unkempt curly coat which fails to shed. This is the most consistent clinical feature of equine HAC.
- Weight loss
- Depression/lethargy
- Laminitis
- Polyuria/polydipsia (PUPD)

Other frequent signs include persistent sweating and some manifestation of infection associated with the concurrent immuno-suppression, e.g. pneumonia, cystitis, or skin infection.

Comment

- A high percentage of patients with HAC develop laminitis, but not all cases of equine laminitis are associated with the development of HAC. However, the onset of laminitis in an older animal, particularly in the presence of one of the other common

clinical signs listed above, merits investigation for underlying HAC.

Clinical pathology

Suspicion of HAC should stimulate a simple clinicopathological investigation. The most consistent (though not invariable) finding is hyperglycaemia which in many cases is sufficiently high to exceed renal threshold, resulting in glucosuria. The basal (resting) blood cortisol concentration may be raised, but this is not a consistent feature and cannot be used diagnostically. Normal adult horses show a diurnal variation in their basal cortisol concentrations, with a peak occurring in the early- to mid-morning.

In patients presenting with PUPD, the differential diagnosis of renal failure should be investigated by checking blood urea and creatinine concentrations. Other differentials of PUPD are covered later in this chapter.

Haematology is non-specific; the erythrocyte parameters are often normal, but a neutrophilia is common.

Dynamic function tests

There are several dynamic tests, largely borrowed from work in other species, which can be used to indicate the presence of a pituitary adenoma. Opinions vary about the suitability of these various tests. The authors currently suggest the thyrotropin-releasing hormone (TRH) response test, but there is no single unequivocal ante-mortem test for HAC in horses.

In all cases, estimation of blood cortisol is required before and after test. This can be undertaken in plasma (heparinized blood) or serum, but in either case the sample should be separated from blood cells before dispatch to the laboratory.

ACTH stimulation test

Adrenocortical hypertrophy can be inferred by demonstrating an exaggerated response of the blood cortisol concentration to an injection of exogenous ACTH. Normal horses will show an approximate 80% increase in cortisol concentration 2 hours after an intravenous injection of 100 iu of synthetic ACTH ('Synacthen': Ciba). In contrast, most — *but not all* — cases of pituitary-dependent HAC will show increases well in excess of this at 2 hours after injection.

Comment

- In patients with laminitis there is a risk of exacerbating the condition by increasing the circulating concentration of endogenous glucocorticoid following ACTH injection.

Dexamethasone suppression test

This test evaluates the adrenal cortex–pituitary axis by demonstrating the capacity for negative feedback of glucocorticoid on the secretion of ACTH from the pituitary gland. Normal horses will show a fall in blood cortisol concentration to some 30% of the resting level within 4 hours of an intramuscular injection of 20 mg dexamethasone. The concentration then remains depressed for at least 24 hours. In pituitary-dependent HAC the depression is much less marked.

Comment

- The dexamethasone suppression test is a more consistent indicator of HAC than the ACTH stimulation test (above). However, corticosteroid administration can precipitate laminitis in horses and its use is questionable in an animal that is already susceptible to laminitis.

Combined dexamethasone suppression/ACTH stimulation test

The above tests can be combined in a protocol conducted over 5 hours which requires only three blood cortisol assays. A basal cortisol sample is collected and an intramuscular injection of 10 mg dexamethasone is administered. A second blood sample is taken 3 hours later, after which 100 iu synthetic ACTH ('Synacthen': Ciba) is given intravenously, and a final blood sample is taken 2 hours later.

Normal horses show a fall in blood cortisol to some 30% of the basal concentration at 3 hours and an increase to approximately twice the basal concentration following ACTH administration. In pituitary-dependent HAC the depression is less marked, but the response to ACTH is exaggerated (Fig. 5.1).

Comments

- Although it is convenient, this combined test does not allow evaluation of the prolonged depression of blood cortisol in response to dexamethasone and it is consequently considered less useful than the individual tests cited above.

- The same concerns about the administration of ACTH and corticosteroid apply as described above under the individual tests.

TRH response test

In many cases of pituitary adenoma there is a significant increase in basal cortisol concen-

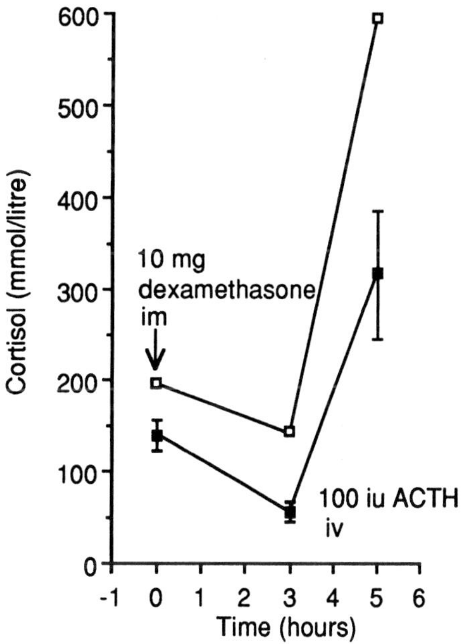

Figure 5.1   Blood cortisol response to a combined dexamethasone suppression/ACTH stimulation test in four normal horses and a case of HAC. ■ Mean of normals; □ case of HAC.

tration within a short time of administering TRH. This presumably results from an aberrant response of the tumour to TRH, in which the release of ACTH and ACTH-like compounds is stimulated. Not surprisingly, the blood cortisol concentration of normal horses should show a minimal response following TRH administration, since no response mechanism exists in the normal pituitary gland.

A heparinized or plain blood sample is taken prior to the intravenous injection of 1 mg TRH (Roche) and a second sample is taken 30 minutes later. In cases of pituitary-dependent HAC, the basal cortisol concentration increases some 50–100% or more.

NB TRH will increase the circulating concentrations of thyroid stimulating hormone (TSH), triiodothyronine (T_3) and thyroxine (T_4), but in this application the assay of these hormones is irrelevant.

Comments

- This test has the advantage of excluding the use of exogenous corticosteroid and the effect on the endogenous cortisol concentration is relatively transient.

- In the authors' experience the response to TRH is less (but nevertheless significant) in Cushingoid patients with high basal cortisol concentrations. Those patients that have a basal cortisol within the normal range show a much greater response. This diminution of response to TRH by high resting cortisol concentrations is also reported in human patients.

Post-mortem examination

A variably sized tumour of the intermediate lobe of the pituitary is seen (access is described under: 'Examination of the head and brain' in Chapter 18: 'Post-mortem examination'). It is usually clearly delineated, though not encapsulated. The mass should be transferred to 10% formalin as soon as possible if histopathological confirmation is required.

Examination of the adrenals reveals hypertrophy of the cortex. Other pathological findings, such as laminitis or various tissue infections, will relate to the presenting clinical signs.

Causes of polyuria/ polydipsia (PUPD)

We have already seen that PUPD in older horses can be caused by HAC — in fact HAC is probably the commonest cause of PUPD in older horses. Less likely causes of PUPD are renal failure, other causes of hyperglycaemia with glucosuria, diabetes insipidus and psychogenic polydipsia.

Hyperadrenocorticism

These cases frequently feature hyperglycaemia with glucosuria, which results in osmotic diuresis. However, some Cushingoid horses have PUPD in the absence of glucosuria. In these patients polyuria may be the result of reduced ADH activity — either by interference of its secretion by the tumour mass, or by inhibition of its activity at the renal tubules by high levels of circulating glucocorticoid. Whenever polyuria occurs in the absence of tangible renal disease, HAC should always be considered as the likely cause and investigated by careful appraisal of clinical signs and dynamic function test (see above).

Renal failure

Renal failure as a cause of PUPD should be investigated by checking a blood sample for azotaemia and pursuing renal function tests (see Chapter 6: 'Urinary diseases').

Hyperglycaemia and glucosuria

Osmotic diuresis as a result of glucosuria is most usually associated with HAC. Other causes of persistent hyperglycaemia are much rarer in horses, but if they are associated with glucosuria then PUPD can be expected (see below under: 'Hyperglycaemia').

Diabetes insipidus

Diabetes insipidus is characterized by the inability of the kidney to concentrate urine due to a lack of ADH (central diabetes insipidus) or an insensitivity of the renal tubules to ADH (renal or nephrogenic diabetes insipidus).

Central diabetes insipidus may be associated with a pituitary adenoma (see above), but it can occur in the absence of tumour activity. Renal diabetes, although very rare, can occur secondary to renal infections, bacterial toxins, or persistent hypercalcaemia and mineralization of tubules.

Where pituitary adenoma, renal disease and glucosuria have been eliminated as causes of polyuria, the remaining possibilities are diabetes insipidus and psychogenic polydipsia. Water deprivation tests should be undertaken first to distinguish between these two conditions (see below). In the case of psychogenic polydipsia, the urine will concentrate (assuming normal renal function), but in the case of diabetes insipidus the urine will fail to concentrate because ADH secretion or activity remains impaired. In these patients an exogenous ADH test is indicated.

Horses afflicted with central diabetes insipidus will show urinary concentration in response to exogenous ADH. Pitressin tannate in oil is given intramuscularly (6 units/50 kg) and the water intake is monitored per 6 hours for 24–36 hours. In central diabetes insipidus the consumption (and output) should decrease, whilst the urinary SG increases.

No response to exogenous ADH suggests either renal diabetes insipidus or psychogenic polydipsia. If psychogenic polydipsia has already been ruled out by deprivation tests (see below), then by elimination the concluding diagnosis is renal diabetes insipidus.

Psychogenic polydipsia and water deprivation tests

Psychogenic polydipsia results from the excessive drinking of water and is presumed to be associated with a psychological problem such as stable boredom. Tubular function and ADH activity are not impaired, so that water deprivation should induce urinary concentration.

NB *Water deprivation tests should not be undertaken in dehydrated horses or those showing azotaemia.*

The deprivation test should begin in the evening to ensure that regular hydration checks can be made during the daylight hours of the following day. The procedure is as follows:

- All feed and water is removed. The bladder is emptied by catheter and the urinary SG determined.
- The SG, blood urea and PCV or total protein are checked per 4–8 hours for a maximum of 20 hours. The test should be stopped when the SG indicates an adequate urinary concentration or, alternatively, if azotaemia or dehydration develop.
- If the SG reaches no more than 1.020 by 20 hours, then deprivation to 24 hours may be considered if it is safe to do so.

An increase in SG above 1.020 following water deprivation indicates psychogenic polydipsia. A low or suboptimal SG suggests either diabetes insipidus or 'medullary washout'. Any longstanding case of polyuria/polydipsia, of whatever cause, may be associated with the 'washout' of sodium and chloride from the medullary interstitium of the kidney. This medullary washout reduces the osmolarity of the renal medulla, causing an inability to concentrate urine. An otherwise healthy kidney may therefore show poor concentrating ability following a water deprivation test. If urine does not concentrate >1.020 at 24 hours, an extended modified water deprivation test should be considered to overcome the confusion in diagnosis caused by medullary washout.

In the modified test, the daily water intake is restricted to 40 ml/kg for several days, after which the SG is reassessed. An increase in SG >1.020 indicates psychogenic polydipsia. A lack of concentration suggests diabetes insipidus, for which an exogenous ADH test is then indicated (see above).

Hyperglycaemia

Hyperglycaemia is an increase in the blood glucose above an accepted 'normal range'. The authors consider this range to be 3.5–6.0 mmol/l (approximately 60–100 mg/dl). Persistent hyperglycaemia is uncommon in the horse and is usually the result of HAC (see above). In contrast, transient hyperglycaemic states are relatively common. Where blood glucose concentrations are found to exceed the normal range it is advisable to obtain several sequential samples, at times which avoid feeding or exercise. This will enable the clinician to distinguish between a transient, reversible hyperglycaemia and a persistent, irreversible state, which is the result of chronic disease.

Causes of transient hyperglycaemia

In healthy horses the blood glucose concentration fluctuates continuously and may increase above the normal range as a result of dietary or other influences as follows:

- Increased carbohydrate intake
- Glycogenolysis (under hormonal influence, e.g. adrenaline)
- Increased insulin resistance — caused by physiological influences such as stress (including strenuous exercise), obesity and pregnancy
- Iatrogenic causes, e.g. corticosteroid or α_2 agonist administration.

In most instances transient hyperglycaemia does not exceed renal threshold and associated glucosuria is unlikely.

Causes of persistent hyperglycaemia (diabetes mellitus)

Persistent hyperglycaemia is uncommon in the horse, but when it occurs it is frequently accompanied by glucosuria. In most instances this is associated with insulin resistance and a resting hyperinsulinaemia. The singular (and extremely rare) exception is hypoinsulinaemic diabetes mellitus in which there is a reduced insulin availability due to pancreatic beta cell disease.

The discovery of persistent hyperglycaemia suggests a condition that is unregulated by insulin and is one of a number of disease features consistent with a diagnosis of diabetes mellitus. However, diabetes mellitus in the horse differs from other species in that primary disease of the insulin producing beta cells is unknown. Almost invariably, equine diabetes is secondary, characterized by the presence of a known or suspected primary disease process which accounts for insulin resistance or, much more rarely, failure of its production. Apart from the most common cause, HAC, these diseases include rare endocrinopathies such as phaeochromocytoma (tumour of the adrenal medulla) and beta cell damage secondary to a generalized pancreatic disease.

Hyperadrenocorticism

HAC is associated with an excess of cortisol secretion which antagonizes insulin activity and promotes gluconeogenesis. Diabetes mellitus in the horse is almost exclusively associated with this condition, which should be investigated as the first differential diagnosis (see above). When HAC is ruled out, the differential causes of persistent hyperglycaemia are narrowed to phaeochromocytoma and pancreatic disease.

Phaeochromocytoma

This is a rare tumour of the adrenal medulla associated with an excessive secretion of adrenaline and/or noradrenaline which antagonize insulin and promote glycogenolysis.

Clinical signs include PUPD (glucosuria and osmotic diuresis), excessive sweating, tachycardia, tachypnoea, muscle tremors and anxiety.

Clinical pathology is unhelpful. Venous noradrenaline concentrations will probably be elevated, but at present there is no commercial laboratory assay for this hormone. A definitive diagnosis is most usually determined at post-mortem examination.

NB Some adrenal tumours can exist as non-functional, asymptomatic lesions in life and are subsequently incidental findings at post-mortem examination.

Pancreatic disease

In general, pancreatic disease is very rare in the horse. Very occasionally, a generalized lesion may cause secondary beta cell damage resulting in hypoinsulinaemia with consequent hyper-glycaemia.

Clinical signs of pancreatic disease will depend upon the nature of the primary lesion:

- *Acute pancreatitis* is a cause of severe colic. In these instances amylase concentrations are likely to escalate in the serum and peritoneal fluid as a result of acute tissue damage. However, acute necrosing pan-creatitis is almost invariably a post-mortem finding since there are no specific clinical signs of pancreatitis to prompt amylase estimation or otherwise differentiate it from other forms of severe colic. In addition, the lesion may not be appreciable at laparo-tomy. Recorded causes include infection, migrating parasites and immune-mediated inflammation.
- *Chronic pancreatitis* may be associated with weight loss, hyperglycaemia and PUPD (as a result of glucosuria). Pituitary function tests for HAC, prompted by the hyperglycaemia, will be normal. Serum and peritoneal amylase may be raised, but enzyme release is much less likely than in the acute case. This is the rare occasion in the horse where a serum insulin assay may reveal hypoin-sulinaemia (secondary beta cell damage) and ketones may be found in the urine.

NB The use of insulin tolerance tests (i.e. the studied effect of exogenous insulin on the hyperglycaemic state) have been shown to be equivocal in horses for diagnosing diabetes mellitus associated with hypoinsulinaemia. In these patients it would seem to be of greater diagnostic value to measure the serum insulin concentration. Equine serum insulin estimation is offered by some commercial laboratories.

Comments

- In all cases of chronic hyperglycaemia featuring insulin resistance, histopathology

of the pancreas is likely to be reported as normal, but with beta cell depletion or degeneration. This is probably the result of hyperstimulation and exhaustion of the islet tissue in the hyperglycaemic state.
- Tumours of the islet cells are exceedingly rare but may be associated with excessive insulin production and a state of persistent hypoglycaemia. A case of recurrent hypoglycaemic seizures is recorded.

Thyroid disorders

The thyroid hormones, thyroxine (T_4) and triiodothyronine (T_3), affect almost every organ system by assisting the regulation of growth, cell differentiation and metabolism. Thyroid dysfunction therefore has the capacity to be associated with an enormous diversity of clinical signs, but as yet these are poorly defined in the horse. With the advent of reliable hormone assays for use by commercial veterinary laboratories, there is the potential for recognizing more syndromes associated with thyroid dysfunction.

Thyroid adenoma

The commonest thyroid disorder of the horse is the thyroid adenoma. It is frequently seen in older horses as an enlarged, palpable, uni-lateral swelling on one or other side of the larynx. *It is non-functional, unassociated with endocrinopathy and rarely merits any inter-ference.*

Hypothyroidism

A definitive clinical state of hypothyroidism in the adult horse is not recognized. It is frequently suspected by clinicians and owners, but is rarely substantiated by hormone assay or dynamic test. The rare cases of hypothyroidism defined by dynamic test are associated with a variety of clinical signs.

Hypothyroidism has been associated with a myopathy in racing Thoroughbreds — clinical signs included erratic appetite, decreased endurance, dullness and a stiffness of gait. A syndrome of progressive hair loss has been described in young horses, but it is exceedingly rare and other causes of non-pruritic alopecia should be considered first (see Chapter 17: 'Skin diseases').

NB Hypothyroidism can stem either from thyroid disease (primary hypothyroidism) or from disease of the hypothalamus or pituitary gland (secondary hypothyroidism).

Dynamic tests of thyroid function

A tentative diagnosis of equine hypothyroidism is made on the basis of abnormally low serum or plasma concentrations of T_3 and T_4, but this must be confirmed by dynamic test.

TSH stimulation test

A heparinized or plain blood sample is collected prior to the intramuscular injection of 5 iu of thyroid stimulating hormone (TSH; bovine origin: Sigma). Subsequent blood samples are collected at 3 hours and 6 hours after injection and the plasma or serum separated for submission to the laboratory. Each sample is assayed for T_3 and T_4 concentrations.

In adult horses with normal thyroid function the basal T_3 concentration rises approximately four-fold at 3 hours after TSH administration and falls to less than twice baseline by 6 hours. In hypothyroidism the low baseline of T_3 concentration is hardly affected by TSH at 3 or 6 hours (Fig. 5.2).

The T_4 concentration of healthy adults rises progressively after stimulation and approximately doubles its baseline value by 6 hours. In hypothyroidism the low basal concentration responds more sluggishly (Fig. 5.3).

Comments

- There appear to be no breed differences in the blood concentrations of thyroid hormones in adults, but some sex differences are recognized. In interpreting results, the advice of the laboratory should always be sought in respect of normal ranges.

- The TSH test determines primary hypo-

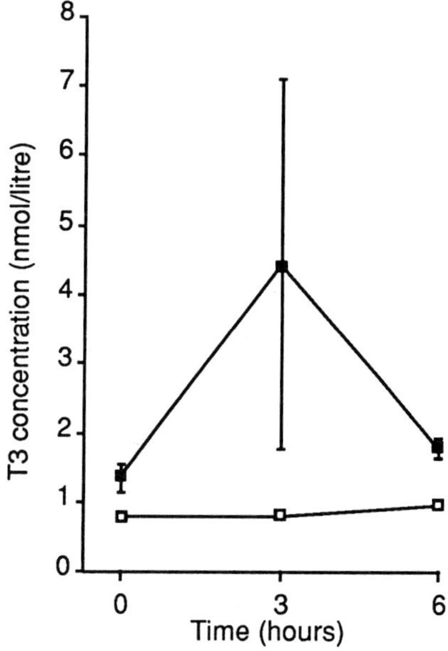

Figure 5.2 Mean blood concentration responses of triiodothyronine (T_3) in the plasma of four normal horses compared with a horse showing alopecia thought to be the result of hypothyroidism. TSH administered at time zero. ■ Mean of normals; □ patient response.

thyroidism only. The diagnosis of secondary hypothyroidism due to hypothalamic or pituitary dysfunction requires demonstration of low circulating TSH concentrations (not available commercially) and/or use of the TRH stimulation test.

TRH stimulation test

Thyrotropin-releasing hormone can be used to stimulate the release of TSH from the pituitary and thence the release of T_3 and T_4 from the thyroid. Whereas the TSH test can only demonstrate normal thyroid activity, or a state of primary hypothyroidism, TRH can additionally test hypothalamic/pituitary function and can therefore be used to differentiate between primary and secondary hypothyroidism.

A heparinized or plain blood sample is taken prior to the intravenous injection of 3–5 mg TRH (Roche, UK). A second blood sample is taken 6–8 hours later, at which time the T_4 concentration of the adult horse should show a

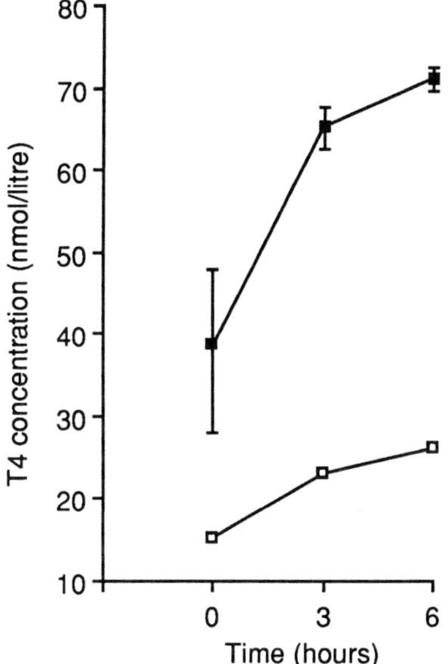

Figure 5.3 Mean blood concentration responses of thyroxine (T_4) in the plasma of four normal horses compared with a horse showing alopecia thought to be the result of hypothyroidism. TSH administered at time zero. ■ Mean of normals; □ patient response.

two-fold increase over baseline. If not, there is a functional problem at the hypothalamus, pituitary or thyroid. If the patient is known to respond positively to TSH stimulation, then by elimination the hypothyroidism is secondary and reflects a problem in the hypothalamus or pituitary.

Disorders of calcium metabolism

Calcium is intimately involved in many diverse physiological processes such as blood coagulation, muscle contraction, hormone release, bone formation, maintenance of the heartbeat and diverse metabolic activities. In the circulation it exists in three states: ionized; chelated and protein-bound. In the laboratory, routine serum or plasma calcium estimation measures the total of all three, but only the ionized portion is biologically active.

Calcium homeostasis is complex and is controlled by:

- The release of parathyroid hormone (PTH) from the parathyroid gland, which is stimulated by a decrease in the blood concentration of ionized calcium. PTH acts to increase calcium and decrease phosphorus in the circulation.
- The release of calcitonin (thyrocalcitonin) from the thyroid C cells, which is stimulated by an increase in the blood concentration of ionized calcium. Calcitonin acts to decrease calcium and phosphorus in the circulation by reducing the rate of bone resorption.
- Vitamin D from ingested sources or endogenous production, which acts to increase calcium and phosphorus in the circulation.

Homeostasis is dependent upon the net activity of these hormones and their influence upon the absorption, excretion and mobilization of calcium. In consequence, the plasma pool of calcium is in a constant state of flux. Other hormones and the intake of phosphorus and magnesium may also influence the maintenance of calcium homeostasis.

Hypocalcaemia

A clinical state of hypocalcaemia develops when the circulating concentration of ionized calcium falls below the homeostatic requirement. It is usually possible to demonstrate a low serum or plasma calcium concentration, but it must be remembered that this laboratory estimation represents total calcium and is not a measure of the biologically available (ionized) calcium. Successful diagnosis and treatment consequently rely heavily on recognition of the circumstances and clinical signs associated with a state of hypocalcaemia.

Clinical hypocalcaemia is uncommon in horses but it tends to occur in particular circumstances which help its recognition. The mechanism(s) associated with its development are poorly understood, but in each case a positive response to treatment is diagnostic.

Lactation tetany

This is a condition seen in mares several weeks after parturition or occasionally just after weaning. Clinical signs include an apprehensive appearance about the eye, sweating, muscle tremors, tachycardia and tachypnoea. In particular, there is a stiffness in the limbs ('tetany'), producing an abnormal gait in which the animal appears to walk on 'tip-toe'. Some cases may also display synchronous diaphragmatic flutter (see below). Untreated cases can proceed to collapse and tetanic convulsion.

Transit tetany

This is probably the same syndrome but is associated with transit fatigue; usually in ponies (of either sex). The clinical signs are as before, but with a marked tetany of all superficial muscles.

Synchronous diaphragmatic flutter ('thumps')

This condition is usually seen in fatigued horses and may consequently involve fluid, electrolyte and acid–base disturbances. In reduced calcium availability the phrenic nerve is stimulated by atrial contraction so that the diaphragm contracts synchronously with each heartbeat. This activity is seen as a twitch or contraction in one or both flanks and heart auscultation reveals that it is synchronized with each heartbeat. In cases of violent diaphragmatic contraction, there is a characteristic 'thumping' sound which is audible at a distance from the animal. Signs of hypocalcaemic tetany may also be present.

Comments

- Retrospective laboratory data is likely to reveal low serum or plasma concentrations of calcium and, occasionally, magnesium and phosphorus. However, the response to treatment (20% Calcium Magnesium Phosphorus diluted 1:4 in saline and given by slow intravenous infusion) is often rapid and diagnostic. However, the amount required for effect varies enormously between cases.
- Cases associated with fatigue are likely to require additional treatment in respect of fluid, electrolyte and acid–base balance, and should be checked accordingly.

- The major differential to the tetany of hypocalcaemia is tetanus itself. Cases of true tetanus show prolapse of the third eyelid at an early stage; cases of hypocalcaemia do not.

Other conditions associated with hypocalcaemia

Acute or chronic renal disease in horses may be accompanied by low, normal or high blood calcium levels (see Chapter 6: 'Urinary diseases'). However, patients with renal failure and low blood calcium do not usually display clinical signs of hypocalcaemia.

Recurrent hypocalcaemia, alleviated but not cured by repeated calcium administration, has been recorded in association with pancreatic disease.

Hypercalcaemia

Persistent hypercalcaemia is a rare disorder of horses, which usually reflects one of the following regulatory problems:

- Hyperparathyroidism — primary or secondary
- Secretion of PTH-like proteins by tumours
- Kidney disease
- Hypervitaminosis D

Primary hyperparathyroidism

Rare though potential causes of primary hyperparathyroidism are parathyroid adenoma, hyperplasia or carcinoma. Persistent hypercalcaemia is likely, but there is no distinctive clinical syndrome.

A definitive diagnosis is obtained by histopathology at post-mortem examination, but there is often difficulty in identifying the parathyroid glands. The upper cervical pair are located dorsolateral to the trachea, near the thyroid gland, but are difficult to identify because of their small size, variable location and similarity to cervical lymph nodes. The larger, lower pair of caudal glands are located on the ventrolateral surface of the trachea near the level of the first rib.

Nutritional secondary hyperparathyroidism

In former times this skeletal disease was common amongst working horses (variously called 'bran disease', 'Miller's disease' or 'big head'), but it is rarely seen nowadays. It is caused by feeding rations containing an excess of phosphorus relative to calcium. The resulting increase in blood phosphorus concentration depresses the blood calcium level which in turn stimulates the secretion of PTH in an attempt to redress the circulating calcium balance. Continued ingestion of the imbalanced ration causes parathyroid hypertrophy, followed by development of a metabolic bone disease owing to persistent calcium loss. Young growing horses are most commonly affected, but pregnancy can also predispose.

NB Although this disease is included here as a cause of hypercalcaemia (owing to persistent PTH secretion), the continued feeding of a high phosphorus ration acts to keep the circulating calcium concentration in check. The net effect is that blood calcium and phosphorus levels may be within normal ranges and diagnosis depends heavily on the recognition of clinical signs and fractional excretion rates.

The early clinical signs may be non-specific with an intermittent shifting lameness and a stiff gait. As more calcium is mobilized from bone, bilaterally symmetrical facial and mandibular swellings appear as a result of fibrous osteodystrophy. This weakening of the skeleton may predispose fractures.

Diagnosis of secondary hyperparathyroidism:

- Clinical signs and feed analysis
- Hypocalcaemia and hyperphosphataemia occur in the early stages, *but serum or plasma calcium and phosphorus concentrations are usually normal once skeletal changes are underway.*
- A high urinary fractional excretion of phosphorus is usual and is indicative of a relatively low, or absolutely low, calcium intake (see 'Rhabdomyolysis and the fractional excretion of electrolytes' in Chapter 13: 'Musculoskeletal diseases').

This is probably the most useful of the clinicopathological tests indicated here.

- Serum alkaline phosphatase (SAP or ALP) may be raised and presumably reflects increased osteoblastic and osteoclastic activity.

Secretion of PTH-like proteins by tumours

In horses, hypercalcaemia is occasionally found in association with various neoplasms such as gastric squamous cell carcinoma, adrenocortical carcinoma and, in particular, lymphosarcoma. In these rare instances it seems that the neoplastic cells can elaborate a PTH-like protein which leads to resorption of calcium from bone ('pseudohyperparathyroidism'). Calcium is then deposited in a variety of soft tissues including the heart, blood vessels and kidney. Mineralization of the kidney leads to hypercalcaemic nephropathy, renal diabetes insipidus and renal failure. At post-mortem examination the heavy depositions of calcium plaque in soft tissues have an 'eggshell' quality.

Kidney disease

Renal failure in horses is accompanied by unpredictable shifts in circulating electrolyte concentrations. Calcium levels may be low, normal or high (see Chapter 6: 'Urinary diseases').

Hypervitaminosis D

Hypervitaminosis D in a horse could result only from oversupplementation. The result is a hypercalcaemia which is associated with limb stiffness and tachycardia. There is a potential for renal complications as a result of mineralization. Post-mortem findings indicate widespread soft tissue mineralization.

Endocrinopathies of the reproductive tract

Granulosa cell tumour

The granulosa cell tumour is the commonest equine ovarian tumour. Since the tumour can produce oestrogens, progesterone or androgens, the main presenting feature is often abnormal sexual behaviour: persistent oestrus; anoestrus or stallion-like behaviour. Diagnostic techniques include rectal palpation, ultrasonography and plasma testosterone assay. For details see 'Differential diagnosis of genital diseases in the mare' in Chapter 7: 'Genital diseases, fertility and pregnancy'.

Cryptorchid

Retention of an inguinal or abdominal testis, or the remnants of testicular tissue following incomplete castration, may lead to stallion-like behaviour in an animal thought to have been castrated. This is not a true endocrinopathy but is considered here for convenience. Diagnostic techniques include external and rectal palpation, ultrasonography and the human chorionic gonadotropin (hCG) stimulation test (for details see 'Cryptorchidism' in Chapter 7: 'Genital diseases, fertility and pregnancy).

Further reading

Beech J and Garcia M (1991) Diseases of the endocrine system. In: Colahan PT, Mayhew IG, Merritt AM and Moore JN (eds) *Equine Medicine and Surgery*, 4th. edn., Vol 2. pp1737–1751. Goleta: American Veterinary Publications Inc.

Hillyer MH, Taylor FGR, Mair TS, Murphy D, Watson TDG and Love S (1992) Diagnosis of hyperadrenocorticism in the horse. *Equine Veterinary Education*. 4: 131–134.

Mooney CT and Murphy D (1995) Equine hypothyroidism: the difficulties of diagnosis. *Equine Veterinary Education*. 7: 242–245.

Taylor FGR and Hillyer MH (1992) The differential diagnosis of hyperglycaemia in horses. *Equine Veterinary Education*. 4: 135–138.

6 Urinary diseases

I. **Practical techniques**

Diseases of the urinary tract are usually indicated by a change in the horse's urination behaviour, such as frequent attempts to urinate (with or without discomfort) and/or a tangible change in the quality or volume of urine passed. This chapter describes the practical techniques and the complementary clinical pathology which can be used for investigating urinary tract diseases.

Examination of the urinary tract per rectum

Kidneys

Only the left kidney is accessible per rectum. Its caudal pole is palpable in the roof of the abdomen to the left of the midline — usually at arm's length. It is normally smooth, pain free and somewhat mobile. The right kidney is palpable only when it is grossly enlarged and/or displaced.

Ureters

The ureters are not usually palpable unless thickened by infection or urinary obstruction.

Bladder

The empty bladder is situated in the midline at the pelvic brim and is usually difficult to palpate. When enlarged with urine it becomes palpable just beyond the pelvic brim, although the overlying uterus may hinder exploration in mares. In chronic cystitis it is likely to be empty, but its wall is then palpably thickened and painful. The presence of a cystic calculus is best appreciated when the bladder is empty, at which time a firm mass, usually oval in shape, is felt at the pelvic brim. In cases of paralysis or obstruction the bladder is grossly distended and the wall feels taut. In cases of chronic paralysis, there may be a pendulous feel to the bladder after the urine has been removed by catheter. This is due to the accumulation of crystalline sediment (mostly calcium carbonate).

Urethra

The pelvic urethra is difficult to identify in either sex. However, in the male a calculus which becomes lodged in the pelvic urethra is palpable per rectum. If obstruction occurs in the distal urethra, the whole pelvic urethra is palpable as a result of urinary distension.

Catherization of the bladder

Passing a urethral catheter demonstrates the patency or otherwise of the urethra and enables collection of a urine sample from the bladder. Catheterized samples are preferable for bacterial culture since environmental contaminants are minimized. The technique is also useful to reduce bladder volume prior to rectal examination or endoscopy (cystoscopy).

The male

It is usually necessary to relax the penis for this procedure using a moderate dose of acepromazine if clinical circumstances permit (0.05–0.10 mg/kg i.m. or slow i.v.). In entires, where penile paralysis is a risk associated with the use of acepromazine, detomidine may be used (0.01 mg/kg slow i.v.), followed by butorphanol (25 mg/kg i.v.), but adequate relaxation of the penis is less predictable.

Once relaxed, the glans and external urethral orifice are cleansed in a warm solution of povidone–iodine. Using aseptic precautions, a horse catheter (Fig. 6.1) is lubricated at the tip with a water-based lubricant and passed into the urethra whilst the body of the penis is held gently in the other hand (Fig. 6.2). The

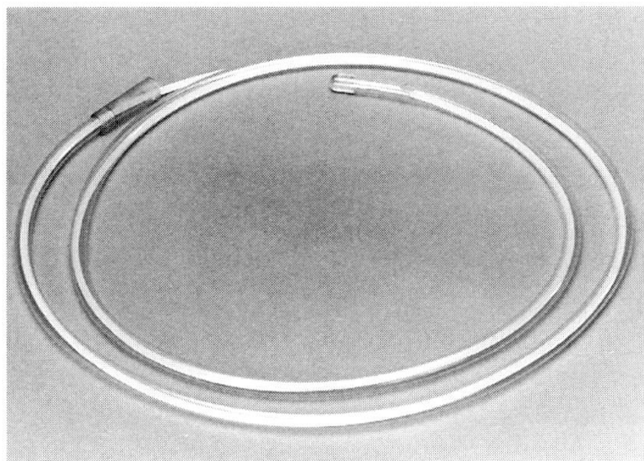

Figure 6.1 Eight mm horse urethral catheter (24 FG x 137 cm), complete with stylet.

catheter passes with ease through the length of the penile urethra, but a slight increase in resistance is felt as it moves around the ischial arch, at which point the tail head is seen to rise. From this position the flexible stylet is gradually withdrawn, preferably by an assistant, as the catheter is advanced over the pelvis and into the bladder — failure to do so renders the stylet immovable once it is beyond the ischial arch. On entry to the bladder, air is often heard being drawn in at the catheter hub.

Unless urine is present under pressure, it is often necessary to start a syphon using a catheter syringe (Fig. 6.3). Even when the bladder is collapsed, it is usually possible to obtain 20–30 ml urine by syringe. If no sample is forthcoming, it is worth standing by with a sample container once the catheter is removed, since the passage of a small volume of urine is

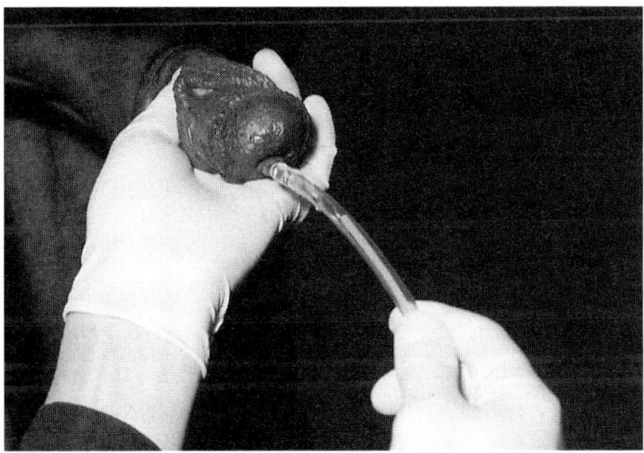

Figure 6.2 Passing the catheter into the urethra.

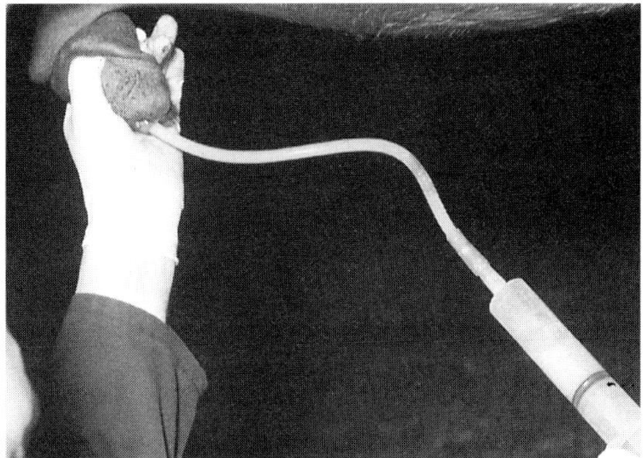

Figure 6.3 Using a catheter syringe to promote urine flow by applying suction.

often stimulated by the presence of the aspirated air.

The female

The external urethral orifice of the mare or filly is highly distensible and is catheterized with ease. The tail is bandaged and the external vulva cleansed. Using aseptic precautions the urethral opening is found by advancing an exploratory finger along the floor of the vulva in the midline. In most cases the opening lies at a distance 10–12 cm from the ventral commissure of the vulval lips beneath the transverse fold (vestibulovaginal fold) which demarcates the entrance to the vagina (Fig. 6.4). The commonest mistake is to miss the

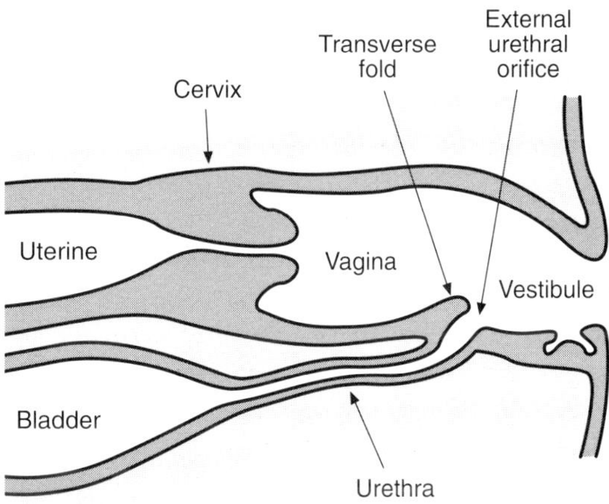

Figure 6.4 Relationship of the external urethral orifice to the transverse fold in the mare.

transverse fold which overlies the opening and thus overshoot the site. The orifice is quite large and, once located, a lubricated catheter is fed through the vulva beneath the hand and directed under the exploratory finger. The urethra is very short (7–10 cm) and the bladder is soon entered. Aspiration by catheter syringe may be necessary to start a urine flow.

Comments

- Following removal of the catheter the animal may adopt a urination stance and expel aspirated air.
- Complications are minimal, but poor technique could result in cystitis. There is also a risk of knotting the catheter if an excessive length is pushed into the bladder.
- Urine samples obtained by catheter are likely to show an increase in trace amounts of erythrocytes, transitional epithelial cells and protein.
- Catheters are distorted by heat sterilization and rendered unsuitable for reuse.

Cystoscopy, ureteral catheterization and urethroscopy

Endoscopy is most appropriate to an examination of the bladder and urethra, but can also be used to catheterize the ureters in order to obtain individual urine samples from either kidney. This is particularly useful where renal lesions are thought to be unilateral. If necessary, the bladder should be drained by catheter prior to endoscopy.

Cystoscopy

In the female, cystoscopy is relatively easy using a standard fibreoptic instrument (1 m length, 1 cm outer diameter). The bladder is drained and, using aseptic precautions, an assistant introduces the endoscope into the urethra in the same manner as described for catheterization. Entrance to the bladder is at a distance of some 10 cm. It is then distended with air until the wall can be seen clearly. Air

will leak out around the endoscope and occasional repeated insufflation is required. Alternatively, the assistant may partially seal the urethra by placing a hand over the transverse fold at the vulvo-vaginal junction to gently compress the external urethral orifice. Overdistension with air causes the mare to strain.

In the male the longer, narrower urethra requires a special endoscope 1.2–1.4 m in length with a maximum outer diameter of 0.9 cm. The technique for passing the endoscope is essentially the same as that described for urethral catheterization in the male. Air leakage following bladder insufflation may be reduced by gently squeezing the body of the penis around the endoscope.

Orientation within the bladder is achieved by identifying the ventral pool of residual urine. The mucosal surface is then explored for anomalies of texture or structure. Inflammation, large calculi or sabulous sludge are easily identified. The volume of sludge (crystalline sediment) is greatly increased by chronic paralysis.

Ureteral catheterization

The ureteral orifices are located by slowly withdrawing the endoscope from the bladder cavity until it is just inside the neck. The openings are then seen as small papillary shaped structures either side of the midline in the dorsal wall, some 2 cm beyond the urethral opening (Fig. 6.5). Frequent pulsatile squirts of urine identify the openings.

Sterile polyethylene tubing (2.0–2.5 mm outer diameter) is passed through the biopsy channel until seen in advance of the endoscope lens. The endoscope is then aligned so that the tubing can be advanced gently into the ureteral orifice for a distance of 5–10 cm. A urine sample is then carefully aspirated by syringe over 2–3 minutes. *Excessive force in either of these procedures will result in ureteral trauma.* Once sampling is complete and the tubing is withdrawn, the biopsy channel is flushed with sterile saline and the procedure is repeated on the opposite side using a fresh catheter.

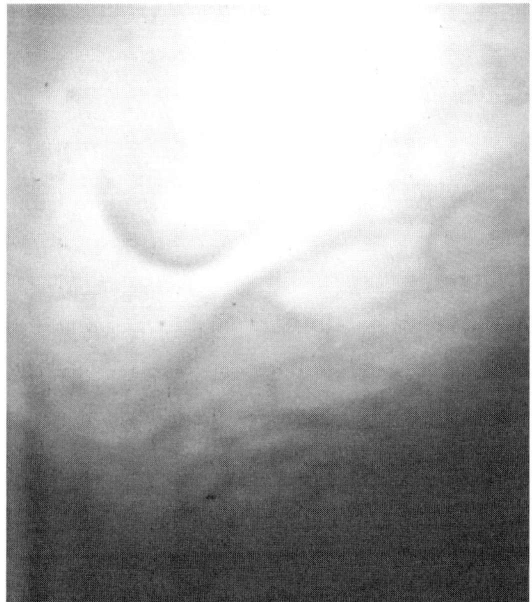

Figure 6.5   Endoscopic view of the ureteral orifice.

Urethroscopy

The urethra is best examined as the endoscope is slowly removed from the bladder unless, of course, it is being examined for obstruction. The male urethra should be kept lightly inflated to give an optimal view of the mucosal lining as the endoscope is withdrawn. It should be noted that the initial forward passage of the endoscope causes the mucosa to appear markedly hyperaemic at withdrawal. The female urethra is extremely short (7–10 cm).

Comment

- Transient stranguria may follow cystoscopy/ urethroscopy.

Ultrasonography of the urinary tract

Kidneys

In the normal horse both kidneys may be imaged or 'scanned' by percutaneous ultra-sonography, but usually it is only possible to scan the left kidney by the rectal approach. Where renal disease is associated with enlargement of the right kidney, both kidneys may be scanned by rectal ultrasono-graphy.

Percutaneous ultrasonography of the kidney

Careful skin preparation is essential for percutaneous ultrasonography and in most cases this involves clipping the hair, cleansing the skin with povidone–iodine and finally degreasing with spirit. Linear array or sector scanners may be used, but as intercostal views are required the sector scanner is preferable since it enables a small transducer/ patient contact area and a wide field of view.

Each kidney is scanned in the dorsal abdomen below the level of the transverse processes. The left kidney is approached through the 17th intercostal space and the paralumbar fossa using a 2.25–3.5 MHz transducer. Here the kidney lies medial to the spleen which is used as an acoustic window, so that a 20–26 cm depth of view may be needed. The right kidney is approached through the 15th, 16th, and 17th intercostal spaces. In this position it lies immediately adjacent to the body wall. It is best visualized with a 3–5 MHz transducer and a 15 cm depth of view is usually adequate.

In chronic renal conditions the scan may be expected to provide evidence of morphologic change. As far as possible the entire kidney should be visualized from pole to pole and the scan should be performed in all planes to verify anomalies. Particular points to note are deviations of kidney position within the abdomen and the kidney's size, shape, surface contour and texture (i.e. relative brightness of tissues).

The overall size may be reduced by chronic disease or enlarged by hydronephrosis and, rarely, neoplasia. The cortex is more echogenic (brighter) than the medulla and a distinct corticomedullary junction should be identi-fiable lying 1–2 cm deep to the capsule. Within the medulla are the pelvic recesses, which are

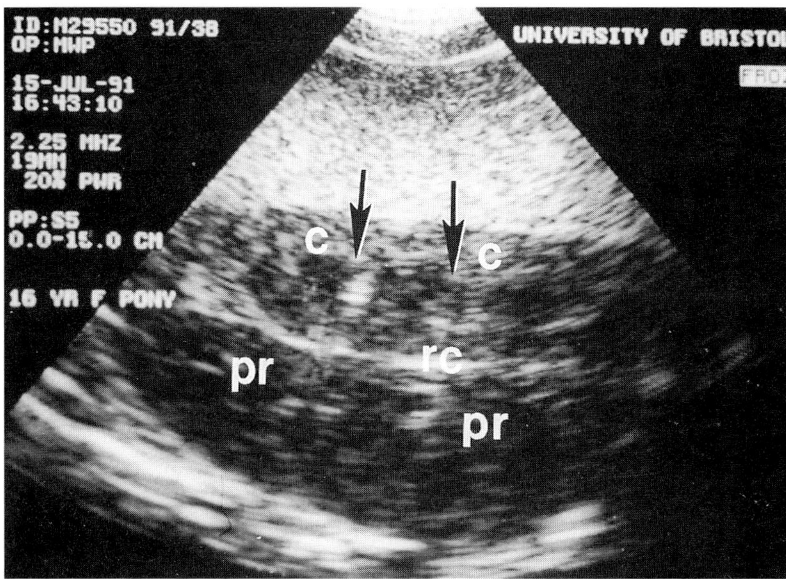

Figure 6.6
Ultrasonogram of a normal kidney showing the cortex (c), corticomedullary junction (arrows), the hypoechoic pelvic recesses within the medulla (pr) and the hyperechoic renal crest (rc).

hypoechoic (darker) areas, approximately 1 cm in size, lying adjacent to the hyperechoic renal crest (Fig. 6.6). The renal pelvis may be identified as an anechoic area on the medial aspect of the kidney, but both this and its associated ureter only become obvious when they are pathologically distended. Dilatations of the pelvis and recesses are seen in hydronephrosis.

Bright, hyperechoic reflections with marked acoustic shadows may indicate areas of mineralization. Small areas of mineralization occur commonly in the recesses of older horses, emphasizing again the need to scan suspected lesions in multiple planes. In the case of renal calculi the passage of ultrasound is totally blocked and an acoustic shadow is cast deep through adjacent tissues (Fig. 6.7).

Rectal ultrasonography of the kidney

Rectal ultrasonography of the left kidney is easily performed with a linear array transducer of 5–7.5 MHz. The transducer is applied to the medial side of the kidney and may be swept along the ventral aspect. The caudal pole is easily accessible and this is particularly useful where a gas-filled bowel prevents the percutaneous examination of this area. The left renal pelvis and both ureters are best examined by the rectal approach.

Ultrasonography of the bladder

The bladder can be visualized in the foal by percutaneous scan, but in the adult it is scanned per rectum using a 5 MHz transducer. The bladder wall is clearly identified as an echogenic structure with abnormalities either appearing as irregularities in the otherwise smooth contour, or as alterations in the wall thickness. Bladder size varies with the volume

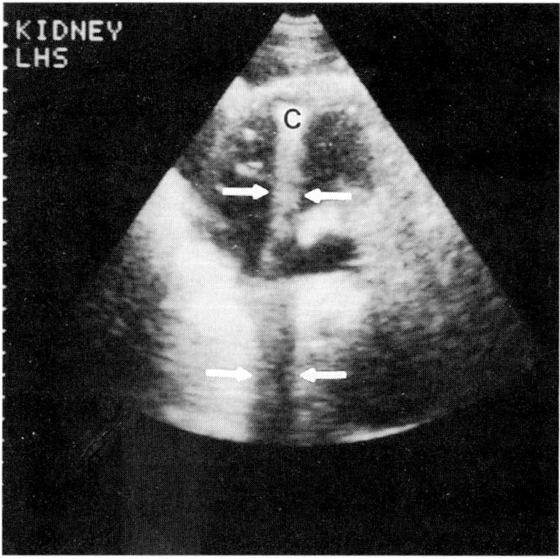

Figure 6.7   Ultrasonogram revealing renal calculi (c). Note the marked acoustic shadow (between arrows).

of urine present and abnormal contents may be identified against the relatively echolucent urine.

Renal biopsy

Renal biopsies are collected using a percutaneous needle technique which may be performed 'blind' or with the aid of ultrasound guidance. Blind renal biopsy is not a safe procedure in the horse and is justified only if histopathology is likely to influence subsequent treatment significantly. The procedure is invariably associated with perirenal haematoma formation and has the potential to cause fatal haemorrhage. Ultrasound-guided percutaneous biopsy offers the safer approach, but the necessary equipment is expensive and tends to be available in specialist centres only.

Needle biopsies are taken from the standing animal and sedation is required only in uncooperative patients. A 14–18 gauge biopsy needle, at least 15 cm in length, is required. The skin overlying the kidney to be biopsied is clipped at the sites described for renal ultrasound (see above) and surgically prepared. A sterile sleeve and biopsy guide are attached to the transducer and a percutaneous scan performed to identify the optimum site for needle insertion. Care should be taken to select a site where the path of the needle is parallel to the interlobular arteries and does not cross any of the arcuate arteries. When the left kidney is biopsied a trans-splenic route is used but this does not appear to be associated with an increased risk of haemorrhage.

Local anaesthetic is then infiltrated into the skin and underlying abdominal wall, and a scalpel is used to make a stab incision through the skin at the selected site. Under ultrasound guidance the needle is inserted through the skin and abdominal wall and directed so that the tip is pressing against the renal capsule. Taking care to avoid major blood vessels, the needle is operated and withdrawn. If the first attempt is unsuccessful a second attempt may be made.

Following this procedure the horse should be kept as still as possible for 2 hours to permit clotting. If bilateral renal biopsies are considered necessary they should not be performed simultaneously; 24 hours should be left between the two procedures.

Comments

- Trace haematuria is inevitable but overt haematuria is a cause for concern and these patients need careful observation. Ultrasonography may allow identification and subsequent monitoring of a subcapsular or parenchymal haematoma.

- Biopsy specimens examined by light microscopy may appear normal despite clinicopathological evidence of severe dysfunction.

II. **Clinical pathology**

Significant diagnostic information concerning diseases of the urinary tract can be obtained by the strategic analysis of blood and urine samples.

Analysis of urine

Urine analysis can provide evidence of upper and/or lower urinary tract disease.

Sample containers should be clean for routine analysis and sterile for bacterial culture. Ideally, samples should be processed as soon as possible after collection to avoid spurious results. Certain urinary constituents are degraded by sunlight and the use of opaque or dark containers will prevent this. Containers with preservatives will inhibit bacterial multiplication, but may interfere with some of the chemical tests.

When collecting a free-flow sample, try to catch a midstream sample. Avoid catching the

Table 6.1. Chemical characteristics of normal urine and changes associated with disease.

Parameter	Normal range	Disease
pH	Range 7.0–9.0 in normal urine Tends to acidity on concentrate feeds	Urine acidity is associated with metabolic acidosis
Protein	Usually <100 mg% in normal urine	Severe proteinuria is associated with glomerular lesions; the protein concentration is also raised by inflammatory lesions of the urinary tract
Glucose	None present usually	Glucosuria occurs when hyperglycaemia exceeds the renal threshold as in some cases of Cushing's disease, stress-related hyperglycaemia or rare forms of diabetes mellitus. Sedation with α_2 agonists may cause transient glucosuria. Alternatively, glucosuria in the *absence* of hyperglycaemia is indicative of tubular dysfunction
Ketones	None present usually	Ketosis is rare in horses; its presence suggests a nutritional stress associated with protein catabolism
Bilirubin	None present usually	It is present during haemolysis or obstructive jaundice
Haemoglobin	None present usually	Haemoglobinuria occurs during intravascular haemolysis; the serum will appear haemolysed*
Myoglobin	None present usually	Myoglobinuria occurs during acute degenerative changes in skeletal muscle (rhabdomyolysis); the serum is not discoloured by myoglobin*

*It is difficult to differentiate haemoglobinuria from myoglobinuria without sophisticated laboratory procedures. However, serum discolouration is only apparent during haemolysis.

first part of the urine stream as it will contain cellular debris, leucocytes and exudate flushed from the urethra, prepuce and genital tract. In addition, it will contain commensal bacteria flushed from the urethra. Similarly, an end of flow sample will contain bladder debris. Catheterized samples are likely to show an increase in trace amounts of erythrocytes, transitional epithelial cells and protein.

Horses will not volunteer urine samples when required, but their behaviour patterns can be exploited to this end. A horse held in a bedding-free box for 2–3 hours will often void urine when transferred to a freshly bedded box after a short walk. This simple ploy may avoid the need for catheterization.

Specific gravity of urine (SG)

This is the only indicator of renal function in the urine analysis. The concentrating ability of healthy equine kidneys will produce a urinary SG of between 1.020 and 1.050. Poor renal perfusion, as for example in dehydration, will produce a more concentrated urine of smaller volume (oliguria). However, if poor perfusion persists then the functional ability of the kidneys is threatened and unless it is reversed the loss of tubular resorptive capacity results in a urine of low SG which is independent of the osmotic pressure of the blood. The SG then assumes that of the glomerular filtrate (isosthenuria) and registers between 1.008 and 1.017. Persistent tubular dysfunction may lead to polyuria and polydipsia.

Chemical characteristics of urine

The chemical characteristics of normal equine urine and the changes associated with disease are shown in Table 6.1.

Sedimentary characteristics of urine

The sedimentary characteristics of normal equine urine and the changes associated with disease are shown in Table 6.2.

Assessing the glomerular filtration rate (GFR)

A fall in the GFR is characteristic of renal failure and eventually leads to an increase in the circulating concentration of nitrogenous waste products (azotaemia). A state of azotaemia is most conveniently defined in the laboratory by measuring the concentrations of urea and/or creatinine in plasma or serum. The fall in GFR precedes these biochemical changes in the blood and its direct measurement is therefore a sensitive indicator of early renal dysfunction. However, GFR is not easily assessed in the horse.

Azotaemia

The development of azotaemia reflects the loss of nephron function which may be caused by:

- Prerenal factors which reduce vascular perfusion of the kidneys
- Intrinsic factors associated with damage to renal tissues
- Postrenal factors which hinder urine excretion

Some 75% of glomerular function is lost before azotaemia becomes apparent. It is therefore an insensitive indicator of the onset of reduced GFR. However, once raised, subsequent increases in the serum concentration of urea or creatinine reflect further decreases in GFR and they then become useful monitors of disease progress.

Comment

- Small increases in the blood urea concentration alone (i.e. up to two-fold, with creatinine remaining within normal range), frequently accompany dehydration and/or wasting diseases associated with increased tissue catabolism. Feeds which are high in protein may also raise blood urea slightly.
- Increases in serum creatinine concentration alone can accompany severe acute myopathies such as exertional rhabdomyolysis.

Table 6.2. Sedimentary characteristics of normal urine and changes associated with disease.

Parameter	Normal content	Disease
Erythrocytes	None present usually	Haematuria reflects: inflammation; trauma; neoplasia or coagulopathy in the urinary tract Trace amounts may be associated with catheterization
Leucocytes	None present usually	Large numbers are associated with inflammation of the tract (pyuria)
Transitional cells	Few present usually	Large numbers reflect: inflammation; trauma or neoplasia of the bladder Numbers increase in endstream urine and catheterized samples
Bacteria	None present usually	Bacteria are significant in the presence of large numbers of inflammatory cells Gram staining of a sedimentary smear or moderate to heavy culture reflect pyelonephritis or cystitis
Crystals	Usually calcium carbonate present — normal Occasionally, triple phosphate and calcium oxalate are seen	Large numbers of triple phosphate crystals indicate infection of the tract; large numbers of calcium oxalate are abnormal but their significance is uncertain
Casts	No cellular casts are usually present but occasional hyaline (mucoprotein) casts appear	Cellular casts reflect tubular damage — the cells are bound together by protein exudate or leakage

Clearance studies

The measurement of GFR by clearance studies is impractical in horses. Inulin, a starch which is excreted in the urine at a rate equal to the GFR, is restricted to laboratory applications. An alternative is the measurement of endogenous creatinine clearance, but this requires long-term collection of urine using special harnesses. A simpler approach is the measurement of sodium sulphanilate clearance which is performed using blood samples alone. This technique is outlined below for interest, but few commercial laboratories will undertake sulphanilate assays.

Sodium sulphanilate clearance

Following intravenous injection, sodium sulphanilate is rapidly distributed throughout fluid spaces and is then cleared, primarily by glomerular filtration, at a linear rate which can be measured. Sulphanilate clearance is not a true measure of the GFR, but does reflect it because renal excretion is a major factor influencing its decay curve.

The patient receives 10 mg/kg bodyweight of the sulphanilate preparation intravenously and heparinized blood samples are taken from the opposite vein at 45, 60, 75 and 90 minutes after injection. The concentration of sodium sulphanilate in blood samples is then determined from a standard curve using a colorimetric assay. The standard curve must be prepared from the batch of sodium sulphanilate used for injection.

The sulphanilate concentrations in the test samples are then plotted against their respective sample times on semilogarithmic coordinates. This should produce a linear clearance curve providing an interval of at least 45 minutes has been allowed between the sulphanilate injection and subsequent blood samples.

The clearance rate of sulphanilate is defined as the time taken for 50% of the salt to be cleared from the blood ($^T1_{/2}$). This can easily be calculated from the curve. In healthy horses and ponies the $^T1_{/2}$ has been found to lie between 26 to 45 minutes. In cases of suspected early renal failure, the clearance times would be expected to lengthen. In cases of established renal failure, clearance times in excess of 200 minutes have been determined.

Comment

- The assessment of GFR offers no advantage in the diagnosis of renal failure once azotaemia is established. Its diagnostic potential lies in detecting and monitoring early renal failure, in advance of azotaemia, in patients suffering nephrotoxicity or circulatory disturbances.

Assessing renal tubular function

Urine concentration

The specific gravity (SG) of urine is an indicator of the renal tubular ability to resorb or excrete water in response to changes in hydration. The presence of persistently dilute (hypotonic) urine in an azotaemic or dehydrated horse is therefore indicative of tubular dysfunction.

Horses with polyuria/polydipsia (PUPD) usually pass urine of persistently low SG. Tubular function in cases of PUPD can be assessed by water deprivation tests. *However, it must be emphasized that these tests are both dangerous and pointless in patients that are already showing signs of renal disease.* Nevertheless, the majority of equine patients with PUPD are unlikely to be suffering renal disease; the most usual differential diagnoses being pituitary adenoma (Cushing's disease), diabetes insipidus, or psychogenic polydipsia. Of these conditions, pituitary adenoma is by far the commonest. The differential diagnosis of PUPD, including the use of water deprivation tests, is detailed under: 'Causes of polydipsia/polyuria (PUPD)' in Chapter 5: 'Endocrine diseases'.

Fractional excretion of electrolytes

In the healthy kidney, the net urinary excretion of an electrolyte is governed by two factors: the GFR and the extent of tubular resorption. In contrast, endogenous creatinine is excreted by glomerular filtration alone and its rate of excretion thus approximates to the GFR, even during renal dysfunction. Creatinine clearance is therefore a useful standard against which the clearance of an electrolyte may be compared in health or disease.

The fractional excretion (FE) of an electrolyte is defined as the percent ratio of its clearance to the clearance of endogenous creatinine. In normal homeostatic balance FE values are very variable, but they are usually within a definable range. With a loss of tubular resorption the excretion of an electrolyte is often increased and its FE rises above the normal range. The percent ratio is derived in Figure 6.8.

The FE of an electrolyte is therefore calculated once the urinary and plasma (or serum) concentrations of both the electrolyte and creatinine are known. This approach eliminates the need for protracted collection of urine, but the urine and plasma samples must be obtained at the same examination time (within 30 minutes of each other). The following FE ranges, determined for healthy horses on a balanced electrolyte intake, serve as a normal guide:

Sodium	0.04–0.52%
Potassium	35–80%
Inorganic phosphorus	0.0–0.2%
Chloride	0.7–2.1%

$$\frac{\text{Urinary concentration of electrolyte } [E]_u}{\text{Plasma concentration of electrolyte } [E]_p} \times \text{Urine flow rate/min} \times 100\%$$

divided by:

$$\frac{\text{Urinary concentration of creatinine } [Cr]_u}{\text{Plasma concentration of creatinine } [Cr]_p} \times \text{Urine flow rate/min}$$

which is simplified to:

$$FE = \frac{[E]_u}{[E]_p} \times \frac{[Cr]_p}{[Cr]_u} \times 100\%$$

Figure 6.8 Calculation of fractional excretion (FE).

Urine should be submitted in capped, sterile containers to avoid artefactual changes in the phosphate and creatinine concentrations as a result of bacterial contamination. The plasma should be separated fairly soon, and both urine and plasma should be analysed as quickly as possible (certainly within 4 days). In cases of delay, high temperatures must be avoided.

In general terms a persistent increase in the FE of one or more electrolytes (frequently sodium and phosphorus) is indicative of tubular dysfunction.

Comments

- In health, the urinary concentrations of electrolytes and their rates of excretion vary between horses and within the same individual throughout the day. This is because clearance is highly influenced by dietary, hydration and endocrine factors. *Tests producing abnormal results should be repeated to confirm the trend.*

- Excessive phosphate intake, or a diet with a low calcium : phosphate ratio (i.e. 2:1), can produce elevated FE phosphate values in animals with normal renal function (see 'Rhabdomyolysis and the fractional excretion of electrolytes' in Chapter 13: 'Musculoskeletal diseases').

- Despite the fact that calcium is precipitated in urinary crystals which may be lost to analysis, its FE value can be of use. However, the colorimetric methods used in most commercial laboratories are unsuitable for urinary calcium estimation and its FE value is not considered here.

- Urine samples delayed in transit and having abnormally low creatinine concentrations (<10,000 µmol/l) are probably contaminated and the FE results will be spurious.

- Measurements undertaken in horses currently receiving intravenous fluids will be spurious.

- Abnormal increases in FE values should never be used as the sole criteria for diagnosis of tubular failure, they are simply part of the cumulative clinicopathological evidence which indicates failure.

Urinary enzymes

Gamma glutamyltransferase (GGT) is found in the liver, pancreas and luminal brush border of the proximal tubular cells. This enzyme is not excreted by glomerular filtration, so that its appearance in urine is indicative of acute tubular damage. It appears before azotaemia develops, therefore offering a sensitive indicator of early tubular disease.

Urinary GGT concentrations are conventionally expressed as a ratio to urinary creatinine concentrations $[Cr]_u$. This approach allows for variations in urine flow rate at the time of sampling, thus standardizing comparisons:-

GGT (iu/l) divided by $[Cr]_u$ (mmol/l)

The normal urinary GGT:creatinine ratio should be less than 0.25.

Comment

- Urinary GGT values fall once the acute insult has ceased, despite the persistence of tubular dysfunction. The value of this assay in signalling progressive failure is therefore dubious.

Urinary indices

It is possible that prerenal azotaemia may be differentiated from renal azotaemia by determining the urinary and plasma (or serum) concentrations of urea and creatinine, and calculating the respective urinary indices as follows:

> Urinary concentration of urea/Plasma concentration of urea

and

> Urinary concentration of creatinine/Plasma concentration of creatinine

In prerenal azotaemia kidney perfusion is reduced but tubular function remains intact and the urine is concentrated, so that urinary concentrations of urea and creatinine are high. In renal azotaemia the tubular ability to concentrate urine is diminished and the urinary concentrations of urea and creatinine are relatively low. It follows that the urinary indices in prerenal azotaemia will be higher than those in renal azotaemia.

Urinary indices greater than 15 for urea and 50 for creatinine suggest prerenal azotaemia, whereas renal azotaemia is suggested by values less than 15 and 37 respectively.

Comment

- These figures were ascribed to a limited study and need further assessment.

Assessing plasma electrolyte concentrations in renal disease

There is no consistent pattern to the changes in plasma electrolyte concentrations which occur as a result of renal disease in horses. The following comments are offered.

Potassium

Since the kidneys are the main site of potassium excretion, conditions of oliguria or anuria are likely to be associated with hyperkalaemia. However, progressive tubular damage will eventually lead to hypokalaemia.

Sodium and chloride

Oliguria or anuria may lead to increased plasma concentrations of sodium and chloride. However, progressive tubular damage will be associated with their loss and plasma concentrations may reflect this.

At a stage when tubular damage is associated with polyuria, the plasma concentrations of potassium, sodium and chloride may fall. However, they could appear to be within their normal ranges as a result of systemic dehydration.

Calcium

The horse is unusual in that its major site of calcium regulation is the kidney rather than the small intestine. Unlike other species, renal dysfunction may be associated with either hypercalcaemia or hypocalcaemia.

Renal failure and metabolic acidosis

In the healthy kidney, tubular cells conserve and generate bicarbonate for the blood alkali reserve. In addition, hydrogen ions are excreted. In renal disease, failure of these mechanisms causes a fall in the alkali reserve and an accumulation of hydrogen ions, leading to a state of metabolic acidosis.

Comment

- Systemic acidosis may accompany a number of disease states and is not pathognomonic for renal disease.

Haematology in diseases of the urinary tract

Haematology provides non-specific information in cases of urinary tract disease. Increases in the PCV indicate dehydration and in chronic disease a non-regenerative anaemia is to be expected. Leucocytosis may accompany gross inflammation of the urinary tract and an elevated plasma fibrinogen concentration is indicative of septic inflammation.

Chapter appendix

Appendix 6.1 suggests some applications of the diagnostic techniques covered in this chapter for the investigation of urinary tract diseases, based upon the presenting signs.

Further reading

Grossman BS, Brobst DF, Kramer JW, Bayly WM and Reed SM (1982) Urinary indices for differentiation of prerenal azotemia and renal azotemia in horses. *Journal of the American Veterinary Medical Association* **180**: 284–288.

Harris P and Gray J (1992) The use of the urinary fractional electrolyte excretion test to assess electrolyte status in the horse. *Equine Veterinary Education* **4**: 162–166.

Rantanen NW (1990) Renal ultrasound in the horse. *Equine Veterinary Education* **2**: 135–136.

Taylor FGR, Hillyer MH and Lowrey PA (1990) The assessment of glomerular filtration rate in ponies and horses by sodium sulphanilate clearance. *Equine Veterinary Education* **2**: 137–139.

Appendix 6.1. Some applications of diagnostic techniques for the investigation of urinary tract diseases.

Observation	Possible cause	Aids to diagnosis	
		Preliminary investigation	Definitive investigation
Frequent attempts to urinate ± pain	Cystitis	Rectal examination Urinalysis Urine culture (catheter)	Cystoscopy/biopsy
	Pyelonephritis/cystitis	Assess cystitis (above) Measure blood urea and creatinine Examine kidney and ureters per rectum	Assess tubular function Renal ultrasonography Ureteral catheterization
	Urolithiasis	Rectal examination Urethral catheterization	Endoscopy
	External pressure on the bladder	Rectal examination Ultrasonography	Laparotomy
Persistent dribbling of urine	Retention overflow:		
	(i) Bladder paralysis	Rectal examination	Evacuate bladder by catheter and reassess function
	(ii) Partial obstruction	Rectal examination Urethral catheterization	Endoscopy
	Ectopic ureter	Endoscopy	Excretory urogram
Anuria/oliguria	Acute renal failure	Measure blood urea and creatinine Urinalysis Palpate kidney per rectum	Assess tubular function Renal ultrasound Renal biopsy
	Obstruction	Rectal examination Urethral catheterization	Endoscopy
	Dehydration	Measure PCV and/or total serum protein	
Polyuria/polydipsia See also Chapter 5: 'Endocrine diseases'	Chronic renal failure	Measure blood urea and creatinine Urinalysis Palpate kidney per rectum	Assess tubular function Renal ultrasound Renal biopsy
	Pituitary adenoma (hyperadrenocorticism)	Measure blood glucose	Dynamic function tests (see Chapter 5)
	Diabetes mellitus	Measure urinary glucose	Eliminate pituitary adenoma (see Chapter 5)
	Diabetes insipidus	Water deprivation/modified deprivation test (Chapter 5); test negative in DI	Exogenous ADH (see Chapter 5)

Appendix 6.1. Some applications of diagnostic techniques for the investigation of urinary tract diseases *(continued)*.

Observation	Possible cause	Aids to diagnosis	
	Psychogenic polydipsia	Water deprivation/modified deprivation test; test positive in PP	
Azotaemia in biochemical profile of patient	Renal failure	See above	See above
	Bladder rupture	Measure creatinine in peritoneal fluid	Cystoscopy

7 Genital diseases, fertility and pregnancy

I. **The mare**

Examination for breeding soundness

Indications

Mares should be examined for breeding soundness in the following circumstances:

- If they are maiden mares
- If they have repeatedly failed to conceive after breeding
- Before being accepted for artificial insemination
- If they are non-pregnant and behaviourally anoestrus
- If they require genital surgery
- Prior to purchase
- After embryonic or foetal loss

It is important to adopt a systematic approach to this examination to avoid compromising the interpretation of later procedures by interference from an earlier one. The sequence of diagnostic techniques described in this section is as follows:

(1) Examination of the vulva and perineal region
(2) Clitoral swabbing
(3) Manual examination of the internal genital tract per rectum
(4) Ultrasonography
(5) Endometrial swabbing
(6) Endometrial cytology
(7) Vaginal examination
(8) Digital examination of the vagina and cervix
(9) Endometrial biopsy

Examination of the vulva and perineal region

The vulval lips should meet evenly in the midline and act as the first protective barrier between microorganisms in the external environment and the uterus. This barrier has been shown to be very important in the prevention of pneumovagina (windsucking). Mares with an ineffective vulval seal have a tendency to develop endometritis and have decreased pregnancy rates. Pneumovagina can also lead to embryonic death in early gestation and placentitis during the later stages of gestation, which can cause abortion or neonatal sepsis. For maximal function, the vulval lips should be vertical or at least have a cranial to caudal slope of no more than 10 degrees from the vertical. At least two-thirds of the vulva should lie below the floor of the pelvis (Fig. 7.1).

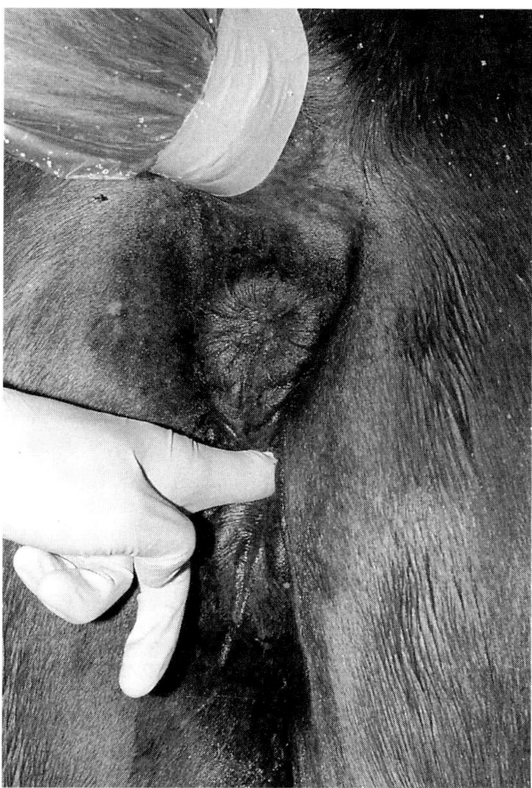

Figure 7.1　Good perineal and vulval conformation with more than two-thirds of the vulva below the floor of the pelvis.

Factors which predispose mares to poor vulval conformation include:

- Increasing age
- Poor body condition
- Thin vulval lips
- Sunken anus
- Foaling trauma

It is possible to test whether a mare is a windsucker or not by placing the palm of either hand on each vulval lip and gently parting them. If the mare is a windsucker a small hole will develop where the lips part and air will be aspirated. In normal mares, all that is heard is a 'click' when the transverse fold (vestibulo-vaginal sphincter) shuts. Appropriate surgery should be performed to correct the vulval seal in mares with pneumovagina.

Clitoral swabbing

The clitoris should be checked for normal appearance. Enlargement can indicate that the mare has received anabolic steroids, or can be suggestive of a chromosomal abnormality — most commonly male pseudohermaphroditism.

Swabs should be collected routinely from all mares at the start of the breeding season. In the UK, the Horserace Betting Levy Board's 'Code of Practice for the Control of Contagious Equine Metritis and Other Equine Reproductive Diseases' recommends that a clitoral swab should be collected before moving the mare to the stallion stud farm. It also recommends that an endometrial swab should be taken on the stud farm at the oestrus prior to mating.

If there is gross contamination of the vulva, it should be wiped with a dry paper towel. The clitoris is exposed using a gloved hand to part the vulval lips, and everted by placing the index finger below the vulval lips. The central and, if present, lateral sinuses are swabbed with a narrow-tipped (paediatric-type) swab (Fig. 7.2). A standard-type swab is used to swab all areas of the clitoral fossa (Fig. 7.3).

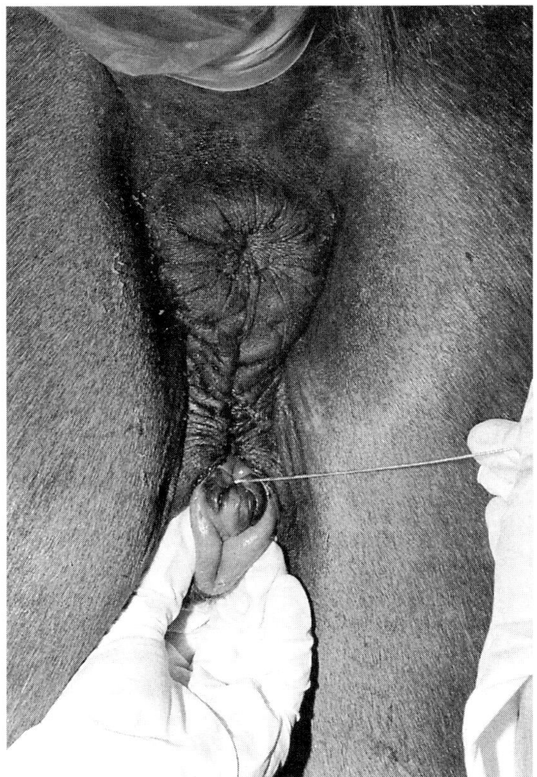

Figure 7.2   Swabbing the central clitoral sinus with a narrow-tipped swab.

Another described procedure is to roll the swab on the ventral aspect of the vestibule before swabbing the clitoris. However, by this method many external contaminants will be picked up, which may overgrow potential pathogens. The swabs should be placed in Amies charcoal-based transport medium and sent to a 'designated' or 'approved' laboratory for the purpose of testing for the contagious equine metritis organism (*Taylorella equigenitalis*). The sample should preferably be kept at 4° C and reach the laboratory within 48 hours.

Comments

- The lateral sinuses may be too shallow to harbour *T. equigenitalis*.
- For all procedures, any assistant holding the mare's tail out of the way should wear disposable gloves and change them between mares.

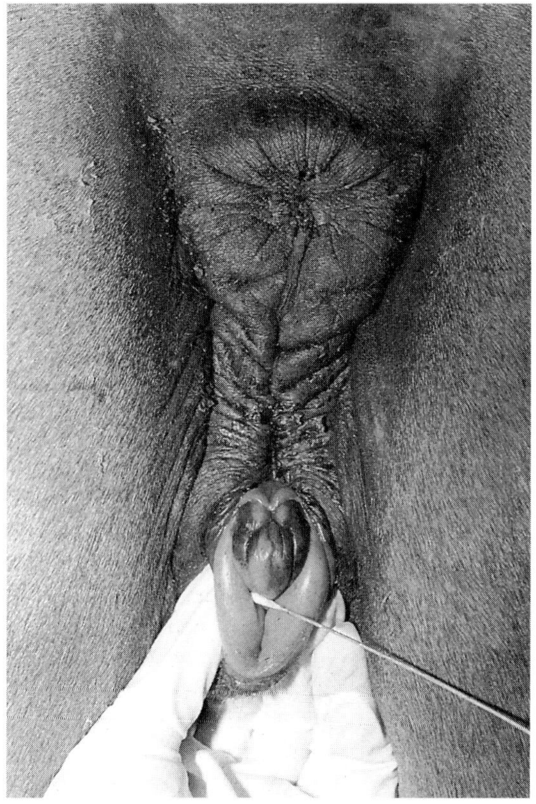

Figure 7.3   Swabbing the clitoral fossa.

Manual examination of the internal genital tract per rectum

This examination should always be performed prior to any internal cervical and/or endometrial manipulations to check that the mare is not pregnant.

Restraint

Ovarian palpation per rectum is a potentially dangerous procedure for the veterinary surgeon. If restraint of the mare is not satisfactory, the clinician should not proceed. As little time as possible should be spent directly behind the mare. It is advisable to stand close to the mare and to one side whenever possible and to reassure her using voice and touch.

There are various options for restraint:

- The mare should preferably be restrained in stocks, but with due attention to the door. If the mare squats she can trap the clinician's arm between her rectum and the top of the door.
- The mare can be positioned such that the examiner can work from behind the door frame of the stable. However, some mares may resent being positioned in this way.
- The mare can be stood half-way through a stable door, which prevents her moving from side to side.
- The mare can be examined in her loose box. The handler should always stand on the same side as the clinician so that when the head is pulled towards the handler the hindquarters automatically move away from the clinician. A bridle with a Chifney bit gives the handler more control.
- If necessary a variety of drugs can be used for chemical restraint, but they may make the mare unsteady and she can still kick out unexpectedly.
- Other procedures include lifting the foreleg on the same side as the examiner, or applying breeding hobbles.

Comment

- When stocks are not used, application of a nose twitch is useful.

Preparation for examination

The mare's tail hairs can abrade the rectal mucosa and the tail should therefore be bandaged or, preferably, placed in a disposable plastic sleeve. A shoulder-length obstetrical sleeve should be worn by the examiner and lubricant should be applied to the back of the hand and the arm. If the mare strains excessively a smooth muscle relaxant such as clenbuterol or propantheline bromide can be administered intravenously. Alternatively, a local anaesthetic can be applied topically to the rectal mucosa.

Comment

- Some veterinary surgeons have reported cases of colic after administration of smooth muscle relaxants for transrectal palpation.

Technique

The mare's rectum tears more easily than that of the cow. If the rectum fills with air ('ballooning'), the fingers should be kept behind a peristaltic wave and withdrawn. The examiner should never push against a peristaltic wave.

Firstly, faecal balls should be removed. The hand is then swept round the floor of the pelvis and up the shafts of the ilium to the sacrum to detect any lesions which may cause dystocia. Specific structures are then located (Fig. 7.4).

Cervix. The cervix is palpated by sweeping the hand from side to side over the floor of the pelvis near the pelvic brim. A thick cord-like structure will be identified, which can then be palpated in more detail by pressing downward with the fingertips. It cannot usually be grasped as is possible in the cow.

Uterus. The body of the uterus may be grasped with a cupped hand just cranial to, and often slightly below, the cranial brim of the pelvis. The uterus feels soft, flat and often flaccid. To confirm that it is the uterus, the tissue is slipped between fingers and thumb to palpate the longitudinal endometrial folds. A check is made for ventral enlargements which can occur at the horn–body junction. These can be endometrial cysts or more usually lymphatic lacunae.

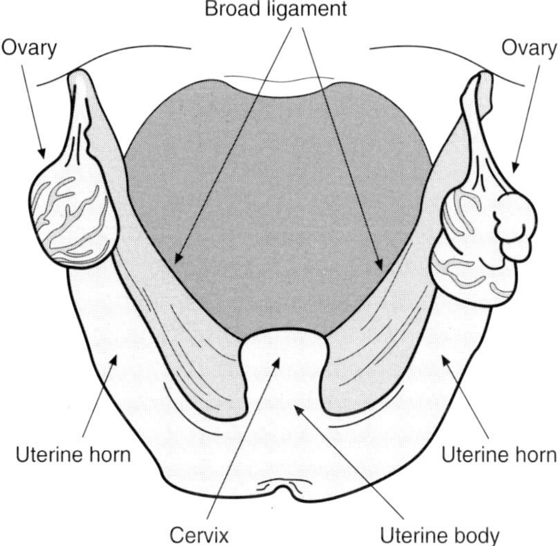

Figure 7.4   Reproductive tract of the mare viewed from in front as if suspended *in situ* during rectal examination.

Ovary. The uterine horns can be followed up to the ovaries. Some clinicians prefer to locate the ovaries first and then follow this with uterine palpation. The location of the ovaries can be quite variable. They are often located cranial and lateral to the mid-shaft of the ilium at '3 and 9 o'clock' or '2 and 10 o'clock'. They measure approximately 5–8 cm in length and 2–4 cm in width. The extent to which the ovaries are mobile is limited by the length of the mesovarium.

The ovaries are kidney-shaped masses orientated longitudinally. The free, concave border containing the ovulation fossa is located ventrally and should always be palpated. The ovaries are considerably less mobile than those of the cow and it is usually necessary to leave them in place and palpate around them. However, they sometimes lie lateral to the broad ligament and it is then necessary to manipulate them onto the cranio-medial aspect for palpation.

As the preovulatory follicle matures, it protrudes from the ovarian surface, creating a shoulder. The follicle reaches an average size of 45 mm on the day before ovulation and usually starts to soften two days before ovulation. After ovulation, the crater becomes filled with blood to form a plum-like corpus haemorrhagicum (CH). The CH feels spongy and non-fluid-filled. The corpus luteum (CL) is formed 4–5 days later and blends into the ovarian stroma. It is difficult to palpate.

Palpable features of the cervix, uterus and ovaries vary with the stage of the oestrous cycle and are shown in Table 7.1.

Ultrasonography

The introduction of transrectal ultrasonography as a diagnostic aid in evaluating the mare's genital tract had a profound effect on the accuracy of detecting ovarian structures and uterine pathology, and facilitated the early diagnosis of pregnancy.

Most of the ultrasound scanners used for transrectal ultrasonography are of the B-mode linear array type. These transducers have a side-by-side arrangement of rectangular piezoelectric crystals along their length. The

Table 7.1. Changes in the mare's genital tract that are palpable per rectum.

Stage of cycle	*Cervix*	*Uterus*	*Ovaries*
Oestrus	Relaxed* Oedematous	Oedematous Flaccid	>25 mm follicle
Dioestrus	Firm Narrow	Increased tone Tubular	Multiple small follicles or a >25 mm follicle
Anoestrus	Moderately firm or thin and open	Flaccid	No palpable structures
Transitional	Not tightly closed until first ovulation	Flaccid	Multiple follicles can be >30 mm

* The cervix may not relax at oestrus in maiden mares.

rectangular picture of the linear-array scan represents a longitudinal view and is oriented lengthwise with respect to the animal. Sector scanners have a pie-shaped examining field, which is oriented crossways with respect to the transducer. The images of both types are in real time, that is, the images move as the structures move.

There are commonly three different transducer frequencies: 3.5; 5, and 7.5 mHz. Lower frequency transducers have greater penetration but poorer resolution. Thus 3.5 mHz transducers are better suited to examining the late pregnant or early postpartum uterus. A higher frequency transducer (most commonly the 5 mHz) is used to examine the genital tract in the non-pregnant and early pregnant mare.

The transducer passes sound waves through tissues. A proportion of these sound waves will be reflected back to the transducer, depending on the density of the tissue being scanned. The transducer converts the sound waves to electrical impulses and an image appears on a screen. The greater the density of the tissue, the greater the strength of echo produced and the whiter the image (the more echogenic) on the screen. In contrast, fluid transmits the sound waves and fluid structures appear black or anechoic on the image. Air is a poor transmitter and therefore it is essential that there is good contact between the transducer and the tissue being scanned.

Technique and image interpretation

Faeces are evacuated from the rectum. Manual examination should always precede ultrasonographic examination to facilitate orientation of the genital tract, and to assess shape, tone and size of the individual components. A disposable plastic sleeve, containing lubricant as a contact gel, can be placed over the probe. The probe should be protected by the hand which forms a cone shape during entry into the rectum. The hand should remain cupped around the transducer and protect the rectal wall during the scanning procedure. The investigation should always be systematic to avoid possible scanning errors. The transducer is held longitudinally with respect to the mare's body, so that the cervix and uterine body are seen sagittally with the cervix to the left of the screen. The uterine horns are then seen in cross-section.

The appearance of the uterus changes during the oestrous cycle. In oestrus, the uterine horns and body have a characteristic pattern of alternating echogenic and hypoechoic areas (Fig. 7.5). This corresponds to oestrual oedema. The hypoechoic areas are thought to be the outer oedematous portions of the endometrial folds. Oedema often, but not always, decreases or disappears within the 24 hours before ovulation. During dioestrus the uterus takes on a much more homogeneous appearance (Fig. 7.6). The uterine lumen is often identifiable by an echogenic line when the uterus is viewed longitudinally (Fig. 7.7).

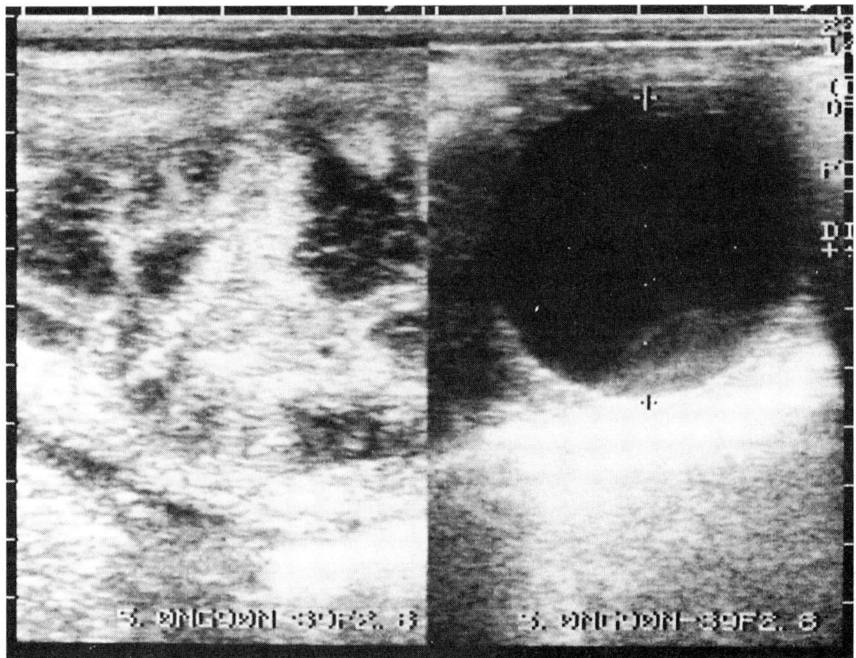

Figure 7.5   Ultrasound images of, left: cross section of the uterine horn during oestrus showing echogenic and hypoechoic areas. Right: anechoic preovulatory follicle.

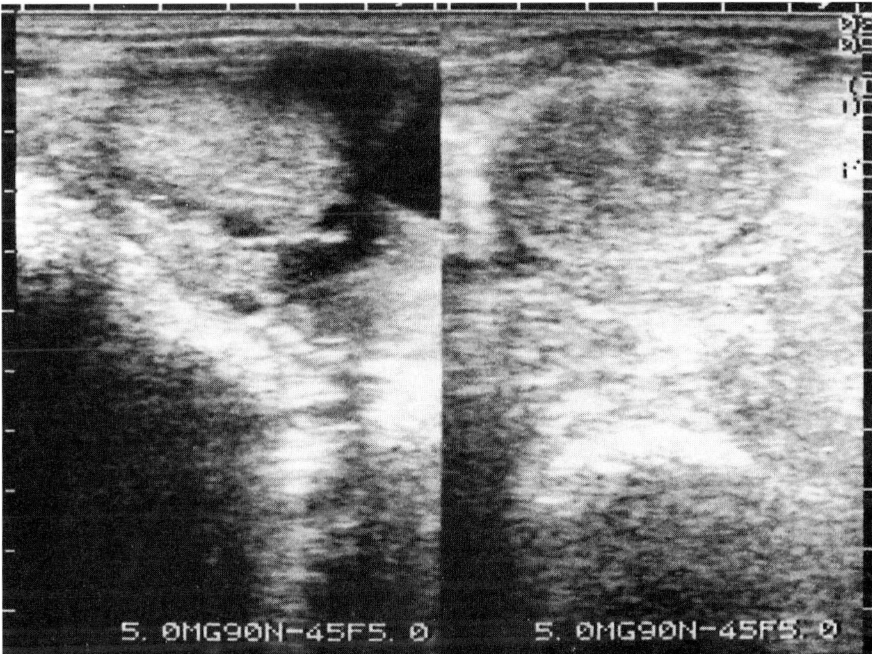

Figure 7.6   Ultrasound images of, right: cross section of the uterine horn during dioestrus, showing a homogeneous appearance. Left: corpus luteum.

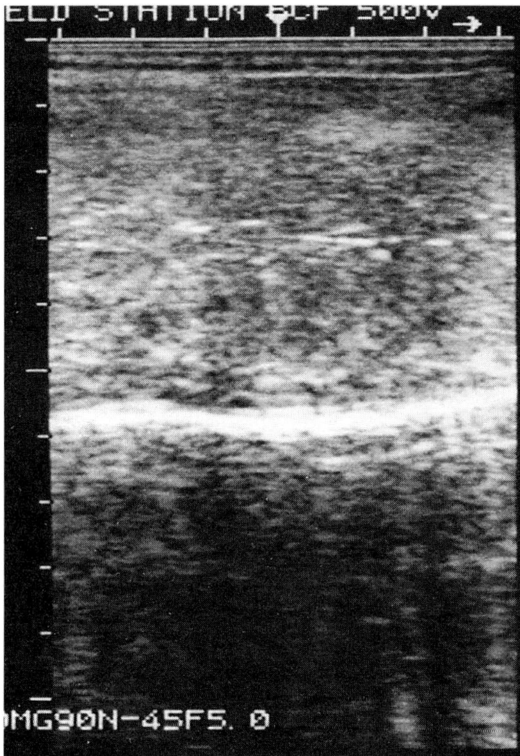

Figure 7.7 Ultrasound image of a longitudinal view of the uterine body. Note the broken echogenic line indicating the lumen.

Ultrasonography of the ovaries is used to provide information on:

- Whether the mare is cycling
- The stage of the cycle
- The predicted ovulation time
- Double ovulations
- Failure to ovulate
- Whether a follicle is of adequate size to induce ovulation by pharmacological means

Follicles appear as black (anechoic) areas (Fig 7.5). Some follicles appear to be an irregular shape owing to compression from surrounding structures or, occasionally, because apposing walls are not detectable. Follicular diameter can be measured by freezing the image and using the calipers on the machine. A 5 mHz transducer can detect follicles as small as 2–3 mm.

Preovulatory follicles attain a mean diameter of 45 mm on the day before ovulation. It is uncommon for ovulation to occur in follicles less than 30–35 mm. Eighty-five per cent of follicles change shape, developing a wedge shape or a neck-like protuberance pointing towards the ovulation fossa on the day before ovulation (Fig. 7.8). The shape change, plus

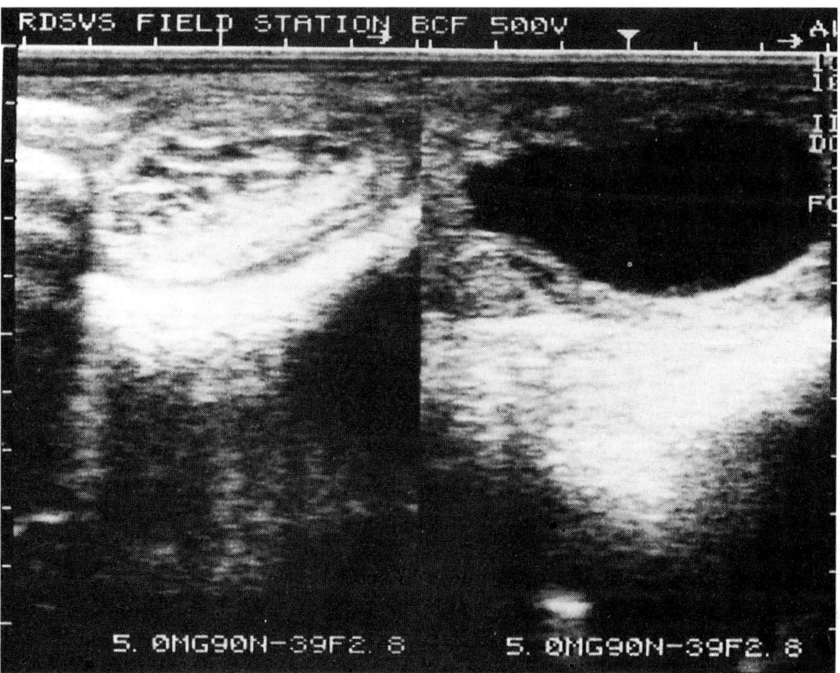

Figure 7.8 Ultrasound image of, right: distortion of the follicle on the day before ovulation as it migrates towards the ovulation fossa. On the left is a corpus haemorrhagicum. Note the mottled appearance representing pockets of serum interspersed with fibrinous bands.

size and soft consistency, are currently thought to · be the best predictors of imminent ovulation.

The occurrence of ovulation is easily diagnosed by ultrasonography based on the disappearance of a large follicle that had been recorded previously, and the appearance of a newly forming corpus luteum, which in most mares is highly echogenic (Fig. 7.9). Sometimes the ovulation crater then fills with blood forming a corpus haemorrhagicum, which appears as mottled hypoechoic areas of serum interspersed with echogenic fibrinous bands (Fig. 7.8). Approximately 50% of corpora lutea develop a central blood clot. In the corpus luteum with a central clot, progesterone production is normal and the central cavity gradually shrinks as the structure ages (Fig. 7.10). The morphology of the remaining 50% of corpora lutea is uniformly echogenic. It can be distinguished from ovarian stroma by its distinct border and by the brighter echogenicity of the denser stromal tissue (Fig. 7.6). There is a tendency for early and late corpora lutea to

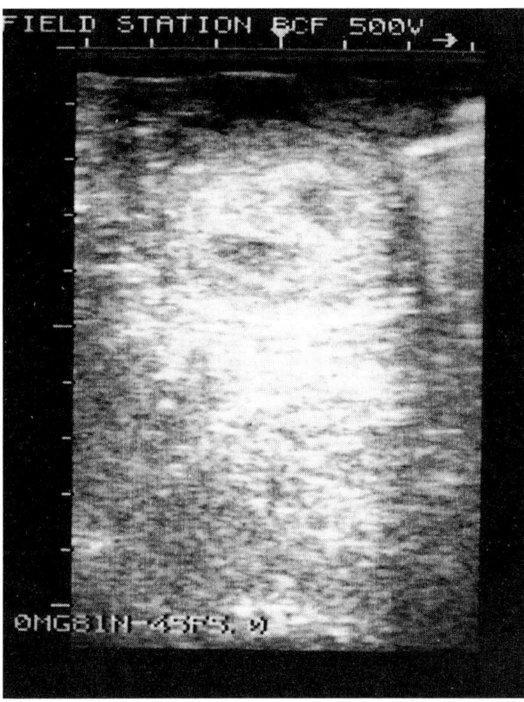

Figure 7.10   Ultrasound image of a mature corpus luteum (day 9) containing cystic cavities.

be more echogenic than mid-luteal corpora lutea.

Endometrial swabbing

The endometrium should be swabbed at the oestrus prior to breeding and at subsequent oestruses if necessary. The perineum should be washed three times with a non-residual soap or povidone–iodine, rinsed thoroughly with warm, clean water and dried with clean paper towels.

Swab samples are highly prone to contamination and therefore careful aseptic procedures are essential. Culture of cervical mucus is thought unreliable in reflecting the presence of bacteria in the uterus. Double-guarded techniques give the most reliable results (Fig. 7.11).

The clinician wears a clean plastic sleeve and sterile glove and cups the end of the culture instrument in his/her hand. Sterile water-soluble lubricant is applied to the back of the hand and arm before entering the vestibule and

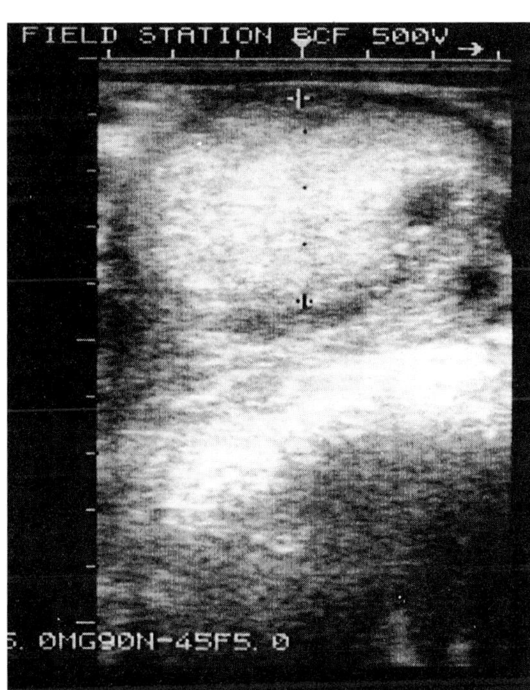

Figure 7.9   Ultrasound image of a highly echogenic newly formed corpus luteum on the day after ovulation.

vagina. The instrument is guided through the cervix by the index finger. The inner tube is then pushed through the opening at the tip of the outer tube and the swab is advanced to contact the endometrium. After 10 seconds the swab is retracted into the inner, and then the outer tube, and withdrawn from the uterus.

Alternative guarded methods have been described where, for example, a standard swab is passed into the uterus under an outer rectal sleeve. Alternatively, the swab can be passed into the uterus on an extension rod via a sterile vaginal speculum (single guarded method: Fig. 7.11).

The swab should be placed in Amies transport medium, labelled clearly and forwarded to the laboratory where it should arrive within 48 hours of collection.

Endometrial cytology

Preparative cleansing of the perineum and vulva for endometrial cytology is the same as described above under: 'Endometrial swabbing'.

There are some instruments available which can provide both culture swabs and cytology smears. More commonly, a second swab is used after the initial swabbing to obtain a sample of endometrial cells. This swab can then be smeared onto a proprietary slide which stains the cells ('Testsimplets': Boehringer Ingelheim, UK), or onto an ordinary microscope slide (Fig. 7.12) which is then stained with Geimsa or 'Diff-Quick' (Baxter Healthcare Ltd, Thetford, UK).

The best, but more time-consuming method of obtaining a sample of endometrial cells is to perform a uterine flush, using a sterile mare embryo flushing catheter or a foal nasogastric tube. Approximately 250 ml of sterile saline is infused and then allowed to run out by gravity or by massage of the uterus per rectum. The recovered fluid is then centrifuged (1000 x g for 10 minutes) and the cell pellet is resuspended in a small volume of saline before smearing onto a glass slide and staining. Alternatively, a small volume can be placed in a cytospin centrifuge and then stained. If the fluid is to be submitted to a laboratory, a portion of the fluid can be placed in an equal volume of cytospin fixing fluid (Shandon Scientific Ltd, UK) for cell preservation.

Comment

● Manipulations involving entry into the uterus are best performed during oestrus. It is inevitable that microorganisms will gain entry to the uterus from the vestibule and vagina, which contain resident populations of microorganisms. Mares can best eliminate this contamination during oestrus.

Vaginal examination

Vaginal examination can be useful in identifying cycle stage and pathological and anatomical changes. This procedure can be performed before or after endometrial swabbing. The advantage of performing speculum examination before swabbing is that the cervix will not have been digitally manipulated prior to viewing. Furthermore, air contact quickly causes artefactual reddening. The disadvantage of performing it before swabbing is that there is an increased chance of contamination of the external os of the cervix, which will then be transferred into the uterus at the time of swabbing.

Various types of speculum have been developed for vaginal examination. A metal trivalve or duck-billed speculum has been used but this is heavy and difficult to sterilize. Disposable specula provide good visibility of

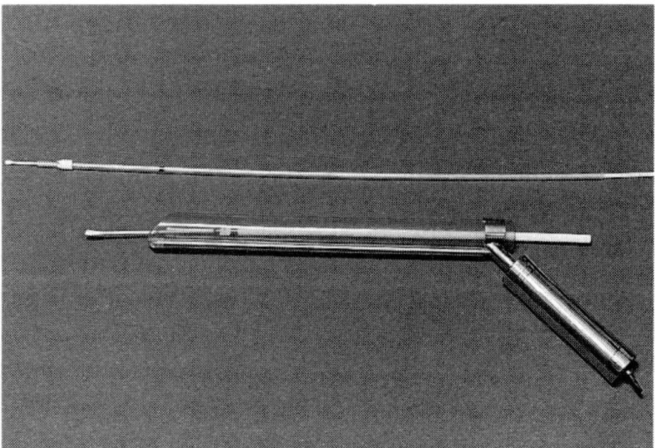

Figure 7.11   Top: double guarded swab for obtaining endometrial culture. Below: extended swab passed through a vaginal speculum.

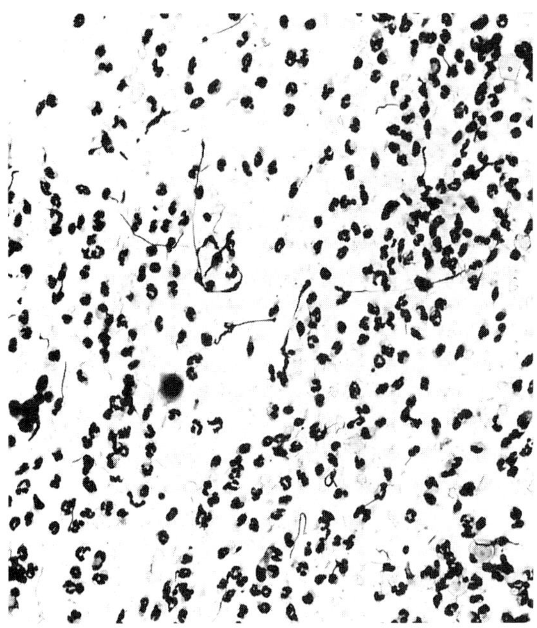

Figure 7.12   Endometrial smear from a mare with acute endometritis showing the presence of many neutrophils (x 25).

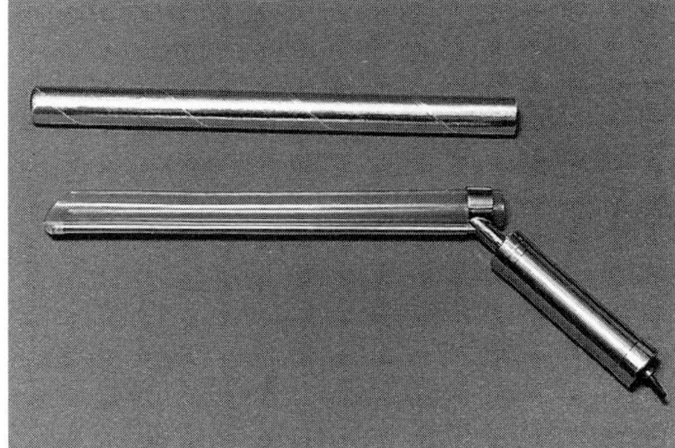

Figure 7.13   Disposable vaginal speculum (top) and autoclavable plastic speculum.

the cervix and can be discarded after each mare, which is ideal when more than one mare needs to be examined. Plastic tubes that fit over a metal template with an integral light source provide good visibility of the cervix and vagina, but need to be sterilized between mares (Fig 7.13).

Sterile, water-soluble lubricant should be applied to the speculum which is then inserted into the vestibule at a craniodorsal angle of 45 degrees with the vulval lips parted. Once the speculum passes through the transverse fold, it can be introduced horizontally. A pen torch or ophthalmic light source can be used to illuminate the cervix and vagina. Various changes can be detected in the cervix according to the stage of the cycle (Table 7.2).

Digital examination of the vagina and cervix

Lesions can be missed in the vagina and cervix if manual examination is not carried out. A clean plastic sleeve with a sterile glove should be worn. The lubricant used should be sterile and water-soluble, such as 'K-Y Jelly' (Johnson and Johnson). The vagina and cervix should be palpated for tears and adhesions. Tears in the

Table 7.2.   Cyclical changes in the cervix detectable by speculum or digital examinations.

Parameter	Oestrus	Dioestrus	Anoestrus	Pregnancy
Number of fingers that can be passed	Three or more	One	One to three (or more)	One
Colour	Red	Pale grey or yellow	Pale white	White
Appearance	Glistening Oedematous Slit-like cervical os	Dry Closed	Dry Can be atonic and open	Dry Closed
Position	On floor of vagina	In mid-vagina	In mid-vagina	In mid-vagina

cervix are most obvious during dioestrus when good tone is present.

Endometrial biopsy

Apart from mares with subfertility problems, mares requiring genital surgery should be biopsied prior to surgery to give an indication of their ability to carry a foal to term. Biopsy can also be used to monitor the response to therapy in mares with uterine infections. However, there is a substantial risk that mares susceptible to endometritis will be reinfected as a result of bacteria being introduced at the time of follow-up biopsy.

Technique

Preparative cleansing of the perineum and vulva prior to endometrial biopsy is the same as described above under: 'Endometrial swabbing'. The biopsy procedure is as follows:

- Large alligator-jaw forceps are available for obtaining endometrial biopsies. These are introduced into the vagina by a lubricated hand covered in a plastic sleeve under a sterile glove. The forceps are guided through the cervix by the index finger. The hand is then withdrawn and inserted into the rectum.
- The jaws of the forceps are kept closed until they are located in the uterus by the hand in the rectum. They are then opened and the uterine endometrium is pushed into the jaws which are then closed. The bite should be taken by pushing the tissue sideways into the jaws of the forceps rather than forwards, in which case it is possible to penetrate the uterine wall.
- The forceps are then removed, keeping the jaws shut. If the tissue has not been completely severed it is sometimes necessary to give the forceps a gentle tug. Very occasionally slight bleeding is seen from the vulval lips after biopsy, in which case the mare should be kept inside for a day until the bleeding stops. No further treatment is usually necessary.

- The biopsy sample should be carefully removed from the jaws with a fine needle or forceps and placed in Bouin's fixative solution. Tissue in Bouin's should be processed within 24 hours of collection. If the biopsy is not likely to reach the laboratory within 24 hours, it should be transferred to 70% alcohol on the day after collection. It is important to include a history and give the stage of the cycle at which the biopsy was obtained.

Interpretation of results

Morphology of the normal endometrium varies with the stage of cycle:

During anoestrus the endometrial glands are inactive and the epithelium is cuboidal or low columnar. Anoestrous mares frequently have groups of closely associated glands owing to coiling of gland branches. No oedema is present.

During oestrus the epithelium becomes columnar to tall columnar. Vacuoles are common in the basal cytoplasm of the luminal epithelium. Neutrophils are often seen in capillaries under the luminal epithelium and at the margin of blood vessels in the lamina propria, but not in the tissue. There may be considerable oedema. Glands appear relatively straight and non-tortuous.

In dioestrus the epithelium varies from cuboidal to columnar depending on the proximity to oestrus. The glandular branches appear highly coiled and tortuous.

Examination for breeding soundness — ancillary techniques

Chromosome analysis

The incidence of chromosomal abnormalities in horses is not known, but in human beings chromosomal abnormalities have been associated with abortion, infertility and congenital defects. The most commonly reported chromosome problems are errors in structure or number of sex chromosomes in infertile or subfertile mares. Errors in sex chromosomes and other chromosomes can cause unthriftiness and growth retardation in either sex. Chromosomal abnormalities have also been reported in infertile stallions.

Karyotyping (chromosome analysis) can be performed on any tissue with dividing cells. Peripheral blood lymphocytes are normally used. Blood samples (10 ml) should be collected into heparin or acid citrate dextrose (ACD) and transported overnight to the referral laboratory.

Progesterone analysis

Serum progesterone assay is a reliable monitor of ovarian function. Serial samples can confirm cyclical ovarian function. If three samples collected at weekly intervals are consistently low (<3 nmol/l), it is likely that the mare is anoestrus. If the samples are consistently >6 nmol/l, it is likely that the mare has prolonged luteal function or has had a late-dioestrous secondary ovulation.

The progesterone assay is also useful in confirming that a mare is in oestrus if she is not displaying overt signs. Analysing a sample collected two days after injection of PGF-2α will confirm whether the mare has experienced luteolysis and can be expected to return to oestrus. The progesterone concentration should be low at this time (<3 nmol/l).

Most laboratories use serum for hormone analysis but specific requirements should be checked before sending the sample. Alternatively, mare-side kits are available for progesterone assay by practitioners.

Comment

● Progesterone is a poor indicator of pregnancy in the mare, with a high false-positive rate. However, basal progesterone concentrations (<3 nmol/l) at around 18–21 days after ovulation are thought to be 100% accurate in detecting *non-pregnancy*.

Endoscopy

Use of endoscopy should be considered when a localized problem within the endometrium has been diagnosed by palpation or ultrasonography, or when the cause of infertility cannot be determined by other means. Flexible fibreoptic endoscopes should be used, at least 1 m in length with an outer diameter of at least 10 mm. A bright light source, preferably 300 W halogen or xenon light is needed. The endoscope should preferably be gas sterilized before use, but failing this the working end can be cleaned using disinfectants recommended by the manufacturer. The endoscope should then be rinsed in alcohol and allowed to dry prior to use.

Technique

● The mare's perineum and vulva should be cleansed as described previously under: 'Endometrial swabbing'.
● The endoscope is introduced into the uterus through the cervix by a lubricated, sterile-gloved hand.
● The lumen should be distended with a non-irritant gas such as CO_2, or using sterile saline. When infusing saline, 1–2 litres can be run through an embryo collection catheter once the endoscope is in the uterus.
● The normal endometrium appears pink and free of exudate. The endoscope is advanced to the uterine bifurcation and then down each horn.

Comment

● This procedure is best performed in dioestrus when the cervix is closed. If the mare is susceptible to endometritis, it may be advisable to infuse antibiotics into the uterus after endoscopy.

Pregnancy diagnosis

Pregnancy diagnosis by transrectal palpation

Rectal palpation for pregnancy diagnosis is

accurate after about 28 days, but is easiest to perform around 42 days of gestation.

Ovarian changes

Numerous follicles are palpable in the ovaries during the first 100 days of pregnancy. Secondary corpora lutea form on the ovaries after day 40.

Cervical and uterine changes

Day 1. The cervix closes and uterine tone increases.

Day 14. There is marked tubularity of the uterus.

Day 21. The cervix is long and tightly closed. The endometrial folds are no longer palpable. The conceptus may be palpated as a ventral swelling (1.5–3 cm in diameter) at the base of one of the uterine horns.

Day 28. The spherical embryonic vesicle (2–3 cm in diameter) is palpable ventrally at the base of the pregnant horn.

Day 42. The enlargement is slightly oval, approximately 5 cm in diameter and occupies one half of the pregnant horn. The non-gravid horn remains tonic.

Day 60. The conceptus measures approximately 12 cm in diameter and fills the gravid horn. The ovaries are now progressively pulled cranially and medially. They are no longer palpable by about day 150.

Day 80. Most of the body and both horns are filled by the conceptus.

Day 90. Decreased pressure in the allantois allows the conceptus to be detected by ballottement. The enlarged uterus begins to descend over the pelvic brim and cannot be retracted.

Day 200. The descent of the uterus is complete. Fremitus in the uterine arteries is present from day 150.

Day 200 plus. The uterus starts to ascend and the fetus is easily palpable.

Comments

● Early pregnancy diagnosis may be difficult in older mares bred at a foal heat in which the uterus is enlarged.

● A filled urinary bladder (located ventral and/or cranial to the brim of the pelvis), or fluctuating pelvic flexure of the colon, can be mistaken for a pregnant uterus. A systematic approach and identification of the cervix and uterus will allow correct diagnosis.

Pregnancy diagnosis by ultrasonography

The embryonic vesicle is first detectable in the pregnant horn as a round, hypoechoic structure of approximately 4 mm around day 10. Detection of the vesicle is aided by the bright specular echoes which are often seen on the dorsal and ventral surfaces of the vesicle. The embryo 'fixes' on day 16 (Fig. 7.14) and changes from a round to a triangular shape by day 18 (Fig. 7.15). On day 21 the embryo is first detected on the ventral surface of the

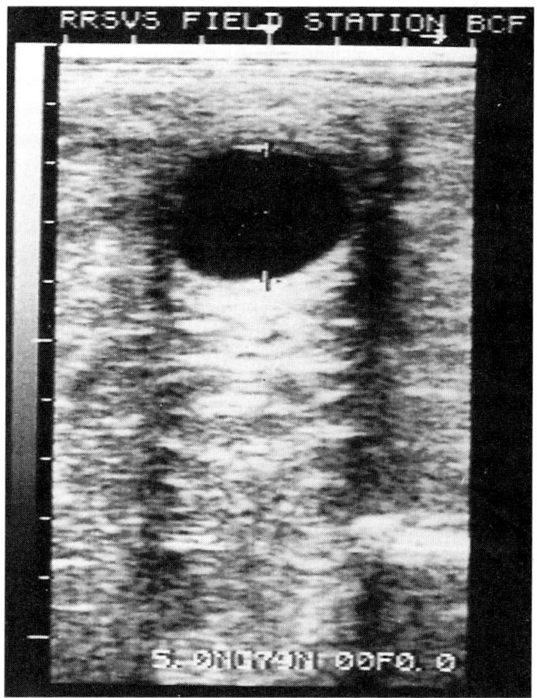

Figure 7.14   Ultrasound image of a sixteen-day-old embryonic vesicle.

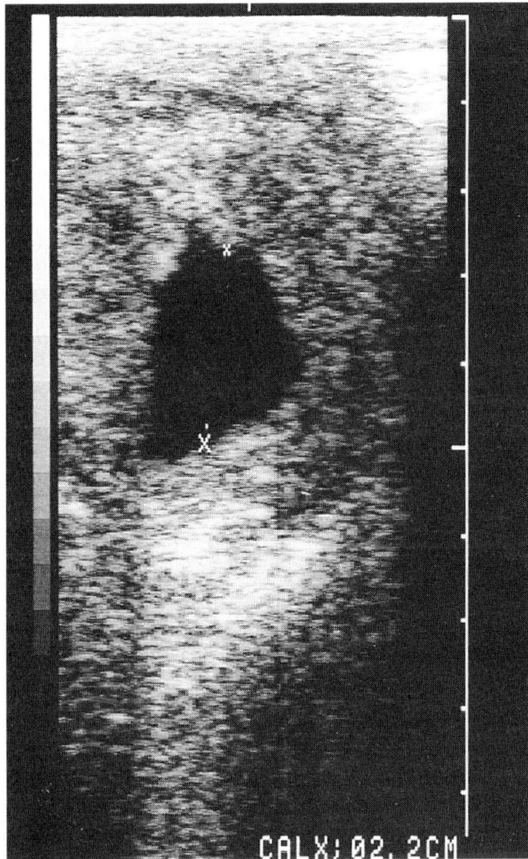

Figure 7.15   Ultrasound image of an eighteen-day-old embryonic vesicle. Note the change to a triangular shape.

vesicle. By day 25 a heartbeat is detectable and the fluid-filled allantoic sac is visible as a non-echogenic area beneath the embryo. At day 30 the allantois occupies the ventral half of the vesicle (Fig. 7.16) and by day 40 the yolk sac has regressed and the allantois fills most of the vesicle (Fig. 7.17). By day 50 the umbilical cord has lengthened and the foetus has descended to the floor of the allantois.

Comments

- Twin conceptuses can be detected reliably at day 14 (Fig. 7.18). A thorough search of both uterine horns and the body should always be performed. Intraluminal cysts can be confused with a conceptus, but they do not move or grow (Fig. 7.19). If there is

uncertainty about diagnosis, the mare should be re-examined at around day 24 when the embryos are easily visible.

- Transabdominal ultrasonography requires a 3.5 mHz transducer and cannot be performed until about day 80. It is useful, but not 100% accurate, for diagnosing twins which are thought to have been missed earlier.

Hormone assays

Serum oestrone sulphate

This is produced by precursors of the foetal gonads, so that high levels confirm the viability of the foetus. It is present in high concentrations from day 90 to term.

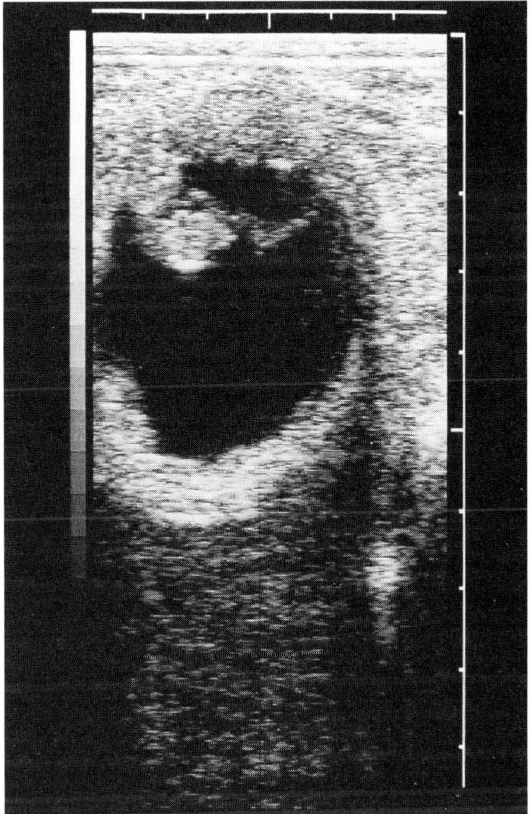

Figure 7.16   Ultrasound image of a 33-day conceptus. The yolk sac is regressing and the allantois fills most of the vesicle.

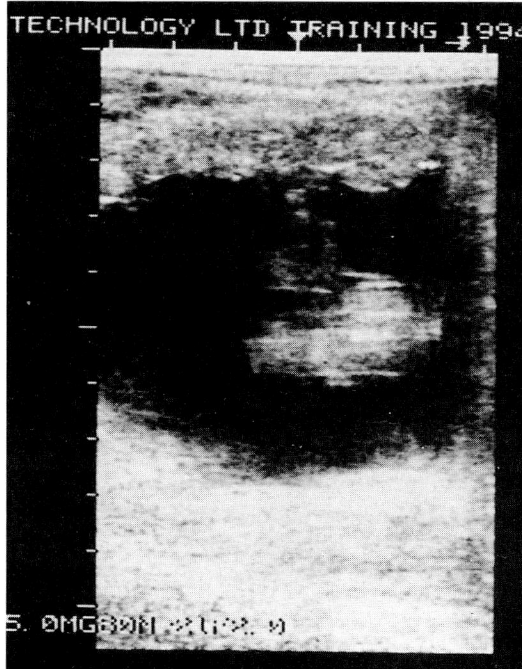

Figure 7.17   Ultrasound image of a 40-day conceptus. The umbilical cord is lengthening and the foetus has moved towards the floor of the allantois.

Equine chorionic gonadotrophin (eCG)

This is present in high concentrations in serum between days 40–120. False positives can be recorded if the foetus dies. NB High eCG concentration indicates the presence of endometrial cups, not a viable foetus.

Investigation of abortion, stillbirth, or birth of a sick foal

Abortion rates for Thoroughbreds have been estimated to be greater than 12%. Strictly speaking, 'abortion' refers to foetuses lost before 300 days and those lost after 300 days are called 'stillbirths'.

Investigative approach

It is necessary to adopt a methodical approach to investigate a cause of abortion. The

Horserace Betting Levy Board's Code of Practice recommends that veterinary intervention should take place in the case of any abortion, stillbirth, or foal death which occurs within 14 days of birth.

Either the whole foetus plus the foetal membranes should be sent to a specialist laboratory along with a serum sample from the mare and a detailed clinical history, or the following procedure should be adopted:

- The crown–rump length is measured to assess foetal age and development.
- The placenta is examined. The recommended method is to lay it flat in an F shape with the cervical star at the bottom of the F, the pregnant horn forming the top arm and the non-pregnant horn the lower arm. A check is made to see whether the foal has exited through the cervical star. The smooth allantoic surface of the allantochorion should be outermost. The length of the cord is measured and cord blood is collected. The placenta is then turned inside out and

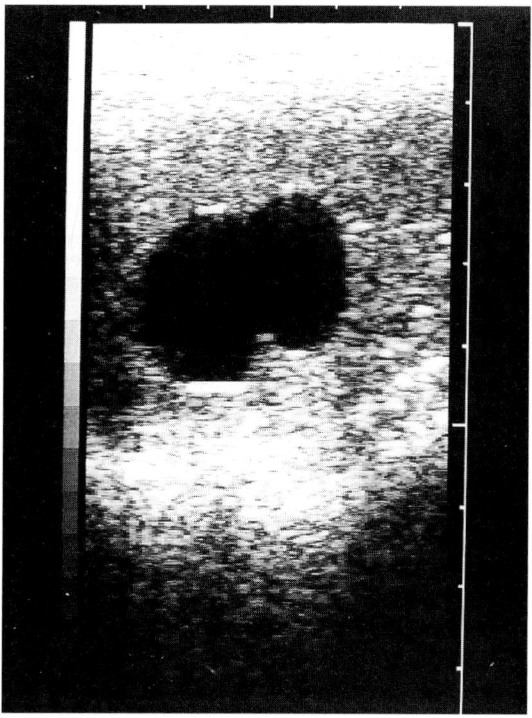

Figure 7.18   Ultrasound image of twin conceptuses at day 14.

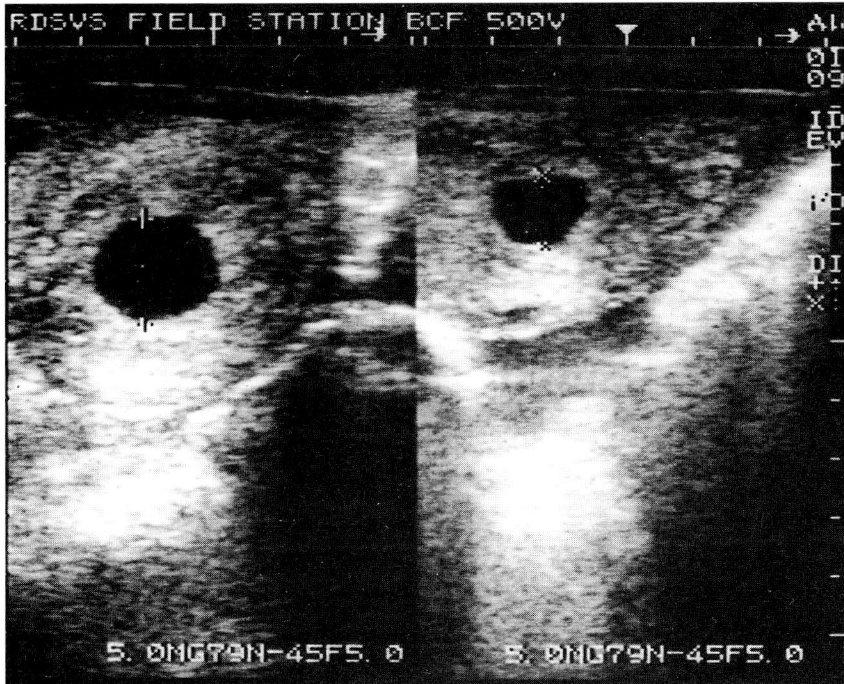

Figure 7.19
Ultrasound image of a fourteen-day embryo (left), compared with intraluminal cyst (right)

the chorionic surface is examined for avillous areas and for areas of discolouration.

- A gross general examination is made of the foetus noting the appearance of organs and any fluid in body cavities. The presence of fractured ribs, haemarthrosis of the shoulder joint or subcutaneous oedema of the head can indicate dystocia.

- Microbiological culture: the liver, stomach contents, lung, allantochorion (near the cervical star) and allantoamnion are sampled aseptically and put in sterile containers packed in ice.

- Virus isolation: the liver, lung and thymus are sampled and put in sterile containers packed in ice.

- Histological examination: the liver, lymph node, adrenal gland, lung, thymus, spleen, allantochorion and allantoamnion are submitted as tissue sections (1 x 2 x 2 cm) in 10% formol-saline or Bouin's fixative.

- Blood is taken from the mare for serology — preferably as paired samples.

If infection is suspected and the foal becomes unwell within 14 days of birth, isolate the mare and foal. Nasopharyngeal swabs and heparinized blood samples should be collected and sent to a specialist laboratory for virological examination.

Infectious causes of abortion — diagnostic features

Infectious causes of abortion are associated with viral, bacterial and fungal agents.

Equine viral rhinopneumonitis (EHV-1)

This abortion is not associated with concurrent maternal illness and tends to occur between 7 months of gestation and term. Abortion at an earlier stage is possible.

Gross examination of the foetus will reveal:

- Recent death (not autolysed)
- Petechiation on mucosae
- Jaundice
- Enlarged liver and spleen
- Focal areas of necrosis in the liver
- Subcutaneous oedema
- Serosanguinous fluid in body cavities

Histopathology will reveal:

- Intranuclear eosinophilic viral inclusion bodies, most commonly in the liver, respiratory epithelium and lymphoid tissues
- Mild multifocal necrotizing inflammation in the liver and adrenal cortex
- Hyperplastic necrotizing bronchiolitis in the lung

NB Where facilities allow, the best diagnostic test is the fluorescent antibody test performed on chilled or frozen samples of lung, thymus, lymph node, spleen and adrenal cortex. Second best is virus isolation, followed by detection of viral inclusion bodies in the liver, lung and thymus.

Equine viral arteritis (EVA)

In the dam, clinical signs range from none at all to severe systemic illness. The typical clinical presentation is fever, lethargy, depression, conjuctivitis, nasal discharge, urticarial rashes and oedema.

The foetus shows no specific lesions but is autolysed.

Paired blood samples from the mare should be submitted for serology. The stallion should also be tested.

Virus isolation is possible from:

- Nasopharyngeal swabs (mare)
- Heparinized blood (mare)
- The stallion's semen
- The stallion's urine

If the stallion is found to be seropositive, he has either been vaccinated or has previously been infected with the virus. Because a proportion of stallions become persistent 'shedders', it is important to ascertain whether virus is present in their semen. This is achieved as follows:

- Isolate the stallion
- Collect two ejaculates of semen at least one week apart and send to a specialist laboratory for virus isolation or detection.
- Test mate the stallion to two seronegative mares and monitor whether the mares seroconvert.

Bacterial infections

Placental examination. Inflammation of the allantochorion is usually most severe around the cervical star (the ascending route of infection). The placenta is oedematous and the chorionic surface tends to be brown with a variable amount of fibrinonecrotic exudate.

Microbiology. Samples of the foetal organs and stomach contents, together with the placenta, should be submitted for bacteriology.

Fungal infections

Placental examination may reveal extensive chorionic oedema and necrosis, originating at the cervical star.

Histopathology of the placenta demonstrates fungal hyphae.

Microbiology. Samples of the foetal organs and stomach contents, together with the placenta, should be submitted for fungal culture.

Non-infectious causes of abortion — diagnostic features

Twinning

One twin is frequently small and autolysed whereas the other is fresh. Placental examination may reveal that areas of placenta–placenta contact are without a normal villous structure.

Placental insufficiency

In these cases the foetal crown–rump length is less than predicted for the gestational length and the foetus appears emaciated.

Endometrial biopsy may reveal endometrial fibrosis or cysts.

Uterine body pregnancy

The foetal membranes are underdeveloped and the foetus shows retarded growth.

Premature placental separation

Full term foetus.

There is an incomplete or complete tear in the middle of the body of the allantochorion.

The placenta is often thickened and the detached areas are dry and brown.

Umbilical cord damage

If the cord is greater than 84 cm in length, it is predisposed to twists. Once occluded, the foetus dies and autolyses.

Differential diagnosis of genital diseases in the mare

The various conditions outlined in this section are associated with a failure to conceive and/or embryo loss. The applied diagnostic techniques which are indicated have already been described above under: 'Examination for breeding soundness'.

Small ovaries

The differential diagnoses for small ovaries include: hypoplasia (congenital); atrophy (acquired), and winter anoestrus.

Diagnostic techniques

Palpation. The ovaries are small and smooth; the uterus and cervix are flaccid.

Ultrasonography. No obvious follicles are present.

Karyotype. The commonest abnormality is 63XO.

Enlarged ovaries

The differential diagnoses include:
- Spring transition
- Haematoma
- Tumour (most commonly granulosa cell tumour)
- Anovulatory haemorrhagic follicle
- Paraovarian cyst
- Abscess

Diagnostic techniques

Palpation. Mares with a granulosa cell tumour usually have one large ovary and one which is very small and hard. The large ovary can be uniformly smooth, knobbly and hard, or soft and fluctuating. The ovulation fossa of the affected ovary is filled in.

A paraovarian cyst can be distinguished from an ovarian-associated structure by palpation.

During the spring transition, ovaries can have multiple follicles which are greater than 30 mm in diameter.

Ultrasonography. Classic granulosa cell tumours are described as having a honeycomb appearance with distinct multilocular cysts. However, the appearance of affected ovaries can vary from being uniformly echogenic to having one (or a few) large fluid-filled cysts.

Haematomas have a mottled appearance. The fluid-filled areas probably represent pockets of serum.

Anovulatory follicles can grow to 100 mm. The follicle becomes filled with blood, and fibrin strands can be seen (Fig. 7.20).

Ovarian abscesses are very uncommon unless there is a history of needle aspiration of fluid from an ovary. Ultrasonographically they appear as thick-walled structures with an echogenic centre.

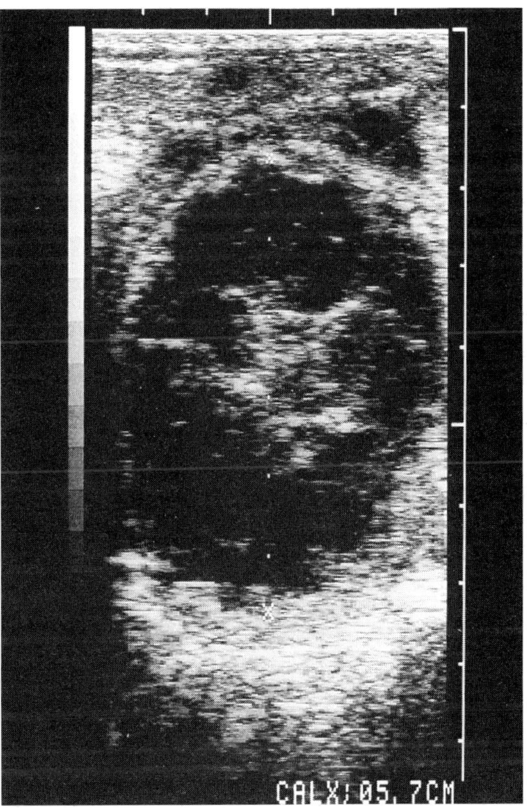

Figure 7.20   Ultrasound image of an anovulatory follicle containing visible fibrin strands.

Hormone assay. Over 50% of mares with a granulosa cell tumour have elevated concentrations of testosterone in the plasma (basal concentration: 0.02–0.5 nmol/l).

Uterine diseases

Diagnostic techniques for the following uterine diseases are indicated below:

- Acute endometritis
- Endometrial cysts
- Endometrial transluminal adhesions
- Endometrosis

Diagnosis of acute endometritis

Ultrasonography. Fluid of variable echogenicity can be found in the uterus and its presence during dioestrus is highly suggestive of endometritis (Fig. 7.21). Pneumouterus (secondary to windsucking) can be seen as hyperechoic reflections caused by air in the uterus.

Vaginal speculum examination. There may be evidence of vaginitis and/or cervicitis with

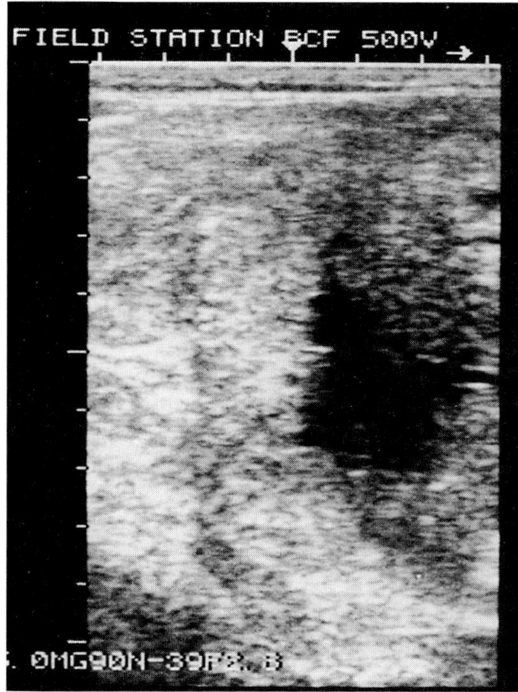

Figure 7.21 Ultrasound image of fluid at the base of the uterine horn.

exudate visible in the vagina or coming through the cervix, especially during oestrus. If the fluid is suspected to be urine, its creatinine and urea concentrations should be analysed and calcium carbonate crystals may be seen on cytology. The finding of debris and air bubbles indicate that the mare is a windsucker. If the speculum falls readily into the vagina, it suggests that the transverse fold is not forming an effective seal.

Microbiology. The growth of known pathogens from an endometrial swab, in the presence of other signs of endometritis, is diagnostic. Pathogens include: haemolytic streptococci, *Escherichia coli*, *Pseudomonas aeruginosa*, *Klebsiella pneumoniae*, *Taylorella equigenitalis*, yeasts and fungi.

Endometrial cytology. The presence of large numbers of neutrophils is evidence of endometritis. The exact proportion of neutrophils to epithelial cells depends upon the method of collection. In general, if more than 2% of the cells are neutrophils, it is likely that the mare has an endometritis.

Biopsy. Infiltration of the biopsy tissue with neutrophils indicates an acute endometritis. These cells are usually found in the stratum compactum (the superficial layer of the lamina propria) and migrating between luminal epithelial cells. In more severe cases, neutrophils will be present in the stratum spongiosum (the deeper layer of the lamina propria). Glands may be dilated and degenerated neutrophils may be present in the lumen.

Diagnosis of endometrial cysts

Palpation. Cysts must be large and/or widespread before they will interfere with pregnancy. It is thought they may be significant if the whole uterus feels spongy.

Ultrasonography. Cysts can be classified as intraluminal (Fig. 7.22) or intramural. They can arise either from endometrial glands (<10 mm) or from lymphatics (>10 mm). They should be differentiated from the early embryonic vesicle by failure to grow, compartmentalization, failure to move and irregular appearance.

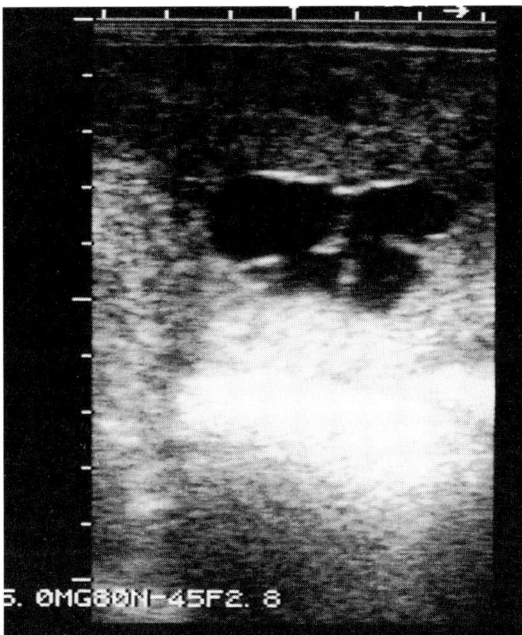

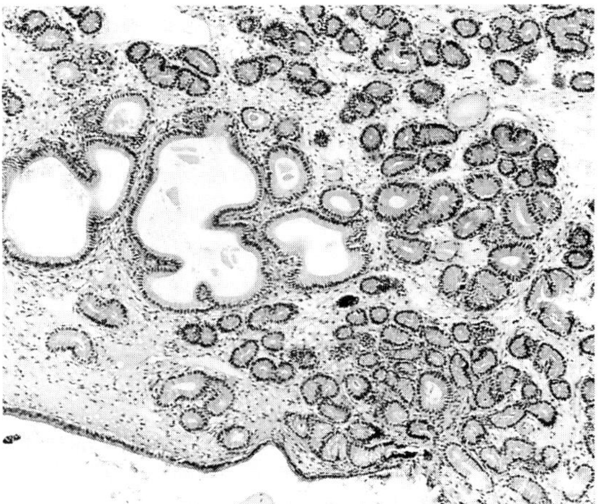

Figure 7.23   Mild periglandular fibrosis around individual gland branches and cystic glandular distension (x 10).

Figure 7.22   Ultrasound image of a complex of intraluminal endometrial cysts.

Endoscopy. Intraluminal cysts can be seen as shiny, fluid-filled structures.

Diagnosis of endometrial transluminal adhesions

Endoscopy. These appear as bands, sheets or tunnels of fibrous tissue.

Ultrasonography. Adhesions are not usually visible. If one uterine horn is completely occluded, infusion of saline into the uterus will enable this to be demonstrated.

Diagnosis of endometrosis by biopsy

Endometrosis is characterized by a number of chronic, irreversible changes which can be defined by histopathological examination of uterine biopsies. Such changes include:

- Degenerative changes of the glands — cystic glandular distension and periglandular fibrosis.
- Fibrosis of the endometrium usually occurs around individual gland branches or around groups of gland branches forming gland nests (Fig. 7.23). Fibrosis is recognized because the stromal cells lose their normal random orientation and become elongated in layers around the glands. The severity is classified by the number of layers present. Two or three layers is classified as mild, whereas 10 or more is classified as severe. The frequency with which fibrotic changes occur in the specimen should be reported by the laboratory, because widespread changes have a more detrimental effect on fertility than localized changes.
- Cystic distension of the glands is usually secondary to fibrotic changes. In anoestrous and transitional endometria, some degree of glandular distension is common. However, this usually resolves with the onset of normal ovarian cyclicity.
- Lymphatic lacunae are possibly associated with myometrial atony in older mares. These must be differentiated from artefactual oedema by identifying an endothelial margin.
- Cellular elements. Chronic inflammation is characterized by infiltration of the tissue with lymphocytes and plasma cells (Fig 7.24). Chronic infiltrations occur most commonly in the stratum compactum, but can also involve the stratum spongiosum. Discrete foci of mononuclear cells can often be seen. The presence of a few scattered mononuclear cells is normal and forms part of the mare's uterine immune system. Acute and chronic cellular infiltrations can be

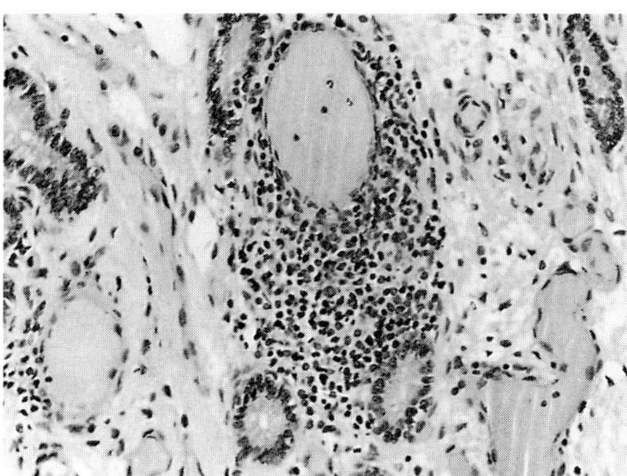

Figure 7.24   Aggregate of mononuclear inflammatory cells in the lamina propria of a mare's endometrium (x 40)

present together. In these mares neutrophils will be visible (Fig 7.25).

Infiltration with eosinophils has been associated with pneumouterus (windsucking) and with fungal endometritis.

Haemosiderophages (macrophages filled with haemosiderin) can be seen in mares that have recently foaled or aborted.

Categorization of biopsy results

Changes within the endometrium have been placed in three or four categories (see Doig *et al.*, 1981, in: 'Further reading'). A good correlation exists between the severity of histological endometrial lesions and the ability

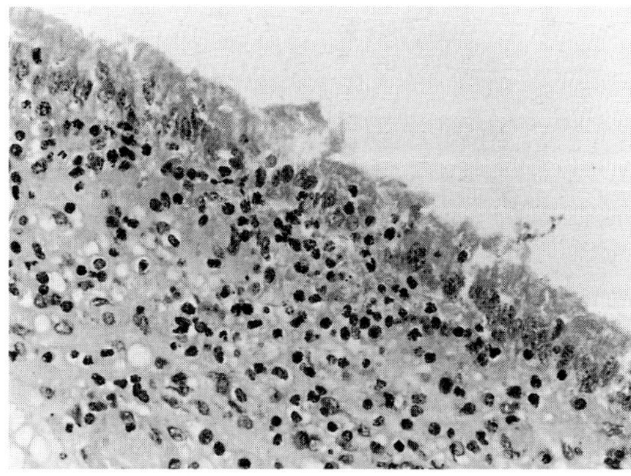

Figure 7.25   Infiltration of the stratum compactum of the endometrium by neutrophils and mononuclear cells (x 40).

of a mare to carry a foal to term.

Category I (normal endometrium, 80–90% foaling rate) — any pathological changes indicating fibrosis and inflammation are slight and scattered.

Category IIA (mild changes, 50–80% foaling rate) — slight, diffuse infiltration with inflammatory cells or frequent and scattered fibrotic changes. If both moderate inflammatory and fibrotic changes are present, the mare is downgraded to Category IIB.

Category IIB (moderate changes, 10–50% foaling rate) — inflammation or fibrosis is widespread and moderate.

Category III (severe changes, 10% foaling rate) — widespread severe inflammation and/or severe fibrotic changes are present.

Interpretation of biopsy results should be modified according to the age of the mare; increased age is associated with decreased fertility. The number of years barren also appears to have a significant effect on foaling probability in mares with a Category IIA or IIB endometrium. If a mare has been barren for 2 or more years, the likelihood of future foaling decreases significantly.

Cervical diseases

Cervicitis and vaginitis

These conditions are diagnosed at speculum examination (see above under: 'Vaginal examination').

Cervical laceration

Cervical laceration should be diagnosed by manual examination of the cervix per vaginam. This should be undertaken during dioestrus when the cervix is likely to have good tone

Vaginal disorders

Apart from vaginitis, the differential diagnoses of vaginal disorders include: pneumovagina; urovagina and persistent hymen.

Diagnosis of pneumovagina

Conformation. The perineum and the vulval seal should be examined (see above under:

'Examination of the vulva and perineal region').

Rectal palpation. In severe cases the uterus may be distended with air.

Ultrasonography. Echogenic air bubbles may be visible if pneumouterus is present.

Speculum examination. Frothy exudate may be seen in the vagina.

Diagnosis of urovagina

Speculum examination may reveal urine in the vagina.

Laboratory analysis. Fluid assay for creatinine and urea may indicate urine. In addition, the fluid deposit should be examined for calcium carbonate crystals.

Diagnosis of persistent hymen

Speculum examination may reveal a membrane visible in the region of the transverse fold.

Rectal palpation and ultrasonography may indicate mucoid secretions accumulated behind the hymen.

II. **The stallion**

An examination of the stallion for breeding soundness should be performed routinely in the following circumstances:

- Before the start of the breeding season
- Before purchasing a stallion to be used as a stud horse
- In stallions with a history of subfertility

Physical examination

Testicular measurement

This is best performed after collection of the first ejaculate. The length, width and height of each testis should be measured. Testicular size is highly correlated with daily sperm output.

Caliper method

Tuberculin calipers can be used to measure testicular size. It is necessary to place the calipers on the testis without distorting the surface and therefore decreasing the diameter. Minimum total scrotal width should be 80 mm before a stallion should be passed as a satisfactory prospective breeder. This measurement

relates to horses; there is little data on smaller pony breeds.

Ultrasonography

More accurate measurements of testis size can be made by ultrasonography using a 5 or 7.5 mHz transducer (see Love *et al.* 1991 in Further Reading).

Testicular consistency

Each testis is examined by passing it between the thumb and fingers after pushing the contralateral testis out of the way. The epididymis, particularly the tail, should also be palpated. Soft or hard testes may indicate some degree of degeneration. If the tail of the epididymis is hard and small it is likely that fibrosis is present, which will reduce the capacity of the tail to store sperm. If any localized lesions are suspected, ultrasonography can be used for further investigation.

Examination of the penis

The penis is best examined when erect, during the washing procedure prior to semen collection.

Swabbing

Stallions are passive carriers of venereal diseases. They are classified as infected if they harbour one or more of the following: *Pseudomonas aeruginosa*, *Klebsiella pneumoniae* (capsule types 1, 2 & 5) and *Taylorella equigenitalis*. In the UK, the Horserace Betting Levy Board's Code of Practice recommends that all stallions and teasers be swabbed after January 1st, but before the start of the breeding season, on two occasions which are not less than one week apart.

Technique

The best way to collect swabs is to tease the stallion with an oestrous mare until he has a full erection. The stallion should be backed away from the mare, preferably into a padded corner. The penis can then be deflected with a gloved hand and the swabs collected. The regions to be swabbed before washing include the urethral fossa and penile sheath. The penis should then be rinsed in clean warm water, with particular attention to removing debris from the glans, and dried with clean, soft paper towels. The washing procedure usually stimulates the release of copious quantities of pre-ejaculatory fluid which can be collected for culture. A swab is then inserted 3–5 cm up the urethra to obtain a urethral sample prior to semen collection. Semen can also be cultured but it is prone to external contamination.

If inflammatory processes are suspected farther up the genital tract, samples for culture are as follows:

Urethra. A postejaculatory urethral swab is obtained. The urethral swab is taken immediately after the penis is withdrawn from the artificial vagina. Normally there should be no growth from this swab.

Vesicular glands. The stallion should be teased to distend the vesicular glands with fluid. A 1 x 100 cm sterile catheter with an inflatable cuff can then be passed up the urethra to the level of the colliculus seminalis (the origin of the excretory ducts of the vesicular glands). The cuff should then be inflated and fluid in the vesicular gland can be expressed manually per rectum for bacteriological and cytological study.

Prostate, ampullae, ductus deferens. The first jet of semen contains secretions which are largely from these sites. An open-ended artificial vagina can be used to collect the first jet and the rest of the ejaculate can be collected separately.

Infections in the epididymis and the testis. These usually cause changes which can be identified on palpation.

Swabs should be placed in Amies transport medium and transported to the laboratory within 48 hours of collection.

Semen collection

Semen from stallions can be collected using an artificial vagina (AV). Several models are available. The most commonly used are the CSU model (Animal Reproduction Systems, Los Angeles) and the Missouri (Arnolds Veterinary Products, UK). The CSU model holds its temperature well but is heavy and difficult to assemble. The Missouri loses its temperature more quickly, but is light and inexpensive (Fig. 7.26).

A disposable plastic liner should be used with the AV as the quality of semen is improved and the chances of transferring infection are reduced. Unfortunately, some stallions do not work well with plastic liners. In these cases the rubber liner needs to be sterilized after use. The liner should be submerged in 70% alcohol for 20 minutes and hung up to dry. Before use it should be rinsed in sterile water to remove any traces of alcohol (which is spermicidal) and dried.

The AV should be filled with water to give an internal temperature of approximately 45° C. At the start of the breeding season or in slow stallions the internal temperature can be increased to around 50° C. Because of the sensitivity of sperm to high temperatures, it is important that the stallion's penis fully enters the AV and that semen does not have to run down a length of hot liner. The semen can be collected in a non-spermicidal plastic bottle or bag, which should be insulated from external

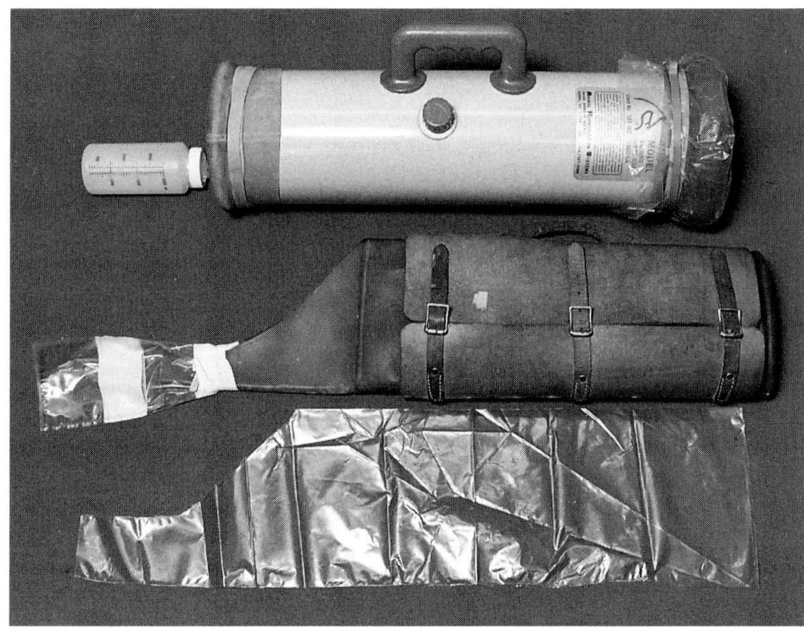

Figure 7.26 Assembled CSU model (top) and Missouri Artificial Vagina (middle) with plastic disposable liner (bottom),

cold temperatures. After the AV is assembled a warm, sterile, water-soluble and non-spermicidal lubricant such as 'K-Y jelly' (Johnson and Johnson, UK) should be applied to the upper two-thirds of the internal surface of the AV with a plastic sleeve. The hand is then withdrawn leaving the sleeve in place to prevent the lubricant from drying out and to help maintain the temperature.

The semen can be collected using a teaser mare or a 'phantom mare'. If a teaser mare is being used, she needs either to be in oestrus, or ovariectomized and oestrogen-treated. Her tail should be bandaged or enclosed in a plastic sleeve so that the stallion's penis is protected from abrasion by tail hairs. If several stallions are using the same mare, her perineal region should be washed with povidone–iodine solution between each stallion. Alternatively, a blanket, which is changed between stallions, can be placed over her hind quarters .

The stallion should be allowed to tease the mare to check that she is receptive and to allow his penis to be rinsed with clean warm water at 42° C. The penis should be dried thoroughly with clean paper towels. Long plastic disposable sleeves should be worn by the person washing the penis and collecting semen from the stallion, in order to avoid transfer of

infection. While the stallion's penis is being washed, the mare can be positioned with a twitch applied.

The stallion can then be allowed to mount the mare. The loose plastic sleeve in the AV should be removed before the penis is deflected into the AV. Pushing the AV upwards against the stallion's abdomen is usually more stimulatory than pushing it down on the penis (Fig. 7.27). The free hand should be placed on the base of the stallion's penis so that the pulsations of ejaculation can be felt. These pulsations will occur at the same time as the tail is seen to flag. After two or three pulsations the anterior end of the AV should be lowered gradually. After ejaculation the stallion will slide off the mare and the collector should follow him and let the penis leave the AV, keeping the AV in the vertical position so that semen flows down into the collecting vessel.

The seminal gel must be removed from the semen before evaluation. This can be done either using a filter built into the AV liner (preferable) or after collection. Nylon filters are more effective than filters used for milk. It is important that semen and all equipment that comes into contact with it be kept at 37° C until the semen is 'extended' with diluent.

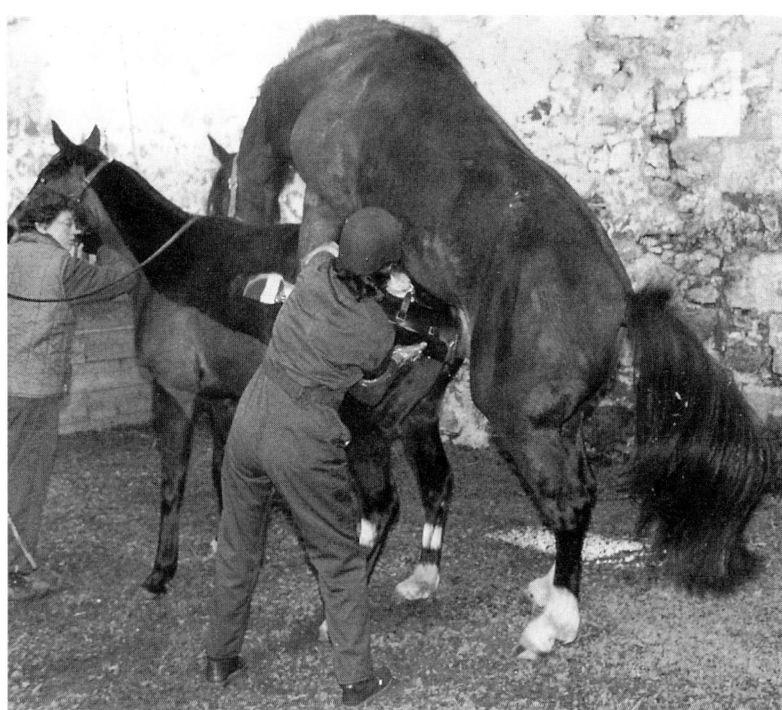

Figure 7.27 Collection of semen from a stallion.

Semen evaluation should be performed as soon after collection as possible.

Semen evaluation

The following parameters should be assessed:

Volume. The mean is 60–70ml.

Colour. Normally whitish.

Motility. One drop of semen is placed on a warm microscope slide and covered with a clean coverslip. To estimate motility accurately, a phase-contrast microscope with a heated stage is essential. An estimate should be made of both the total per cent motile and the per cent progressive motile. For sperm to be classed as progressively motile they must be moving rapidly across the field and, with each lash of the tail, the head must rotate 360 degrees. If the head does not rotate, many of the sperm will move in circles as 50% of stallion sperm have abaxial heads. More than 60% should be progressively motile.

pH. Normal range = 7.2–7.6. If the pH is raised, it is possible that the semen is contaminated with urine, or that infection is present.

Concentration. The number of sperm per ml must be determined. The quickest way to perform this is with a densimeter or calibrated spectrophotometer. However, a haemocytometer is commonly used. The semen is diluted 1:100 (10 µl semen +990 µl formol-saline). The haemocytometer chamber is filled with diluted semen and the chamber is placed on moistened tissue in a covered petri dish for 10 minutes to allow the sperm to settle. The sperm heads in five small squares in the large central square of the Neubauer chamber are counted. Only the heads on the left and top lines of each square are counted. Those on the right and bottom lines are excluded. The number obtained is multiplied by 5×10^6 to give the number of sperm per ml. For samples of very low concentration, the semen is diluted 1:10 rather than 1:100. The average total sperm in an ejaculate is 8×10^9. This falls to approximately 3×10^9 if the stallion is collected frequently, and represents the daily sperm output.

Morphology. This examination can be performed using buffered formol-saline (one drop in approximately 2–3 ml) and phase-contrast microscopy, or by staining with nigrosin–eosin. To stain with nigrosin–eosin, a drop of stain is mixed with a drop of semen on the end of a slide. The resulting drop is then smeared along the slide using a second slide (as for a blood film) and allowed to dry. Another smear should then be made with the residual fluid on the second slide. Morphology should be assessed under the oil immersion lens of the microscope. Two hundred sperm should be counted and specific types of abnormal morphology are recorded. There should be more than 60% of sperm which are morphologically normal.

Total number of morphologically normal, progressively motile sperm. This number is derived from the total number of sperm in the ejaculate multiplied by the % progressively motile x the % morphologically normal. This figure is much more important than individual figures for motility, morphology, volume or density. The minimum acceptable number of usable sperm is 1 billion in the second ejaculate. This figure should be approximately 50% of that of the first ejaculate.

NB This figure probably represents an underestimate of useable sperm as many morphologically abnormal sperm will not be progressively motile.

Longevity of motility. A portion of the ejaculate can be placed in semen extender (approximately 1:2) and, together with an aliquot of raw semen, is kept in airtight, dark conditions at 23° C. Motility should be evaluated hourly for 6 hours, and then evaluated at 24 hours. At least 10% sperm should be progressively motile at 6 hours in the raw semen sample and at 24 hours in the extended semen. The value of this test may be questionable as a means of reflecting how long sperm live in the female tract. However, if a stallion is being evaluated for a chilled, transported semen programme, it would be essential to test longevity of motility at 4° C in different extender/antibiotic combinations.

Comment

- Morphology and motility of stallion semen is not affected by season, but volume and

total sperm numbers increase in spring and summer.

Cryptorchidism

This is a fairly common condition in which one or both of the testes fail to descend into the scrotum. If the testis has passed through the vaginal ring but not the external inguinal ring, the horse is referred to as an inguinal cryptorchid. Subcutaneous testes which cannot be displaced into the scrotum are termed ectopic. If the testis and epididymis are retained within the abdomen the horse is termed a complete abdominal cryptorchid. If the testis is within the abdomen but a portion of the epididymis is in the inguinal canal the horse is called a partial abdominal cryptorchid.

Diagnosis

Palpation

The presence of only one scrotal testis (occasionally none) can be detected on palpation of the scrotal contents and external inguinal ring. Tranquillization may relax the cremaster muscles making subcutaneous or inguinal testes more accessible. The scrotum should be palpated and inspected visually for the presence of a scar which would indicate previous surgery.

If the testis cannot be found by external palpation, rectal palpation can be performed. However, this should only be undertaken if adequate facilities for restraint are available. Abdominal testes are small, flabby, mobile and difficult to identify. It is usually more informative to palpate the vaginal ring on the appropriate side; if this is identifiable it is likely that the testis or the epididymis has descended into the inguinal canal. The vaginal ring is located by placing the wrist laterally on the brim of the pubis near the pubic symphysis. The fingertips are then pressed against the abdominal wall. By flexing and extending the middle finger in a cranio-ventral direction it is possible to enter the slit-like vaginal ring. The left hand is used to identify the right ring and the right hand to identify the left ring.

Ultrasonography

Scanning is started at the pubic brim and then continued cranially using lateral movements between the midline and the lateral abdominal wall. *This procedure is more useful than palpation in locating inguinal and abdominal testes and estimating their size.* The retained testis tends to be less echogenic than a descended testis.

Blood hormone tests

A human chorionic gonadotrophin (hCG) stimulation test can be performed to stimulate testosterone production by the retained testicular tissue. A blood sample is collected and then 6000 iu hCG is administered intravenously. A second blood sample is collected approximately one hour or 24 hours later. A significantly elevated concentration of testosterone in the second sample is diagnostic for the presence of testicular tissue. This test is considered to be approximately 95% accurate.

Serum oestrone sulphate

Serum oestrone sulphate can be measured in a single sample from horses >3 years old and is reported to be 95–96% accurate. The test should not be used on horses <3 years of age and donkeys, as these give a high incidence of false-negative results.

Further reading

Acland HM (1987) Abortion in mares: diagnosis and prevention. *Compendium of Continuing Education* **9**: 318–324.

Doig PA, McNight JD and Miller RB (1981) The use of endometrial biopsy in the infertile mare. *Canadian Veterinary Journal* **22**: 72–76.

Love CC, Garcia MC, Riera FR and Kenney RM (1991) Evaluation of measures taken by ultrasonography and caliper to estimate testicular volume and predict daily sperm output in the stallion. *Journal of Reproduction and Fertility* **Suppl. 44**: 99–105.

8 Blood disorders

This chapter covers the diagnostic techniques for investigating blood disorders and includes clinical examination, the interpretation of haematology and any associated clinical pathology (e.g. coagulation tests), and bone marrow aspiration/biopsy.

I. **Diagnosis of anaemia**

Anaemia is a decrease in the oxygen carrying capacity of the blood, which is caused by an absolute reduction in the number of circulating red cells. The associated clinical signs vary with the onset and severity of the condition. In general terms these include one or more of the following:

- Depression and weakness
- Pale mucous membranes
- Tachycardia and tachypnoea at rest
- Reduced exercise tolerance

Confirmation of anaemia is usually based on the evaluation of red cell parameters in a peripheral blood sample (EDTA). However, the interpretation of results must take into account the normal physiological variations of individuals which are, associated with breed, excitability and fitness (see 'Interpretation of haematology' in Chapter 1: 'Submission of samples and interpretation of results'). In particular, the clinician should be aware that a state of anaemia can be masked if excitement at sampling causes elevation of the PCV as a result of splenic contraction. In addition, anaemic patients suffering dehydration may show erythrocyte parameters which appear normal. Table 8.1 shows typical erythrocyte parameter ranges for different groups of horses. Values below the normal ranges are indicative of anaemia.

Once it has been established that a state of anaemia exists, the underlying cause needs to be determined. This will be one or a combination of the following events:

- Absolute blood loss
- Haemolysis
- Decreased red cell production

Of these, decreased red cell production (dyserythropoiesis) is the commonest cause of anaemia in horses.

Before considering the diagnosis of these causes of anaemia, it is important to realize a limitation of haematology in the horse. In the blood samples of other domestic species, regenerative changes (such as reticulocytosis, polychromasia, macrocytosis, anisocytosis and the appearance of nucleated red cells), are indicative of increased erythropoiesis associated with blood loss or haemolysis. These are termed 'regenerative' or 'responsive' anaemias, in contrast to 'non-regenerative' anaemias, which are associated with decreased erythropoiesis. *In contrast, juvenile red cells mature within the bone marrow of the horse and are rarely found in the circulation.* Because of this, erythrocyte indices are not particularly useful for characterizing anaemia in the horse and erythropoietic activity is best defined by bone marrow aspiration or biopsy (see later). However, a moderate increase in mean corpuscular volume (MCV) is usually apparent during the course of a regenerative anaemia and an associated anisocytosis may be seen on occasion.

Table 8.1. Typical erythrocyte parameter ranges* for different groups of adult horse.

Parameter	Thoroughbred	Hunter	Pony
PCV%	40–46	35–40	33–37
RBC x 10^{12}/l	7.2–9.6	6.2–8.9	6.0–7.5
Hb g/dl	13.3–16.5	12.0–14.6	11.0–13.4
MCHC g/dl	34–36	34–36	33–36
MCV fl	48–58	45–57	44–55
MCH pg	14.1–18.1	15.1–19.3	16.7–19.3

*Adapted from data supplied by the Clinical Pathology Diagnostic Service, Department of Clinical Veterinary Science, University of Bristol.

Blood loss anaemia

Blood loss may be acute and potentially life-threatening, or chronic and barely detectable.

Acute haemorrhage

The blood volume of a healthy horse represents some 6–10% of its body weight. An acute loss of 25–30% is tolerated, but greater losses induce hypovolaemic shock. This situation must be judged on clinical grounds alone since the early haematological parameters will appear normal despite impending shock. Assuming survival, there is a compensatory increase in plasma volume by 12–24 hours, causing a dilution of the total protein concentration and a drop in the packed cell volume (PCV), red blood cell count (RBC) and haemoglobin concentration.

Diagnosis

- The clinical signs reflect hypovolaemic shock and include tachycardia, tachypnoea, weak pulse, dry pale mucous membranes, cold extremities, profound weakness and eventually, cardiovascular collapse.

- The erythrocyte parameters and total plasma protein reflect acute blood loss some 12–24 hours after the event. A PCV less than 20% suggests that red cell reserves have been depleted. However, a stable PCV between 12–20% does not usually warrant transfusion.

- The possibility of an internal abdominal haemorrhage may be investigated by abdominal paracentesis (see Chapter 2: 'Alimentary diseases'). In such circumstances a defibrinated (non-clotting), platelet-free, bloody fluid is obtained.

- A proliferative response by the bone marrow is usually demonstrable after 4–7 days.

Chronic haemorrhage

Chronic haemorrhage can be quite protracted before the problem is recognized because the bone marrow has a chance to regenerate erythrocytes as they are lost. Anaemia becomes apparent only when regeneration falls behind loss.

Early on there is an erythropoietic response by the bone marrow that continues until the iron reserves are depleted by persistent blood loss. After this, there is the potential for an iron deficiency anaemia to develop. However, assuming the horse continues to eat, the quantity of dietary iron usually compensates the loss.

Diagnosis

- Because of the physiological adaptation to chronic blood loss, clinical signs are generally masked until the PCV falls below 10–15%. However, signs will appear earlier if the animal is required to exercise.

- Chronic blood loss is indicated by long-term depression of PCV, RBC count and haemoglobin concentration, together with evidence of bone marrow regeneration.

- Unless a site of blood loss is obvious, investigation should include analysis of urine, faecal and peritoneal fluid samples for detection of blood. A number of coagulopathies, the diagnoses of which are covered later in this chapter, can also be associated with chronic blood loss.

- Severe and persistent redworm infection can result in chronic blood loss. Faecal egg counts are indicative.

Haemolytic anaemia

Haemolytic anaemia is uncommon in the adult horse. It occurs in acute or chronic forms and can be caused by infectious agents, but it is most usually the result of an immune-mediated disease (immune-mediated haemolytic anaemia). More rarely, it is associated with erythrocyte damage within lesions involving the microcirculation (microangiopathic haemolytic anaemia). Haemolysis is also a component of the terminal stages of liver failure.

Diagnostic characteristics of haemolysis

A haemolytic crisis is characterized by discolouration of the plasma with haemoglobin (haemoglobinaemia) and, if the renal threshold is exceeded, haemoglobinuria. Because haemoglobin is rapidly cleared from the plasma and converted to bilirubin, jaundice (icterus) may be the only obvious clinical evidence of recent haemolysis. Jaundice first appears in the mucous membranes some 12 hours after the initial crisis and is most pronounced in the sclerae.

The absence of jaundice does not preclude haemolysis since a more gradual destruction of red cells may be matched by the clearance of bilirubin by the liver. This is often the case in 'extravascular haemolysis', which is probably the commonest form of haemolysis in horses.

In haemolytic patients a haematology sample reveals subnormal PCV, RBC count and haemoglobin concentration. In a crisis the plasma is discoloured by haemoglobin. An increase above range in the mean corpuscular haemoglobin (MCH) also indicates the presence of free haemoglobin and a state of haemolysis. However, increases in plasma haemoglobin or MCH could reflect haemolysis as a result of sample spoilage and should be interpreted with this caution in mind.

Serum biochemistry reflects haemolysis by demonstrating raised bilirubin concentrations. However, hyperbilirubinaemia is not of itself pathognomonic for haemolysis. Anorexia, for whatever reason, is probably the commonest cause of hyperbilirubinaemia (and jaundice) in horses. Unlike the anaemia of acute haemorrhage, the total plasma protein concentration is maintained during haemolysis, despite a fall in erythrocyte parameters.

Infectious causes of haemolytic anaemia

These are rare in horses:

- Several bacteria such as clostridia, staphylococci and *Leptospira* are capable of producing haemolysins during the infective process, but these are seldom encountered in practice.
- Equine infectious anaemia is a viral disease transmitted by biting flies (or contaminated needles). The disease has a world-wide distribution but most outbreaks occur in warm, wet areas where the blood-sucking vectors are abundant.
- *Ehrlichia equi* is a rickettsial organism believed to be transmitted by ticks.
- *Babesia caballi* and *B. equi* are protozoal parasites transmitted by ticks.

Leptospirosis

Leptospirosis is known to be associated with a variety of overt clinical signs in horses including uveitus, intermittent pyrexia and abortion. Since some leptospira produce potent haemolysins that may be implicated in haemolysis. Serological evidence indicates that leptospiral infection is relatively common in the horse, but clinical signs of infection are often inapparent. Moreover, the horse does not seem to harbour a specific serotype, but rather reflects those of the wildlife in its environment. Consequently, the association of infection with a specific disease process is often uncertain.

Diagnosis

- Culture of leptospires is difficult, costly and rarely attempted. The organisms can be demonstrated directly by dark-field microscopy of urine or aqueous humour, but serology is the most useful technique.
- In the UK, serum antibodies to mixed leptospiral antigens are assayed by the Central Veterinary Laboratory at Weybridge. Titres greater than 1:100 are regarded as suspicious.

Comment

- Because of the high prevalence of leptospiral titres in healthy horses, confirmation of active disease depends upon the demonstration of rising titres during the acute phase.

Equine infectious anaemia (EIA)

Equine infectious anaemia is a notifiable disease in many countries, including the UK and others in the EU, Canada, Sweden and some Australian states. Although it is not endemic to these countries it is liable to importation and the clinician should be aware of its diagnosis. It is caused by a virus which is transmitted by biting flies.

Diagnosis

- In the acute form there is depression, fever and petechiation of the mucous membranes. At a later stage this is followed by jaundice, anaemia and oedema of the lower abdomen and legs. Any horse showing these clinical signs should be viewed with suspicion and tested for EIA, especially if there is a history of importation from an infected area or contact with imported horses.

- Infection is confirmed by an agar-gel immunodiffusion test (the Coggins' test) which identifies EIA virus neutralizing antibodies in a serum sample. In the UK this diagnostic test is undertaken by the Central Veterinary Laboratory at Weybridge.

- Other clinical pathology is non-specific. Haematology will show anaemia with possible neutropenia and lymphocytosis. Serum biochemistry will show hyperbilirubinaemia.

Comment

- The petechiation and oedema associated with EIA are thought to be the result of a hypersensitivity vasculitis. The anaemia is the result of immune-mediated haemolysis associated with the attachment of viral particles to erythrocytes. In terms of petechiation and oedema the clinical expression may be similar to ehrlichiosis, purpura haemorrhagica and equine viral arteritis (see later). In terms of haemolytic anaemia, the clinical signs may be similar to ehrlichiosis and immune-mediated haemolytic anaemia (see below). The importance of excluding EIA from these differential diagnoses is self-evident.

Equine ehrlichiosis

Ehrlichiosis is caused by a rickettsial organism, *Ehrlichia equi,* which parasitizes the white cells of the blood and is believed to be transmitted by ticks. Isolated cases of *E. equi* have been reported in the UK but it is believed to be rare.

Diagnosis

- The clinical signs are of pyrexia, depression, jaundice (mild haemolytic anaemia), mucosal petechiation and oedema of the extremities. NB The resemblance in clinical presentation to EIA.

- Definitive diagnosis is based on demonstrating *E. equi* morulae in the cytoplasm of neutrophils and eosinophils in a peripheral blood smear. In the laboratory, routine staining with Giemsa or Wright's stains reveals blue-grey inclusions which have a 'mulberry-like' appearance.

- Other clinical pathology is non-specific. Haematology may reveal a transient, mild to moderate anaemia as a result of haemolysis. Leucopenia, including thrombocytopenia, is seen during the period of pyrexia. Serological confirmation is possible using an indirect fluorescent antibody test, but this is not available commercially.

Babesiosis

Babesiosis is an intraerythrocytic parasitic disease of horses which is widely distributed the Americas and parts of eastern and southern Europe. The distribution probably reflects the suitability of habitat for the tick vector. Despite the occurrence of ticks in the UK, it is not thought to be a problem in the indigenous horse population.

Diagnosis

- The clinical signs are of pyrexia, depression, jaundice and haemoglobinuria. In endemic areas the indigenous horses often carry *Babesia* without showing clinical signs, but newly introduced stock can be expected to succumb.

- Blood samples show evidence of acute haemolysis. Parasitized erythrocytes may be seen in smears during the febrile period, but these are often absent once haemolysis develops. In consequence, diagnosis may have to be confirmed serologically by complement fixation or indirect fluorescent antibody tests.

Immune-mediated haemolytic anaemia (IMHA)

Immune-mediated haemolytic anaemia is not common in horses, but it remains the commonest cause of equine haemolytic anaemia in the UK.

IMHA is usually secondary to some event which alters the surface of erythrocytes, making them susceptible to immune recognition. The subsequent attachment of antibodies or complement components results in haemolysis. The effect is either lysis within the circulation by activation of the complement cascade ('intravascular haemolysis'), or removal from the circulation and gradual destruction by the mononuclear phagocytic system (MPS) of the spleen ('extravascular haemolysis'). Both forms of haemolysis can occur concurrently.

An immune-mediated haemolytic anaemia occurs in neonatal foals and is termed 'isoimmune haemolytic anaemia'. During pregnancy the dam becomes inadvertently sensitized to 'foreign' paternal antigens on the foal's erythrocytes and antibodies are produced. Because there is no transplacental antibody exchange during gestation, the foal is healthy at birth but suffers haemolysis following the passive transfer of colostral antibodies. The diagnosis of neonatal disease is outside the scope of this book and the reader should consult appropriate texts.

The clinical history in cases of IMHA may be diagnostically useful since the condition is usually secondary to an earlier disease or treatment regime, or alternatively, to some chronic intercurrent disease. Predisposing causes of immune-mediated haemolysis in adult horses are thought to include the following mechanisms:

- Antigenic components of bacteria, viruses, parasites and tumours coat red cells and provoke an immune response which results in erythrocyte destruction.
- The erythrocyte surface may be altered by drug components acting as haptens. This provokes an antibody response to the 'foreign' component with the same results as above.

- Several weeks after an acute infection, circulating immune complexes may be formed from the antigenic remnants of the infectious agent, coupled to the antibodies they generated. On rare occasions these immune complexes may bind non-specifically to erythrocyte surfaces and activate the complement cascade, thereby lysing the cells as 'innocent bystanders'.
- In some cases of lymphosarcoma, a clone of lymphocytes is activated which produces an immunoglobulin with a non-specific binding capacity for red cells, i.e. it acts as a weakly bound 'antibody'.

On occasion, 'idiopathic' forms of IMHA occur in the absence of any apparent causation and are thereby regarded as a true autoimmunity. However, this diagnosis is somewhat arbitrary since some form of predisposition is difficult to disprove.

In horses, antibodies of the IgG class are most often involved and these are usually associated with extravascular destruction of red cells by the mononuclear phagocytic system. In this case the cells are sequestered and destroyed in the spleen. Less frequently, antibodies of the IgM class are involved. These readily fix complement and activate the cascade, resulting in rapid intravascular haemolysis.

Diagnosis of intravascular haemolysis

- This is the most aggressive form of the disease in which there is an acute haemolytic crisis. The clinical signs of acute haemolysis may be accompanied by fever.
- Autoagglutination in anticoagulant (EDTA) is often seen in the blood of IMHA patients shortly after sampling. Resuspension of the sample by gently turning the tube is much more difficult than usual. This can be confused with the normal phenomenon of 'rouleaux' formation in which the red cells stack like a pile of coins. In addition, autoagglutination of red cells can occur non-specifically in any severe inflammatory state. To differentiate, dilution of the sample 1:4 in isotonic saline will disperse rouleaux and

prevent non-specific agglutination, but it will not disrupt immune-mediated haemagglutination. In the latter instance, scanning a diluted smear under low power microscopy will reveal groups of erythrocytes bounded together at their circumference.

- Haematology during the haemolytic crisis reveals a drop in PCV, RBC count and haemoglobin concentration, as well as transient discolouration of the plasma by haemoglobin. Haematology reports may indicate erythrocyte abnormalities such as anisocytosis (abnormal variations of size), and the presence of spherocytes (red cells in the process of lysis: small, globular, hyperchromic cells lacking the usual central pallor).

- A high proportion of the erythrocytes left in the circulation following intravascular haemolysis have an increased fragility, i.e. their cell surface is damaged or compromised and they are prone to haemolysis. This tendency can be measured in the laboratory using the *osmotic fragility test*. Samples of blood are pipetted into a series of tubes containing decreasing concentrations of saline and the sequential haemolysis is measured by spectrophotometer. Compromised cells suffer 100% lysis at significantly higher concentrations of saline than healthy cells. A particularly useful application of the test is monitoring the return of normal fragility values to circulating erythrocytes once treatment is underway. Despite its simplicity, the osmotic fragility test is not available at commercial veterinary laboratories. However, this probably reflects the low incidence of intravascular haemolysis in horses.

- The definitive diagnosis of immune-mediated haemolytic anaemia is detection of erythrocyte-bound immunoglobulin by the *Coombs' antiglobulin test*. Specialist veterinary laboratories will undertake this test on samples submitted in anticoagulant (EDTA). Essentially, the cells are washed in isotonic solution and reacted with an anti-equine immunoglobulin reagent. The reagent binds to erythrocyte-bound immunoglobulin and by cross-linking causes agglutination of the patient's cells (direct Coombs' test). Healthy erythrocytes do not react in this way. By using class-specific antisera the immunoglobulin class can be identified.

Comments

- Because the end point of the Coombs' test is agglutination, the assay is inappropriate if immune autoagglutination has already been demonstrated in the blood sample (see above).

- The Coombs' test may be negative following a severe haemolytic episode in which all the affected RBCs have been destroyed. False negative results are also likely during periods of corticosteroid treatment.

- The reactivity of the erythrocyte-bound immunoglobulins is often temperature sensitive and laboratory tests conducted at inappropriate temperatures can produce false negative results. For this reason and those given immediately above, a negative Coombs' test does not preclude a diagnosis of immune-mediated haemolytic anaemia.

- The acute phase of EIA is also Coombs' positive. *In cases of uncertainty, the clinician must rule out the possibility of EIA by submitting serum for a Coggins' test.*

Diagnosis of extravascular haemolysis

Extravascular haemolysis is the commonest of the two forms of immune-mediated haemolytic anaema in the horse and presents a greater diagnostic challenge. This is because the splenic sequestration of erythrocytes is not associated with a haemolytic crisis; they are instead destroyed gradually by cells of the mononuclear phagocytic system. The clinical consequence is anaemia without a preceding haemoglobinaemia or obvious mucosal jaundice. Rectal examination will reveal a greatly enlarged spleen, but splenic enlargement is not of itself pathognomonic for extravascular haemolytic anaemia. Diagnostic pointers are as follows:

- As in the case of intravascular IMHA, blood samples in anticoagulant may show autoagglutination. Dilution of the sample 1:4 in isotonic saline will indicate whether the agglutination is immune-mediated or not (see above under: 'Diagnosis of intravascular haemolysis').
- Haematology reveals a reduction in PCV, RBC count and haemoglobin concentration. This can often be quite marked and in the absence of clinical signs of hypovolaemia it indicates a gradual rather than a sudden removal of erythrocytes from the circulation. A laboratory report of profound anaemia is not diagnostic of extravascular haemolytic anaemia, but coupled with the finding of a persistently enlarged spleen, it is at least suspicious.
- A blood sample will not reveal haemoglobinaemia, but serum biochemistry may show an increase in total bilirubin concentration as a result of gradual erythrocyte destruction. However, such an increase will not be apparent if the rate of production is matched by the rate of hepatic clearance.
- Definitive proof of extravascular haemolytic anaemia requires the demonstration of erythrocyte-bound immunoglobulin using the Coombs' test. However, in the authors' experience the conventional test often fails to show positive haemagglutination in anaemic patients that subsequently respond to treatment for extravascular IMHA. There are three possible reasons for this:
  (1) the bulk of affected cells are sequestered in the spleen and are unavailable to peripheral blood sampling;
  (2) the test is conducted in the laboratory at a temperature which is inappropriate to the immunoglobulin involved;
  (3) the immunoglobulins are weakly bound to the erythrocytes and are too few in terms of surface concentration to be identified by the conventional Coombs' test.

Comment

- In the absence of a positive Coombs' test, a diagnosis of extravascular haemolytic anaemia is indicated by profound anaemia, hyperbilirubinaemia, persistent splenic enlargement and the elimination of other causes of haemolysis.

NB If an immune-mediated haemolytic anaemia has been diagnosed, but the cause is not apparent, then investigation must turn to identifying an occult infection or neoplasia before the condition can be judged 'idiopathic'. In addition, the possibility of EIA should be ruled out by Coggins' test (see above under 'Equine infectious anaemia').

Microangiopathic haemolytic anaemia

This form of haemolysis is secondary to some other disease process in which erythrocytes are physically damaged during their journey through abnormal vasculature or turbulence of flow. As such, the resultant low grade haemolysis is likely to be masked by the enormity of the primary disease. Examples are disseminated intravascular coagulation, hypersensitivity vasculitis (e.g. purpura haemorrhagica) and arteriovenous shunts (e.g. laminitis).

Diagnosis

- Clinical pathology is non-specific. Haematology may be unremarkable or reveal irregularly shaped red cells (schistocytes), but these can be a feature of any haemolytic condition. Gross anaemia is unlikely. Serum biochemistry may show hyperbilirubinaemia, even in the absence of positive haematological findings, but it is not of itself pathognomonic of haemolysis.

Decreased red cell production

Decreased red cell production or dyserythropoiesis is the most common form of anaemia in equine practice and is usually secondary to some other condition such as:

- Chronic inflammatory disease
- Nutritional or other deficiency
- Neoplasia
- Toxicity

Of these, chronic inflammatory disease is the most usual cause.

The slow onset of anaemia usually allows plenty of time for physiological adaptation by the patient and it may not be clinically apparent until an exercise intolerance develops.

Chronic inflammatory disease

Long standing inflammatory, infectious or malignant diseases depress erythropoiesis. Because of the lengthy life span of the equine erythrocyte (some 140–155 days), there is a prolonged time lapse before clinical anaemia is apparent. In consequence, signs of mild anaemia are frequently seen to follow in the wake of a chronic disease process.

Diagnosis

● The anaemia is generally mild to moderate with a PCV of 20–30% and there is a clear association with a primary disease process.

Comment

● Inflammation associated with tumour necrosis depresses erythropoiesis, but there are other mechanisms by which neoplasia can cause chronic anaemia. These include: blood loss secondary to ulceration of a tumour; immune-mediated haemolytic anaemia (which is sometimes associated with lymphosarcoma); bone marrow neoplasia (see below), and microangiopathic haemolytic anaemia.

Deficiency anaemias

Theoretically, deficiencies of iron, cobalt, copper or folate will cause anaemia, but in reality they are exceedingly rare in horses; particularly if there is access to grazing.

The commonest is probably iron deficiency anaemia secondary to chronic external blood loss. In these cases the serum iron concentration is decreased and the total iron binding capacity (TIBC) may be increased.

Diagnosis

● The clinical signs of iron deficiency anaemia are the same as those of chronic blood loss.

● Blood should be taken into iron-free tubes for estimation of serum iron and TIBC and the serum must be separated before submission to the laboratory. Haemolysed samples are quite unsuitable for analysis. The referral laboratory should be consulted before taking samples for these specialized procedures.

● Bone marrow aspiration/biopsy reveals arrested maturation of erythrocytes and reduced iron stores (see later).

Neoplasia

Primary myeloproliferative diseases and secondary neoplastic invasion of the bone marrow result in proliferation of abnormal cells at the expense of normal cell lines (*myelophthisis*). Because of this anaemia is usually accompanied by leucopenia and thrombocytopenia.

Diagnosis

● Clinical signs may include spontaneous haemorrhages (due to thrombocytopenia) and local or systemic infections (due to leucopenia), as well as lethargy and pallid mucous membranes.

● Haematology indicates *pancytopenia*, with anaemia, leucopenia and thrombocytopenia. Leucopenia and thrombocytopenia precede anaemia because the life span of these cells is shorter than that of red blood cells.

● Bone marrow aspiration/biopsy reveals neoplastic cells and depressed erythropoiesis.

Toxicity

Toxic depression of bone marrow activity may be caused by: the persistent use of drugs at high dosage (e.g. phenylbutazone; potentiated sulphonamides); heavy metals (e.g. chronic lead ingestion), and insecticides. The usual result is depression of erythropoiesis without effect on leucocyte production.

Diagnosis

- Bone marrow aspiration/biopsy reveals depressed erythropoiesis.
- Toxic concentrations of lead may be reflected in a blood assay, but not invariably. Estimations in topsoil from the grazing or, in fatalities, liver and kidney assays, are more indicative.

Comment

- On rare occasions an *aplastic anaemia* is described in which the development of all marrow cell lines is inhibited. This is reflected in the peripheral blood as a pancytopenia. This rare disease may be idiopathic rather than the result of toxic depression. Bone marrow aspiration/biopsy shows generalized hypoplasia and replacement by fatty tissue.

Bone marrow aspiration/biopsy

As indicated at the beginning of this chapter, non-regenerative anaemias are difficult to differentiate from regenerative anaemias in the horse because juvenile red blood cells are confined to the bone marrow and do not usually enter the circulation. In consequence, both types of anaemia usually have a similar appearance in a blood smear and erythropoietic activity is best judged on examination of a bone marrow aspirate/biopsy.

Bone marrow aspirates/biopsies may be obtained from a number of skeletal sites in the horse, but the most accessible are the sternum and the ribs. Aspirates for cytology can be obtained from the sternum or the ribs, whereas core biopsies must be taken from the ribs.

The marrow sample must be correctly processed as soon as it is obtained and accurate histological interpretation requires considerable experience. For these reasons an experienced haematologist is best available at aspiration/biopsy and the technique therefore tends to be confined to specialist centres. However, providing the clinician has experience of preparing good air-dried smears, the technique can be used in the field.

Sternal aspiration of marrow

Technique

- A small area of skin in the ventral midline is clipped at the crossing point of an imaginary line drawn between the two points of the elbow. This is scrubbed with povidone–iodine, rinsed and swabbed with spirit.
- Two to three ml of local anaesthetic are placed subcutaneously at the midline site between the deep pectoral muscles.
- A bone marrow collection needle, or a 3.5 inch x 18G (90 x 1.2 mm) disposable spinal needle with stylet, is inserted through a small stab incision in the skin and advanced until its tip reaches the bone. The tip is then rotated using firm upward pressure against the hub while the body of the needle is steadied with the fingers of the other hand (Fig. 8.1). The sternal cortex is very thin and there is no obvious loss of resistance as the medullary cavity is entered.
- Once the needle is self-retaining within the sternum, the stylet is removed and a 20 ml syringe is attached. Clotting of the sample may be prevented by including a few drops of 15% tripotassium EDTA in the syringe. While the needle is steadied with one hand, the other rapidly pulls the plunger down to the 10 ml mark and releases it (Fig. 8.2).

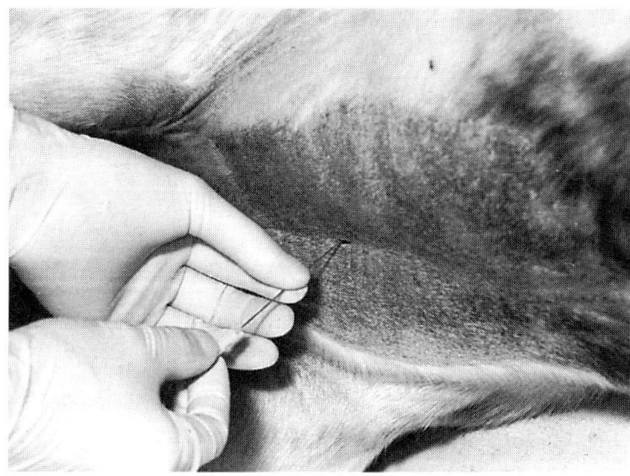

Figure 8.1   Placement of needle at the sternum for bone marrow aspiration.

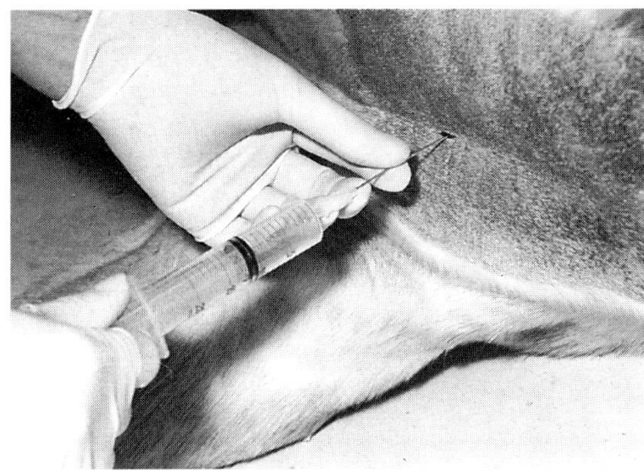

Figure 8.2   Suction applied to aspirate bone marrow at the sternum.

This is repeated 2–3 times until blood is seen at the hub of the syringe. The purpose of this activity is to break apart marrow stroma without allowing free blood to enter the site. As soon as blood is seen at the hub, suction must be released immediately.

- The needle and syringe are removed together and the sample is transferred through the syringe hub to a glass slide. Marrow has a granular, fatty appearance and does not flow in the manner of peripheral blood. If marrow is not obtained, the sampling process may be repeated at a slightly removed site.
- Thin smears must be prepared immediately to preserve cellular morphology. A drop of marrow is placed at the end of a clean glass slide and overlaid with another, causing the material to spread in a thin layer between them. The slides are then pulled apart to create a thin smear on each (Fig. 8.3). Suitable samples have a gritty feel on smearing owing to the presence of marrow spicules. Several smears may be produced from one sample to increase the chances of one good specimen.
- The specimens are promptly air dried and should be fixed in methanol for 20 minutes. Fixing should be undertaken within 12 hours of preparation, in order to preserve cell morphology. The slides can then be stained after arrival at the laboratory (Wright's stain for cell morphology; methylene blue for identifying reticulocytes,

and Prussian blue for semiquantitation of iron storage).

Rib aspiration/biopsy

Rib aspiration or biopsy requires the use of a larger bone marrow collection needle. A 2 inch x 13G (50 x 2.2 mm) bone marrow needle is suitable. In general, core biopsies allow a more complete histopathological assessment of bone marrow activity. Specially machined needles are available for this purpose.

Technique

- The hair over the upper third of a rib, between numbers 9–15, is clipped and the skin is scrubbed with povidone–iodine, rinsed and swabbed with spirit.
- Two to three ml of local anaesthetic are placed subcutaneously over the middle of the rib width.
- The biopsy needle is introduced at right angles to the rib through a small skin

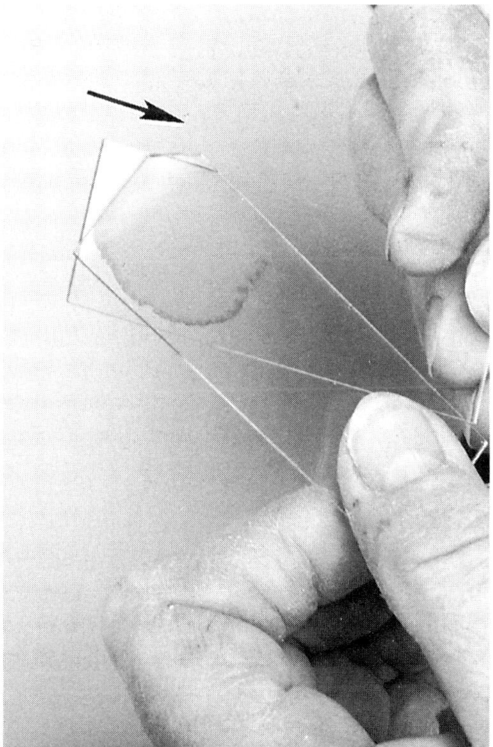

Figure 8.3   Creating a bone marrow smear.

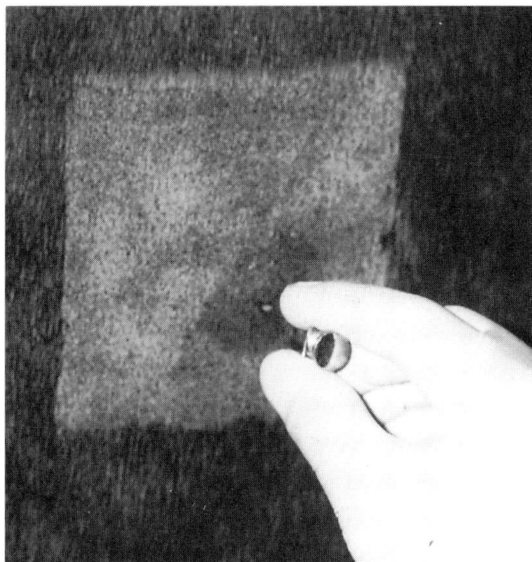

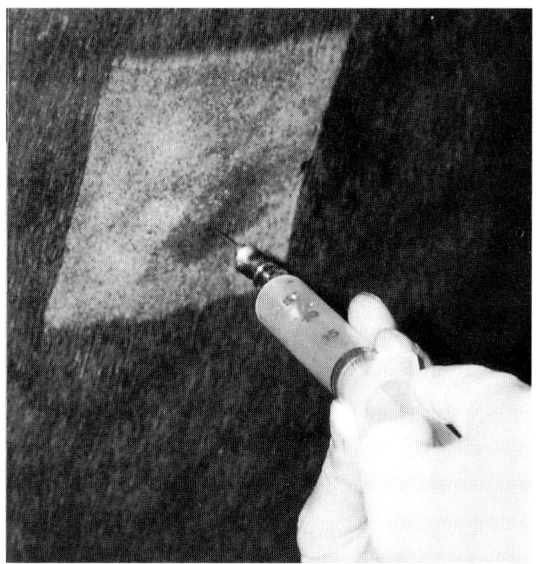

Figure 8.4 Placement of bone marrow aspiration/core biopsy needle at the rib.

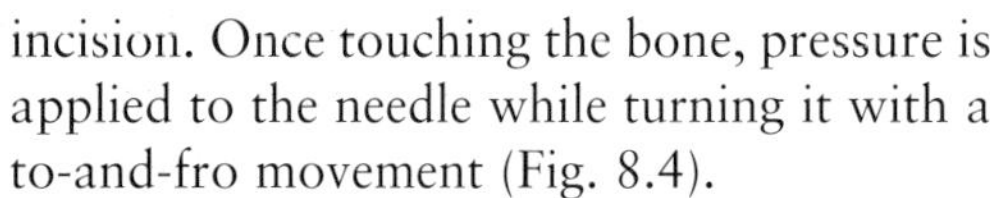

Figure 8.5 Suction applied to aspirate bone marrow at the rib.

incision. Once touching the bone, pressure is applied to the needle while turning it with a to-and-fro movement (Fig. 8.4).

- There is a slight release of resistance as the marrow cavity is entered. At this point either a biopsy or an aspirate may be obtained.
- *For biopsy:* the stylet is removed and the needle is advanced further into the bone. Once a core of tissue has been cut, the needle is rocked to break the core attachment and is then removed. Some designs of needle have particular requirements for manipulation of the core and the manufacturer's instructions should be followed closely. The core is pushed out with a probe and can be rolled on a microscope slide to produce an impression smear. The remainder is placed in 10% buffered formalin for histopathology.
- *For aspiration:* the stylet is withdrawn, and a 20 ml syringe attached. As with sternal aspirates, clotting of the sample is prevented by including a few drops of EDTA in the syringe. The plunger is rapidly pulled down to the 10 ml mark and released (Fig. 8.5). If no marrow appears in the syringe after 2–3 attempts at suction, the needle should be withdrawn slowly to check that it has not

re-entered bone after passing through the marrow cavity. If this manoeuvre fails and a decision is taken to advance the needle again, the stylet must be replaced to prevent the needle blocking with bone. If necessary, a further attempt to obtain a sample may be made at an adjacent rib, repeating all the sterile precautions. An air-dried smear is prepared immediately as described above under 'Sternal aspiration of marrow'.

Comment

- Contamination of core samples with free blood is difficult to avoid, but the marrow portion can still be useful for interpretation providing it is not excessively diluted.
- Pleural puncture is a potential hazard of rib aspiration/biopsy, but it is unlikely to cause complications.

Interpretation of sample analysis

Normal erythropoiesis is indicated by a myeloid to erythroid cell ratio of less than 1.5 and a regenerative response often produces a ratio less than 0.5. The haematologist will also report on cell morphology and reticulocyte counts within the marrow. Reticulocyte counts greater than 2% are indicative of erythroid regeneration.

A report of megakaryocytes in marrow is indicative that platelets are being adequately produced by the bone marrow, despite any peripheral evidence of thrombocytopenia.

II. Diagnosis of coagulopathies

Coagulopathy may be associated with either obvious or occult bleeding and often results in petechial or ecchymotic haemorrhages, or both.

In the healthy horse, haemorrhage is controlled at three fronts:

(1) the reaction of a blood vessel to limit injury;,
(2) the formation of a platelet plug at the site of injury, and
(3) coagulation of the blood.

Accordingly, an investigation of coagulopathy must consider:

- Vascular disorders
- Thrombocytopenia or platelet function defects
- Coagulation disorders

Vascular disorders

Coagulopathies resulting from vascular disorders are characterized by petechiation of the mucous membranes, dependent oedema, lethargy and occasionally fever. The usual causes are infectious agents and the vascular inflammatory response (vasculitis) may be immune-mediated. Potential causes are as follows:

- Purpura haemorrhagica
- Equine viral arteritis
- Equine infectious anaemia

Purpura haemorrhagica

This is probably the most commonly recognized vasculitis of horses and is believed to be a hypersensitivity reaction within blood capillaries to antigenic remnants from a previous bacterial or viral infection. Where implicated, *Streptococcus equi* infection ('strangles') precedes clinical signs of purpura by 2–3 weeks.

The presentation and severity of clinical signs varies greatly between cases, but consistent features are some form of oedematous swelling with petechiation of the mucous membranes. The oedematous swellings can vary from diffuse urticarial plaques to a marked oedema of each limb which terminates as an abrupt ridge in the upper leg ('bottle neck leg'). In some cases there is oedema of the muzzle and face. There is often, though not invariably, a history of recent infection.

Diagnosis

- Diagnosis is largely based on the clinical signs of oedema with petechiation. If there is no obvious petechiation of the oral mucous membranes, the clinician should carefully check the membranes of the intranasal septum and, in mares, the vulva.

- Haematology is non-specific and usually reveals mild progressive anaemia with neutrophilia and a left shift. NB Thrombocytopenia is not a feature of purpura, but platelet numbers may be reduced as a result of extravasation. The plasma fibrinogen concentration is raised within 48 hours of onset.

- Skin biopsies of oedematous areas reveal vasculitis, but these should not be necessary in the diagnostic work up.

Equine viral arteritis (EVA)

EVA is a highly contagious viral disease, spread by respiratory and venereal routes. The virus replicates in the tunica media of small arteries throughout the body and the resultant vascular damage can lead to lung oedema, pleural effusion, limb swelling, conjunctivitis and placental separation. The result is respiratory disease with widespread tissue inflammation, which causes abortion in mares. The causal virus has a world-wide distribution and entered the UK in 1993.

Clinical diagnosis can be difficult because the presenting signs vary greatly in their severity; infection is more common than clinical disease. As with other viral respiratory infections in horses, infection may be obvious or inapparent.

The arteritis is associated with petechiation of the nasal mucosae and conjunctivae, but as the only clinical sign this could be confused with purpura haemorrhagica (see above). However, most clinical cases of EVA feature a marked keratoconjunctivitis and photophobia, with swelling of the eyelids — this is not usual in purpura.

Diagnosis

- In acute disease, viral isolation is possible from:
    Nasopharyngeal swabs
    Heparinized blood (the virus is isolated from buffy coat cells)
    Urine/semen
    The spleen and lung of an aborted foetus (if possible the entire foetus and membranes should be submitted).
- Viral antibody can be detected in serum, but the EVA vaccination status of a horse must be determined and reported to the laboratory when the sample is submitted. Rising titres within 10–14 days of the onset of illness are diagnostic.

In the UK, laboratory diagnosis is undertaken by the Animal Health Trust in Newmarket. The disease became notifiable in 1995.

Equine infectious anaemia

EIA was considered earlier in this chapter under causes of 'Haemolytic anaemia'. In the chronic, recurring conditon the virus can stimulate a continuous hyperimmunity which may result in hypersensitivity vasculitis as well as recurrent immune-mediated anaemia. In terms of petechiation and oedema, EIA is therefore a differential diagnosis for other causes of vasculitis; in particular, purpura haemorrhagica and EVA. It also has clinical similarities to ehrlichiosis (see under: 'Haemolytic anaemia' above).

Thrombocytopenia

Thrombocytopenia is uncommon in horses and is usually associated with the excessive consumption of platelets by coagulation processes (e.g. disseminated intravascular coagulation). More rarely, neoplastic infiltration of the bone marrow (e.g. lymphosarcoma) may also cause thrombocytopenia. In both cases the clinical presentation reflects the primary disease and thrombocytopenia is often an incidental finding in a sample submitted for haematology.

Another well documented cause is immune-mediated destruction of platelets by the mononuclear phagocytic system, but the exact aetiology is unknown and it is frequently termed 'idiopathic thrombocytopenia'. In this case the affected animal is bright and alert, but shows petechiation of the mucous membranes. If the platelet count is sufficiently low (<20 000/µl), haematomas may be noticed following minor trauma. Spontaneous haemorrhage (e.g. epistaxis) is rare.

Diagnosis

- In all forms of thrombocytopenia, haematology indicates depression of the platelet count (<90 000/µl).

- Clinical signs of petechiation and severe thrombocytopenia in an otherwise healthy horse suggest a tentative diagnosis of idiopathic thrombocytopenia.

- In idiopathic cases the bleeding time is prolonged and clot retraction is abnormal, but the coagulation times and plasma fibrinogen concentrations are normal (see later under: 'Coagulation tests').

- A definitive diagnosis of immune-mediated destruction in idiopathic cases requires the demonstration of immunoglobulin or complement components bound to thrombocytes, and/or the presence of plasma antiplatelet activity. These tests are not commercially available for horses.

- In cases of bone marrow pathology, aspiration/biopsy will reveal a low megakaryocyte count. However, the megakaryocyte count is normal or increased in idiopathic thrombocytopenia.

Comments

- In summary, the criteria for a diagnosis of immune-mediated (idiopathic) thrombocytopenia are: (1) persistent thrombocytopenia in the presence of a normal (or increased) number of megakaryocytes in bone marrow; and (2) the exclusion of other disorders associated with the consumption of platelets, e.g. disseminated intravascular coagulation. A subsequent response to corticosteroid therapy will also support the diagnosis.

- The discovery of thrombocytopenia in the blood sample of a horse that shows no signs of petechial haemorrhage should be viewed with caution. Spuriously low platelet counts may be associated with poor sampling technique, inadequate anticoagulant in the sample, or the phenomenon of 'platelet clumping'. Platelet clumping is peculiar to EDTA samples and if in doubt, a fresh sample should be submitted in sodium citrate.

Coagulation disorders

Coagulation disorders are uncommon in the horse. The commonest is probably disseminated intravascular coagulation, which can occur secondary to a number of diseases which promote hypercoagulable states. Less common disorders of adults are liver disease and vitamin K deficiency.

Disseminated intravascular coagulation (DIC)

DIC is characterized by widespread deposition of fibrin in the microcirculation, with subsequent ischaemic injury to many body tissues. As a consequence, defensive fibrinolytic mechanisms are triggered to restore vascular patency and *fibrin degradation products* (FDPs) are released into the circulation to act as potent anticoagulants, preventing further fibrin formation. This fibrinolytic effect, together with the excessive consumption of platelets and clotting factors, results in widespread haemorrhages. Fibrinolysis is thus activated concurrently with coagulation and the patient may present clinical signs within a spectrum of two extremes: a thrombotic crisis and/or a haemorrhagic disease.

DIC is always secondary to any severe systemic disease in which a hypercoagulable state has been reached. *It is associated most frequently with diseases causing endotoxaemia, such as septic processes and, in particular, acute gastrointestinal disorders.* These diseases promote DIC by generating excessive procoagulant activity within the blood and by endotoxic injury to vascular endothelium.

DIC is a state of affairs that tends to be inferred on the basis of the clinical circumstances, i.e. the patient is seen as being 'at risk' of DIC. Unfortunately, the early signs of microvascular thrombosis are not sufficiently specific for diagnosis, and are more difficult to recognize than the later development of haemorrhage. In consequence, DIC is not usually diagnosed until late in its course.

Diagnosis

There is no definitive test for antemortem diagnosis of a state of DIC. Only post-mortem examination with histopathology can define disseminated fibrin thrombi in the microcirculation of organs. However, the cumulative evidence indicated below can suggest that a state of DIC may be developing:

- Any clinical condition where endotoxaemia is suspected and there is a tendency to thrombosis following intravenous treatments (usually at the jugular veins), is highly suspicious. As the syndrome develops, there is a tendency for haemorrhage, characterized by petechial or ecchymotic haemorrhages in the mucosae and sclerae, and a tendency to bleed after venepuncture or minor trauma. At this stage the prognosis is poor.
- Platelet counts are usually lowered in acute DIC due to excessive consumption. Serial analysis will reveal decreasing numbers during the course of the disease.
- Coagulation tests (prothrombin time and/or partial thromboplastin time) tend to be extended (see later).
- The concentration of fibrin degradation products increases in the circulation once DIC is established and fibrinolysis has commenced. FDP detection is a service offered by a limited number of veterinary laboratories. Special blood collection tubes are available from referral laboratories who should be consulted before samples are taken.

Comment
- Most coagulation tests are likely to be abnormal during DIC, but no single test can specifically provide a definitive diagnosis. *A careful clinical appraisal to identify the hypercoagulable patient that is at risk is often more helpful than any laboratory data.*

Liver disease

All coagulation factors except III, IV and VIII are produced by the liver. In conditions of terminal liver failure a coagulopathy develops.

Diagnosis
- The clinical observation is usually haematoma formation following venepuncture. Coagulation tests (see later) will demon-

strate coagulopathy, but the clinical and clinicopathological evidence of liver failure will be obvious by the time this stage is reached (see Chapter 4: 'Liver diseases').

Vitamin K deficiency

Vitamin K is essential to the production of coagulation factors II, VII, IX and X. In horses, deficiency is usually associated with the therapeutic use of warfarin as an anti-thrombotic in navicular disease. Warfarin inhibits the synthesis of these vitamin K-dependent factors.

Clinical signs are of spontaneous haemorrhage during therapy: epistaxis; haematoma formation following minor trauma; ecchymoses in mucous membranes; haematuria; gastrointestinal bleeding; anaemia.

Diagnosis
- Clinical signs in association with warfarin therapy indicate the diagnosis, irrespective of subsequent laboratory findings.
- Factor VII has the shortest half-life of all vitamin K-dependent clotting factors and its deficiency leads to an abnormality in the extrinsic clotting pathway. The prothrombin time (PT) is a measure of extrinsic pathway integrity and provides the earliest indication of warfarin toxicosis.

Comments
- PT should be monitored routinely during warfarin therapy in order to prevent toxicity.
- Toxicity is potentiated in conditions of reduced vitamin K intake, hypoalbuminaemia, or concurrent use of other protein-bound drugs such as phenylbutazone.

Coagulation tests

Blood coagulation is generated by an enzymic cascade of reaction steps which culminate in fibrin formation. The reaction pathways can follow alternate routes depending upon the initiating factor.

The *extrinsic pathway* of coagulation is initiated by tissue thromboplastin (factor III), which is released from damaged tissues. The coagulation test used to evaluate this pathway is the prothrombin time (PT), also known as the one-stage prothrombin time (OSPT).

The *intrinsic pathway* is initiated by contact of blood with subendothelial collagen. The coagulation test used to monitor this pathway is the partial thromboplastin time (PTT), also known as the activated partial thromboplastin time (APTT).

Both pathways lead to the activation of factor X and proceed along the *common pathway* to the formation of a fibrin clot.

Prothrombin time (PT) or one-stage prothrombin time (OSPT)

Prothrombin time assesses the integrity of the extrinsic pathway and detects a deficiency of one or more of the specific coagulation factors II (prothrombin), V, VII, X and fibrinogen.

A blood sample must be taken in the correct proportion of sodium citrate (9:1) for submission to the laboratory. Citrated 'Vacutainers' (Becton Dickinson) are available; alternatively, the referral laboratory should be able to supply suitable sampling tubes. Ideally, the sample should be delivered to the laboratory within four hours, but postal samples should be satisfactory providing the delay does not exceed three days. As a laboratory control, it is advisable to send a sample from a clinically normal horse, together with the patient's sample, in order to assess any artefacts induced by transit delay.

In the laboratory, tissue thromboplastin is added to plasma and the mixture is recalcified to assess clotting time. The laboratory procedure and the reagents used will have a marked bearing upon the clotting time. The result must therefore be judged against the laboratory's 'normal range', which should be reported with an in-test control for 'normal prothrombin time'.

Prothrombin time will be extended in:

- Vitamin K deficiency

- Advanced liver failure
- Reduced fibrinogen concentrations (e.g. late DIC)

Partial thromboplastin time (PTT) or activated partial thromboplastin time (APTT)

Partial thromboplastin time assesses the intrinsic clotting activity of whole blood and detects deficiencies of the specific coagulation factors II, VIII, IX, X, XI, XII and fibrinogen.

As with PT, a sample in sodium citrate is submitted to the laboratory, together with a healthy control sample, as rapidly as possible. In the laboratory, a source of partial thromboplastin is mixed with the plasma and the time to clotting after the addition of calcium is recorded. Once again, the laboratory's 'normal range' and a suitable in-test control should be reported.

An extended PTT indicates a coagulation defect of whole blood, such as DIC. In particular, it indicates a deficiency of one of the thromboplastic factors listed above and modifications of this test may be used to identify a specific factor deficiency, e.g. factor VIII deficiency in foals (Haemophilia A).

Bleeding time

This simple though imprecise test can be used to evaluate the capillary–platelet aspect of haemostasis. A relatively hairless area is chosen and a small, deep skin puncture is made with a medical lancet. A stopwatch is then started as the first drop of blood appears. As drops accumulate, they are removed every 30 seconds with a filter paper which should not touch the skin. When blood no longer appears, the endpoint is reached. The normal bleeding time in horses is 2–5 minutes.

Bleeding time will be prolonged in:

- Vascular disorders
- Thrombocytopenia or platelet function defects
- Advanced liver failure
- Vitamin K deficiency

Clot retraction time

Clot retraction time can be used as a crude indication of thrombocytopenia or a platelet defect. Normal blood drawn into a plain glass tube will form a clot which draws away from the vessel wall in 1–2 hours at room temperature. This retraction is a function of *thrombosthenin*, a protein released by platelets.

Extended retraction time (or poor retraction) suggests thrombocytopenia or a platelet defect.

III. Blood tumours

Tumours of the haematopoietic system are rare in horses. The commonest is lymphosarcoma, but this rarely takes a leukaemic form. Much rarer conditions include: erythrocytosis; myelogenous leukaemia and plasma cell myeloma.

Lymphosarcoma

Lymphosarcoma is the commonest haematopoietic tumour in the horse and is probably the commonest internal tumour. The clinical presentation depends upon the organs affected and techniques for its diagnosis are considered in detail under 'Investigating specific diseases' in Chapter 10: 'Lymphatic diseases'.

A definitive antemortem diagnosis of lymphosarcoma requires identification of neoplastic lymphocytes in the peripheral blood, bone marrow, pleural or peritoneal fluids, or in the biopsy sample of a tumour mass. However, neoplastic cells are rarely found in the peripheral blood of horses with lymphosarcoma and although the total lymphocyte count can be variable, it is often normal.

Erythrocytosis (polycythaemia)

On occasion, haematology may show an increase above the expected values for PCV, RBC count and haemoglobin concentration. Most usually this is the result of a 'relative erythrocytosis' associated with dehydration, endotoxaemia or splenic contraction. Much more rarely it indicates 'absolute erythrocytosis' in which there is persistent elevation of red cell parameters.

Primary absolute erythrocytosis

Primary absolute erythrocytosis, or *polycythaemia vera*, is a myeloproliferative disease of red cell precursors in bone marrow.

Secondary absolute erythrocytosis

Secondary absolute erythrocytosis is a non-myeloproliferative disease resulting from an increase in erythropoietin production. This can be a normal response to chronically decreased arterial oxygen tension, or an inability to deliver oxygen normally to tissues. Non-physiological increases in erythropoietin production may be associated with neoplasia or some forms of chronic renal disease.

Diagnosis

- Clinical signs of erythrocytosis are non-specific, but include erythema of the mucous membranes. Relative erythrocytosis is usually associated with clinical conditions causing dehydration and/or endotoxaemia.

- Absolute erythrocytosis is indicated by a persistent elevation of PCV, RBC count and haemoglobin concentration, which is unresponsive to treatments for dehydration or endotoxaemia. If necessary, a suspicion of relative erythrocytosis caused by splenic contraction at sampling can be investigated by resampling after sedation with xylazine.

- A diagnosis of primary absolute erythrocytosis is finally derived by eliminating the causes of secondary absolute erythrocytosis, i.e. by careful evaluation of cardiopulmonary and renal systems.

Comment

- Bone marrow biopsy is unlikely to be abnormal in cases of erythrocytosis.

Myelogenous leukaemias

Myelogenous leukaemias are extremely rare in horses and are classified on the basis of the predominant neoplastic cell type which is present in the bone marrow.

Clinical signs are non-specific and include depression, weight loss, mucosal petechiation, hindlimb oedema and pyrexia. Anaemia and thrombocytopenia may accompany this marrow neoplasia.

Diagnosis

- Haematology may reveal pleomorphic, poorly differentiated leucocytes in a peripheral blood smear. Anaemia and thrombocytopenia may also be noted.

- Definitive diagnosis requires critical examination of bone marrow cytology.

Plasma cell myeloma

Plasma cell myelomas are primary diseases of the marrow and are extremely rare in horses. Those recorded are usually *multiple myelomas* in which the myeloma cells invade bone and other organs such as liver, spleen and lymph nodes.

The uncontrolled proliferation of a clone of plasma cells characteristically produces a plasma protein (often termed a 'paraprotein') in excessive amounts. On analysis the protein is found to consist of a whole immunoglobulin molecule or its constituent fragments.

Clinical signs are variable and bizarre, reflecting tissue infiltration by neoplastic cells, or the systemic effects of the immunoglobulin produced. For example, weight loss and anorexia are usual, but lameness and neurological deficits are reported secondary to osteolysis caused by an osteoclast-activating factor produced by the myeloma cells. Chronic infections can follow the obliteration of cellular defences by neoplastic cells in the bone marrow. This bone marrow pathology also results in chronic anaemia.

Diagnosis

- Haematology may reflect the bone marrow pathology, e.g. anaemia, a reduced total white cell count and the presence of mature plasma cells.

- Serum protein biochemistry demonstrates an elevated total globulin concentration and serum protein electrophoresis reveals a monoclonal γ-globulin peak that characterizes the myeloma. Most commercial laboratories can demonstrate this peak, but characterization of its protein content requires reagents which are only available in specialized laboratories.

- Bone marrow aspirates reveal an abnormal increase in plasma cells.

- In patients displaying lameness, radiography of long bones may reveal 'punched-out' areas of radiolucency.

IV. **Blood culture**

Blood culture is a useful diagnostic test in patients with suspected bacteraemia, although it is rarely indicated in adult horses. The technique offers identification of the organism and production of a sensitivity profile. However, in most cases the number of organisms within the circulation is likely to be transient and of a low order. Consequently, a relatively large volume of blood is required for the inoculum (e.g. 10 ml) and samples should be taken on at least three occasions to increase the chances of isolation. *Strict aseptic precautions must be used to avoid contaminating the sample.*

Technique

- A site over the jugular vein is clipped, cleansed with povidone–iodine, rinsed and swabbed with spirit. The skin should be allowed to dry before taking blood.
- A sterile syringe and needle are used to withdraw an appropriate volume of blood in an aseptic manner.
- The protective covering is removed from the blood culture bottle and the injection port is swabbed with spirit. If the bottle has been removed recently from cold storage, it should be warmed to ambient temperature before use.
- The sample in the syringe is injected into the medium using a new sterile needle to avoid contamination of the bottle with organisms from the skin. Both aerobic and anaerobic bottles should be inoculated (Fig. 8.6). Some manufacturers produce a single bottle system which is suitable for both aerobe and anaerobe recovery.
- The bottle contents are then gently swirled or inverted several times to mix the blood and medium.

In the laboratory, positive results are usually recognized within 24 hours by turbidity or haemolysis in the medium.

Comments

- A negative culture could be the result of a fluctuating bacteraemia rather than the absence of bacteraemia. If the disease is associated with fluctuating pyrexia, the patient should be resampled as the rectal temperature starts an intermittent rise.
- Repeat cultures should be undertaken if the condition appears refractory to treatment.
- If the patient is on a course of antimicrobial treatment, blood samples for culture should be obtained before a treatment is due.

Chapter appendix

Chapter appendix 8.1 shows a number of clinical situations which suggest an associated blood disorder: anaemia; the presence of petechial or ecchymotic haemorrhages; thrombocytopenia, and jaundice. Further investigations are suggested, details of which are available within the text of this chapter.

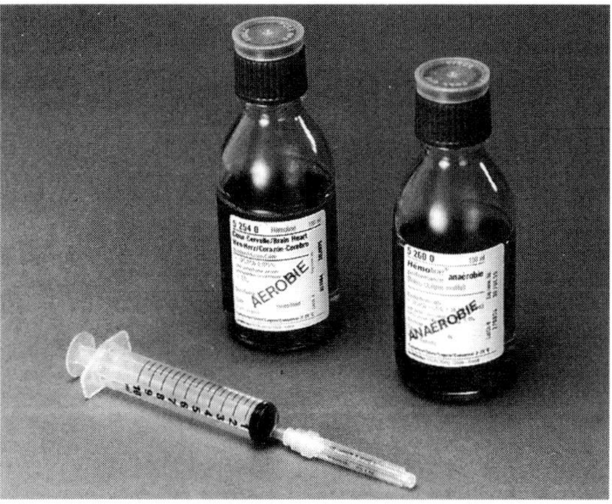

Figure 8.6   Aerobic and anaerobic blood culture bottles suitable for use in horses.

Further reading

Korbutiak E and Schneiders DH (1994) First confirmed case of equine ehrlichiosis in Great Britain. *Equine Veterinary Education* 6: 303–304.

Mair TS, Taylor FGR and Hillyer MH (1990) Autoimmune haemolytic anaemia in eight horses. *Veterinary Record* **126**: 51–53.

Morris DD (1991) Hematopoietic diseases. In: Robinson NE (ed) *Current Therapy in Equine Medicine* 3rd edn, pp. 487–520. Philadelphia: WB Saunders.

Appendix 8.1. Some applications of diagnostic techniques for the investigation of blood disorders.

Possible cause	*Aids to diagnosis*
Anaemia	
Haemorrhage	
Acute external loss	Assess cardiovascular parameters; check haematology 12–24 hours later
Acute internal loss	Assess cardiovascular parameters; abdominocentesis; thoracic auscultation; thoracic radiography
Chronic occult loss	Check urine, faeces and peritoneal fluid for blood; investigate parasitism
Coagulopathy	Check for haematomas and petechial/ecchymotic haemorrhages (see differentials below)
Haemolysis	
Immune-mediated haemolysis	
Intravascular	Assess cardiovascular parameters including jaundice; check blood for autoagglutination and haemoglobinaemia; Coombs' antiglobulin test
Extravascular	Check blood for autoagglutination; Coombs' antiglobulin test; rectal examination (persistent splenic enlargement)
Infection	
EIA	Coggins' test
Leptospirosis	Serum antibody
Ehrlichiosis	Cytoplasmic inclusions in neutrophils and eosinophils
Dyserythropoiesis	
Chronic inflammatory disease	Investigate chronic infection/inflammation/tumour; bone marrow aspirate/biopsy shows dyserythropoiesis
Deficiency disease	Bone marrow aspirate/biopsy shows dyserythropoiesis
Iron deficiency	Check serum iron concentration and total iron binding capacity; iron stores in bone marrow reduced
Bone marrow neoplasia	Check blood for pancytopenia; bone marrow aspirate/biopsy shows infiltration by neoplastic cells (myelophthisis)
Toxicity	Bone marrow aspirate/biopsy shows dyserythropoiesis; check recent drug therapy, lead poisoning, exposure to insecticides

Appendix 8.1. Some applications of diagnostic techniques for the investigation of blood disorders. *continued*

Possible cause	*Aids to diagnosis*
Petechial/ecchymotic haemorrhage	
Purpura haemorrhagica	Check for associated oedema
Equine viral arteritis	Virus isolation (nasopharyngeal swab/buffy coat); serum antibody
Ehrlichiosis	Cytoplasmic inclusions in neutrophils and eosinophils
Equine infectious anaemia	Coggins' test
Thrombocytopenia	Check platelet count; see other investigations below
Disseminated intravascular coagulation	Investigate predisposing disease (endotoxaemia in association with thrombosis)
Terminal liver failure	Check liver enzymes and function test (Chapter 4)
Vitamin K deficiency	Check concurrent warfarin treatment; prothrombin and bleeding times extended
Thrombocytopenia	
Platelet clumping in sample	Resubmit in sodium citrate
Platelet consumption	
DIC	Investigate predisposing disease (endotoxaemia in association with thrombosis)
Loss in haemorrhage	See above under 'Haemorrhage'
Neoplastic infiltration of the bone marrow	Check blood for pancytopenia; bone marrow aspirate/biopsy shows infiltration by neoplastic cells (myelophthisis)
'Idiopathic' thrombocytopenia	Check bleeding time and clot retraction; bone marrow aspirate/ biopsy is normal or shows an *increase* in megakaryocytes
Jaundice	
Haemolysis	See under 'Haemolysis' above
Reduced feed intake	Check food consumption
Liver disease	Check liver enzymes (chapter 4)

9 Cardiovascular diseases

I. Examination techniques

This section describes the techniques that can be used to aid diagnosis and prognosis in horses with suspected cardiovascular disease. It centres on cardiac disease and those techniques which are of most practical value in the field. The principles of each technique, suitable equipment and a guide to its practical use will be described.

Techniques for evaluation of the cardiovascular system include:

- General clinical examination
- Auscultation
- Electrocardiography
- Echocardiography
- Radiography
- Phonocardiography
- Exercise tests

General clinical examination

Irrespective of whether an animal is known to have cardiac disease, a general examination is essential because it provides useful information about cardiovascular function and ensures that no other abnormalities are missed.

Mucous membranes

Examination of the mucous membranes should include an assessment of their colour and the capillary refill time. The oral mucosa is the most easily examined. The mucous membrane colour may be pale (e.g. in animals with anaemia), or injected (dark red) (e.g. in animals with a septicaemia or toxaemia). Cyanosis due to cardiac disease is a rare finding, more often shades of grey or a bluish tinge are found in animals with circulatory collapse owing to endotoxaemia.

The capillary refill time (CRT) can be measured by blanching the mucous membranes with light digital pressure. The refill time is usually around 1.5–2.5 seconds, but this is a somewhat subjective measurement. It is a guide to peripheral perfusion and is dependent on cardiac output and local factors affecting the peripheral distribution of blood.

The most likely findings of significance in horses with cardiac disease are: (1) pale mucous membranes and a slow capillary refill time in patients with congestive heart failure (CHF), and (2) injected mucous membranes in rare patients with endocarditis. However, colour and CRT are crude indicators of cardiac disease.

Arterial pulse

The arterial pulse should be palpated in order to assess its rate, regularity and quality. The facial artery is the most easily assessed. Some experience is required in order to identify abnormal findings from the wide range of normality. Apart from arrhythmias, in which pulse quality is often reduced following a short diastolic interval, severe heart disease is usually present before any changes in pulse quality can be detected. However, a weak pulse may be found in animals with reduced cardiac output such as those with CHF due to mitral regurgitation (left atrioventricular valve regurgitation) or severe myocardial disease. In horses with aortic regurgitation, pulse quality is a very useful guide to severity. If aortic regurgitation is severe, there is a strong initial pulse quality because of a large stroke volume; thereafter the aortic diastolic pressure declines rapidly because of valvular insufficiency and the pulse pressure is not maintained.

It may be helpful to palpate the median artery at the same time as auscultating the heart in order to detect pulse deficits (i.e. contraction of the heart without a palpable pulse). However, pulse quality is difficult to assess from the median artery and the facial artery is preferable. The digital pulse quality should not be used because it is affected by many factors other than cardiac disease.

Jugular distension

Jugular vein distension can be caused by obstruction to flow (e.g. a thoracic mass), raised intrathoracic pressure (e.g. severe pleural effusion), or raised central venous pressure due to CHF. If the horse's head is raised to a normal upright position, the veins should not fill for more than a few inches at the thoracic inlet.

A raised central venous pressure is found in right-sided CHF. However, many horses will be presented with signs of right-sided CHF even when the primary cardiac abnormality is present on the left side of the heart, because pulmonary hypertension is a common sequel to left-sided heart failure. Raised central venous pressure is often associated with dependent oedema formation. Distension of the jugular veins is a useful guide to the presence of significant heart disease: the more marked it is, the higher the central venous pressure and the more severe the CHF. However, many horses have significant heart disease without jugular distension.

Jugular pulse

Changes in central venous pressure during the cardiac cycle result in pressure changes in the jugular vein at the thoracic inlet. The result is an apparent pulsation of the vein; however, some pulsation is normal and should not be termed a 'jugular pulse'. A true jugular pulse results from blood being ejected in a retrograde fashion from the right atrium into the jugular veins. This can be due to severe right atrioventricular (AV) valve insufficiency and also occurs with some uncommon arrhythmias. Most commonly, a jugular pulse is found when severe CHF has resulted in distension of the veins and right AV valve incompetence. A distended vein can also appear to pulsate owing to transmission of impulses from the underlying carotid artery.

Dependent oedema

There are many causes of dependent oedema, including hypoproteinaemia, local obstruction to flow and right-sided CHF (see above). Even if there is evidence of heart disease, it is wise to rule out hypoproteinaemia as a potential cause. Dependent oedema owing to CHF usually extends along the ventral abdomen and includes the penile sheath in males; however, it may be present only at the brisket in mild cases. It may also develop in all four distal limbs.

Respiratory sounds and pattern

The most common presenting sign of both cardiac and pulmonary disease is exercise intolerance. It is therefore very important to examine both systems in detail, even if cardiac disease is known to be present. The entire lung field should be auscultated. A re-breathing bag is essential for full evaluation of lung sounds (see 'Auscultation' in Chapter 12: 'Respiratory diseases'). Coarse crackles may be auscultated in horses with left-sided CHF, and fluid sounds may be heard in those with frank pulmonary oedema. Often, detailed examina-tion of the respiratory tract is justified in these cases (see Chapter 12: 'Respiratory diseases').

Severe left-sided heart disease may result in the formation of pulmonary oedema. This causes tachypnoea, hyperpnoea and dyspnoea. Similar signs may also be seen in horses with primary pulmonary disease. *Dyspnoea following exercise is a common finding in horses with cardiac or pulmonary disease.* However, although coughing is common in horses with marked pulmonary disease, it is uncommon in left-sided heart disease — even in moderate to severe forms.

Palpation of the apex beat

Palpation of the apical impulse (the point at which the left ventricular free-wall is in contact with the chest wall, rather than the true cardiac apex) is helpful because it gives some indication of the force of ventricular contraction, and because it allows identification of the position of the heart in relation to external landmarks. The strength of the impulse is normally greater in fit, thin Thoroughbreds than in horses such as fat cobs, but it can also be weak in horses with myocardial disease or a pericardial effusion. Identification of the position of the apex acts as a reference point for auscultation (see below). It is usually found in the 4th or 5th intercostal space on the left side of the chest, but may be displaced caudally in horses with marked cardiomegaly or intrathoracic masses.

Auscultation

Auscultation is the basis of the diagnosis of cardiac conditions and careful use of the technique is essential before considering further diagnostic aids. There is no substitute for time spent practising this important technique and every effort should be made to auscultate the chest carefully in suitable surroundings and to record the findings accurately.

Auscultation allows the detection of the normal heart sounds that mark the mechanical events in the cardiac cycle, and abnormal sounds, such as murmurs, which result from turbulent blood flow. In addition, identification of the heart sounds allows the clinician to appreciate heart rhythm.

Auscultation should be performed in a quiet environment, preferably indoors to avoid wind noise.

Equipment

A good quality stethoscope is essential for auscultation. There is little point spending a great amount of money on sophisticated ultrasound equipment, but compromising auscultation by the use of a cheap and unsuitable stethoscope.

Both a bell and a diaphragm are essential; the bell for listening to low frequency sounds and the diaphragm for listening to high frequency sounds. A standard diaphragm should always be used since a paediatric size is unsuitable for equine auscultation. A relatively flat bell is helpful because bulky heads are difficult to position sufficiently far forward in the axilla to auscultate over the entire heart area. Sound transmission is compromised once the length of the tubes exceeds 35 cm and extra length is not necessary for examining the horse. Double tubes are somewhat better at transmitting sound but should be fastened together to avoid movement artefact.

Heart sounds

The beginning of systole is marked by the closure of the atrioventricular valves (mitral and tricuspid), and to a lesser extent by the opening of the semi-lunar valves (aortic and pulmonary) which closely follows. The deceleration and acceleration of blood associated with this process results in the generation of a low frequency sound designated S1. Because this sound is principally caused by deceleration of blood as the AV valves close, it is best heard towards the apex beat area of the heart.

The second heart sound (S2) marks the end of systole and is more high pitched in nature. Because it results from the deceleration of blood in the aorta and pulmonary artery, S2 is best heard over the semi-lunar valves at the heart base.

The third heart sound (S3) is a low frequency sound associated with the deceleration of blood in the ventricles at the end of early diastolic filling. It is best heard over the apex on the left side and is often more noticeable in fit, athletic horses or in animals with volume overload.

The fourth heart sound (S4) is heard towards the end of diastole and marks atrial contraction. It is sometimes difficult to distinguish it from S1 if the P–R interval is short (i.e. the conduction period from the beginning of the P wave to the beginning of the QRS complex). Because it is perceived as being the first of the sounds on auscultation, the term S4 is sometimes confusing and the term atrial contraction (A) sound is often used.

Heart rate

Heart rate is one of the primary factors governing cardiac output. When demands for increased output are present, the heart rate will rise above the normal range of 24–40 beats per minute (bpm). If cardiac disease is so severe that forward stroke volume is reduced (i.e. the heart is not pumping enough blood per beat), the resting heart rate will be elevated in order to maintain cardiac output. Measurement of heart rate is therefore an important part of examination of the cardiovascular system.

When a raised heart rate is detected, other causes of tachycardia must be discounted before the change is interpreted as resulting from cardiac disease. Pain, fever, toxaemia and anaemia are examples of other potential causes; however, excitement is by far the most common cause. It is therefore very important to allow a horse time to settle and become used to the presence of the examiner before a meaningful measurement of heart rate can be made.

Cardiac rhythm

Assessment of cardiac rhythm is an important part of auscultation which is often overlooked. Some minutes should be devoted to identification of heart sounds with the stethoscope positioned at the left cardiac apex,

in order to establish the cardiac rhythm and identify intermittent arrhythmias. One of the most important findings is identification of S4. This indicates that atrial contraction has occurred and helps to identify the most common arrhythmias. In second degree atrioventricular block (2°AVB), S4 can usually be identified during the long diastolic interval as an isolated 'bu' sound. In atrial fibrillation the absence of coordinated atrial contraction means that S4 is absent. Other identifying features of arrhythmias are discussed later under: 'Murmurs and arrhythmias'.

Cardiac murmurs

Cardiac murmurs are abnormal sounds which are heard during a usually silent period of the cardiac cycle. They are caused by turbulent blood flow and the vibrations that result. *In horses these vibrations are often found in association with normal blood flow.* This is because of the substantial stroke volume associated with the size of the heart and the large great arteries which allow turbulence to occur. It is important that the characteristics of these murmurs are understood so that those associated with pathological change can be identified. To help this process, murmurs are characterized according to a number of different criteria:

- Timing and duration
- Character (change in intensity, pitch, quality)
- Intensity
- Point of maximal intensity and radiation

Timing and duration

Murmurs should be identified as being systolic or diastolic. The duration of the murmur should also be noted. Murmurs may be early systolic, early–mid systolic, late systolic, holosystolic (from the end of S1 to the beginning of S2) or pansystolic (from the beginning of S1 to the end of S2). Diastolic murmurs can be classified as early diastolic (between S2 and S3), presystolic (between S4 and S1) or holodiastolic (between S2 and S1).

Character

The character or quality of a murmur refers to the change in intensity during the murmur, the pitch of the murmur and other descriptive terms such as 'harsh' or 'musical'.

Intensity

The intensity of a murmur is graded on a scale of 1–6. Each grade should be given in relation to the range used (e.g. grade 3/6). The grades are:

> Grade 1: A quiet murmur that can be heard only after careful auscultation over a localized area.
> Grade 2: A quiet murmur that is heard immediately the stethoscope is placed over its localized point of maximum intensity.
> Grade 3: A moderately loud murmur.
> Grade 4: A loud murmur heard over a widespread area, with no palpable thrill.
> Grade 5: A loud murmur with an associated precordial thrill.
> Grade 6: A murmur sufficiently loud that it can be heard with the stethoscope raised just off the chest surface.

Point of maximal intensity and radiation

The point of maximal intensity (PMI) helps to identify the source of a murmur. It must be remembered that vibration from the turbulent source is best transmitted to the body surface by more rigid tissues. Therefore murmurs associated with the AV valves are often transmitted down the ventricular walls and are best heard over the apex beat area where the walls are in closest contact with the body surface. In addition, the murmur may radiate over a localized area or more widely. The areas of auscultation are shown in Fig. 9.1.

The practice of auscultation

A methodical technique is required to avoid missing important findings:

- Place the stethoscope over the apex beat area on the left side. S1 is loudest at this point.

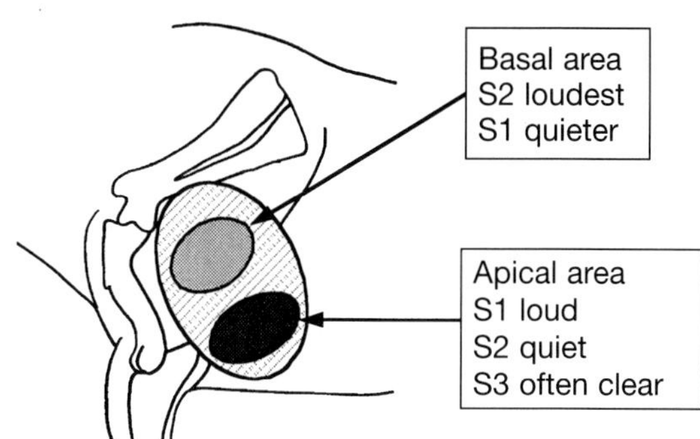

Figure 9.1   The areas of auscultation.

- Measure the heart rate and ensure that it is a true resting rate.
- Evaluate the heart rhythm, it may be helpful to palpate an arterial pulse if an arrhythmia is detected.
- Identify systole and diastole (diastole long and systole short at resting heart rates, identify S1 and S2).
- Identify S3 and S4 (if present).
- Listen for heart murmurs. It may help to concentrate first on systole and then on diastole, and then on sounds of different pitch.
- Gradually move the stethoscope cranially and dorsally, listening to changes in the heart sounds. Identify the PMI and radiation of murmurs.
- Identify the heart base area. In this region S2 will be heard relatively louder than in other areas.
- Repeat the process on the right side.

NB It may help to draw the leg forward so that the stethoscope can be pushed well into the axilla.

Electrocardiography (ECG)

Principles

In man and small animals, the Einthoven limb lead system is widely used to provide useful information about cardiac chamber size and rhythm. In these species the process of depolarization spreads through the myocardium in characteristic wave fronts. The contribution of these wave fronts to the surface ECG depends on the amount of myocardium which is being depolarized. As a consequence, characteristic changes in the size of complexes are seen in the different limb leads when there is enlargement of the cardiac chambers as a result of an increase in muscle mass.

The Einthoven limb lead system is also used for equine ECGs by some clinicians, but is not a valuable technique for detecting chamber enlargement. A number of systems such as vector electrocardiography and heart score were developed to try to derive further information about the size of heart chambers, but they have found little use in general practice. The reason for the lack of correlation between the surface ECG and cardiac enlargement in the horse is the way in which the ventricles are depolarized. In large animals the Purkinje network, which carries electrical impulses to the myocardium, is much more extensive than in man or small animals. The vast majority of the myocardium therefore depolarizes almost simultaneously, no wavefronts are created and the depolarization does not contribute to the surface ECG. The early part of the QRS complex in horses represents the depolarization of the apical region of the septum. The second part of the complex results from the depolarization of the basal region of the heart, so that the complex is likely to show little change if the mass of the ventricles alters. *The principal purpose of electrocardiography in the horse is therefore investigation of cardiac rhythm.*

In order to record the cardiac rhythm all that is required is a clear trace in which the P, QRS and T waves are easily seen (Fig. 9.2). Only one lead is required, with a positive and negative electrode (bipolar lead).

Equipment

Because a bipolar lead is all that is required for equine electrocardiography, a single channel machine is ideal.

Techniques

For a clear bipolar lead trace all that is required is that one lead is placed in front of the heart and the other level with, or behind it. Most single channel machines are labelled for use with the Einthoven lead system and a bipolar lead can be created by using the right arm (RA) and left arm (LA) leads and switching the selector to lead I. The polarity of the leads is unimportant but it is helpful to use a consistent lead system and the following methods are suggested:

- Base–apex lead: For this lead system attach a positive electrode (use the LA lead) over the cardiac apex and a negative electrode (use the RA lead) over a basal position such as the right or left jugular furrow, or just cranial to the right or left scapula. If the RA and LA leads are used, switch to lead I.
- Y lead: This lead is derived from the orthogonal vector system and is also convenient in use. Attach a positive electrode (use the LA lead) over the xiphoid and a negative electrode (use the RA lead) over the most cranial part of the sternum (see Fig. 9.3). Switch to lead I.

The same information that can be derived from these leads can be obtained from limb leads, but the limb leads are more prone to movement artefact and are of no extra benefit.

For mains powered machines, a neutral lead must also be used to earth the machine and can be attached to any convenient point on the animal. The loose skin in front of the scapula is suitable.

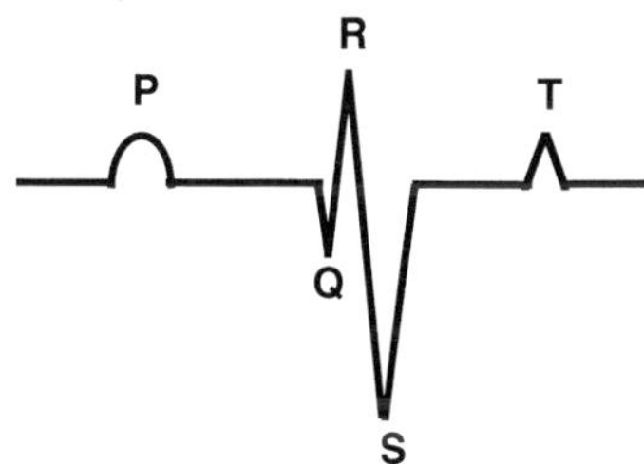

Figure 9.2   Illustration of the typical P wave, QRS complex and T wave in a normal equine ECG (Y lead).

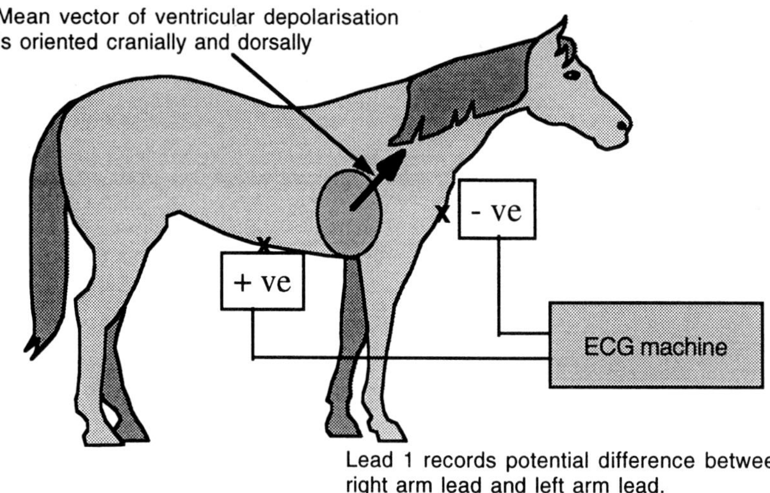

Lead 1 records potential difference between right arm lead and left arm lead. The lead system used above is a Y lead and produces a negative QRS complex

Figure 9.3 Y lead technique: position of electrodes.

Electrical contact between the leads and the skin can be established using surgical spirit or electrode gel. Ideal electrodes are crocodile clips, which should always be kept scrupulously clean to avoid rust and potential artefact. Crocodile clips are not usually supplied with machines and if possible silver/nickel rather than plated clips should be obtained. The teeth can be filed off and/or the clip bent to avoid hurting the animal by excessive pressure.

Always ensure that rechargeable machines are left to charge. Too often the batteries are run down when an ECG is most urgently required.

Interpretation of ECGs

A methodical technique is essential for the accurate interpretation of an ECG. A recording should be made at a paper speed of 25 mm/sec, and also at 50 mm/sec if the heart rate is high or the complexes are of an unusual shape. If intermittent arrhythmias are present, recording for a prolonged period at a slower paper speed is helpful. This also saves paper, but not all machines have this facility. A suitable technique is as follows:

- Assess the quality of the ECG trace. Check the calibration of the amplitude of deflection, the paper speed and whether the AC interference filter was on or off. Look for artefacts.
- Calculate the heart rate. Establish whether it is fast, slow or normal, and whether it is variable.
- Assess the overall rhythm. Establish whether changes in rhythm are intermittent or persistent and whether they are induced or terminated by excitement.
- Assess each wave/complex in turn. Measure the duration and amplitude of the P wave and QRS complex and the duration of the intervals. Establish whether all the complexes are similar or not.
- Examine the relationship between the complexes. Check whether each P wave is followed by a QRS complex, and whether there is a P wave before each QRS complex.
- Define the heart rhythm and plan further diagnostic investigations and treatment if necessary.

Radiotelemetry

The use of radiotelemetry is for the most part confined to specialist centres, but the principles are outlined here.

Arrhythmias that develop during exercise can be an important cause of poor athletic performance and can be difficult to detect and diagnose. Auscultation is possible immediately after exercise when some arrhythmias are most likely to occur, but interpretation of heart sounds can be difficult at elevated and changing heart rates, particularly when S3 and S4 merge to create a 'gallop rhythm'. Vagally mediated physiological arrhythmias, such as sinus arrhythmia and second degree atrioventricular block, may occur during the post-exercise period as the heart rate slows, a situation termed 'autonomic imbalance'. This is particularly common after sub-maximal exercise. These arrhythmias are not associated with any significant problems.

Although portable ECG machines can be used to obtain a recording of the rhythm on these occasions, radiotelemetry is the best method for evaluation of the ECG during and immediately after exercise. It is also useful for the monitoring of critical care patients, e.g. those undergoing treatment of arrhythmias such as atrial fibrillation. Evaluation of ECGs at exercise also requires suitable facilities which will allow maximal exercise. A high-speed treadmill is ideal for these studies.

Outdoors, the range of cheaper radiotelemetry machines is often limited to approximately 50 m, but this may be sufficient under most circumstances. Good electrical contact can be maintained using a surcingle and small pads or sponges soaked in electrode gel, saline or even water. A 'Z lead' system is suitable and consists of one electrode placed over the sternum and one over the withers. Movement artefact is a problem unless the electrodes are well secured. Interference from the electric motors of a high-speed treadmill does not appear to be a problem.

Holter monitoring

Twenty-four hour 'Holter' ECG recordings are useful in selected cases in which arrhythmias are intermittent and may be missed during the relatively brief period over which a standard, resting ECG is recorded. An example is the animal with occasional atrial or ventricular premature beats and clinical signs that are thought to be cardiovascular in origin. Other examples are syncopal episodes or poor athletic performance which are sometimes related to paroxysmal arrhythmias. Such patients should be referred to a specialist centre which has access to suitable facilities. The monitors themselves can be reasonably priced but they must be compatible with the computer used for reading the tape.

Echocardiography

Principles

Echocardiography is now an invaluable part of the evaluation of the horse with suspected heart disease. It is particularly useful for assessing the clinical significance of cardiac murmurs suspected to be related to pathological change. However, its usefulness depends upon the purchase of a suitable ultrasound machine with a low frequency sector scanner and the development of practical skills in the manipulation of the transducer and the interpretation of findings. Meticulous attention to detail is necessary when measurements are made.

The principles of ultrasound are now well established but are largely outside the scope of this book. It is important to appreciate that the best images can be obtained only with appropriate equipment. M-mode and two-dimensional echoes (2DE) are strongest when the beam is perpendicular to the interface between structures of different acoustic impedance, principally between myocardium and blood.

The sternum, ribs and lung prevent transmission of ultrasound and limit positioning of the transducer to a few specific locations from which the beam can be directed through acoustic windows to image the heart. In the horse the apex of the heart sits on the sternum, preventing a true apical image which is obtainable in man and small animals.

A variety of different modalities of ultrasound can be applied, but 2DE and 2DE guided M-mode measurements are the most useful clinically. The following section concentrates on their use.

associated with poor athletic performance. Occasionally arrhythmias usually associated with pathological change, such as ventricular premature beats, are abolished at higher heart rates. While this makes them less likely to be a significant problem, it is important that they are recognized. The abolition of an arrhythmia by an increase in the heart rate is not in itself a diagnosis of a vagally mediated arrhythmia. All arrhythmias should be recognized by their other characteristics and if necessary by electrocardiography. A portable ECG machine can be rushed to the side of the horse immediately that the animal comes to a halt. A base–apex lead is the easiest to use under these circumstances, although the exact positioning of the leads does not matter provided that a clear trace is obtained. Often this is sufficient to confirm the identity of an arrhythmia suspected on auscultation during the post-exercise period. However, for optimal assessment of the significance of an arrhythmia, it is necessary to record an ECG during exercise, for example by radiotelemetry (see above).

Exercise and murmurs

It is a commonly held belief that murmurs which are inapparent after exercise are insignificant. In the author's view this rule of thumb, although not wholly without foundation, is dangerous. Numerous factors may affect the intensity of the murmurs, including stroke volume, blood pressure and blood viscosity. Functional murmurs associated with ejection of blood through the semi-lunar valves are of variable intensity at different heart rates. Sometimes these murmurs are less obvious or absent at higher heart rates. On other occasions they may become apparent in animals during excitement or exercise although they were absent at rest. Quiet holosystolic plateau-type murmurs associated with mitral insufficiency may be more difficult to hear at higher heart rates. While a quiet murmur of this type may not always be significant at the time of examination, it is important that it is detected and not attributed to normal flow.

Unfortunately, auscultation after exercise is often hampered by extraneous noise and respiratory sounds. Under these circumstances it is easy to miss murmurs that may be of significance to the future performance of the horse.

Exercise and heart rate

The speed of recovery of the heart rate of animals with suspected heart disease is helpful in some cases. However, it is very difficult to know the normal rate of recovery, which depends on numerous variables such as the fitness of the horse, the state of the ground and presence of other abnormalities. For example, the heart rate of a lame horse may be higher than that of a sound animal at an equivalent level of exercise. As a rough guide, the heart rate should return to within 10% of the normal level within 15 minutes of the end of moderate exercise, and within 30 minutes of more rigorous exercise.

Standardized exercise tests using a high-speed treadmill

The use of a high-speed treadmill allows graded exercise. Usually the heart rate (and often ECG) is monitored during the exercise so that the speed and incline of the treadmill can be altered depending upon the response of the horse. It is somewhat easier to know what constitutes the expected rate of heart rate slowing under these circumstances. The technique is often used for investigation of poor athletic performance in racehorses where the level of fitness is more predictable and uniform than in pleasure horses.

II. **Murmurs and valvular disease**

Murmurs

The haemodynamics of normal and abnormal blood flow results in recognizable characteristics which are associated with functional or pathological heart murmurs. These can be defined by their timing, duration, intensity, character and point of maximal intensity (see above under: 'Auscultation'). Identification of these characteristics enables the clinician to pinpoint the cause of the murmur, an essential step in assessing its significance.

Alterations in blood flow frequently result from valvular heart disease. Abnormal flow is also found with congenital structural defects. In horses, valvular narrowing of sufficient severity to obstruct the outflow of blood (stenosis) is very uncommon. However, valvular incompetence leading to regurgitation of blood is common.

Systolic murmurs

Functional systolic murmurs

The most common murmur heard in horses (approximately 50% of all horses) is an early–mid systolic ejection-type murmur, usually of grade 1–3/6, with a point of maximal intensity (PMI) over the left and/or occasionally the right heart base. These murmurs are often most striking in foals and in young fit horses, but are a common finding in any breed. They are often variable at different heart rates and may become quieter or more intense after exercise. These murmurs are often called 'flow murmurs' because they are associated with normal blood flow through the semi-lunar valves. They are of no clinical significance, except that they must be distinguished from other systolic murmurs resulting from abnormal blood flow. The most distinctive feature is that they end well before the end of systole and that they have a crescendo–decrescendo or decrescendo character.

Systolic murmurs due to valvular disease

Systolic murmurs of clinical significance most commonly result from valvular regurgitation or congenital heart defects.

The most common congenital defect in horses is a ventricular septal defect (VSD). This usually causes a grade 5–6/6 harsh, pansystolic, plateau-type murmur with a PMI just above the sternum on the right side of the chest (see below under: 'Congenital heart disease in the growing/adult animal').

Regurgitation through the AV valves results in a grade 2–6/6 plateau-type holo- or pansystolic murmur. *Mitral regurgitation* (left AV valve regurgitation) has a PMI over the left apical impulse area, while *tricuspid regurgitation* (right AV valve regurgitation) is best heard on the right side of the chest, often well underneath the triceps muscle. In some instances, the murmurs associated with these conditions are late systolic with a crescendo character. Mitral regurgitation is the most common cause of CHF in the horse, but more commonly results in poor athletic performance. Tricuspid regur-gitation is often an incidental finding, and is particularly common in large fit Thoroughbred racehorses. However, in a few cases, it is associated with poor athletic performance or even CHF. Rupture of the chordae tendineae usually results in a loud harsh murmur with a precordial thrill. The prognosis for horses with mitral regurgitation owing to ruptured chordae tendineae is poor.

Clinical guides to the severity of pathological systolic murmurs are the presence of signs indicating heart failure, including dependent oedema, jugular distension and tachycardia. Most often these signs are not present and judgement of severity is then more difficult. The more widespread and louder the murmur, the more likely it is to be significant. Murmurs due to AV regurgitation which are associated with a thrill are usually sufficiently severe to prevent future athletic use. The presence of abnormal arrhythmias such as atrial premature complexes or atrial fibrillation are also a cause for concern (see below).

Further investigation can also be helpful in assessing the severity of the condition. ECGs are of little value except for identification of arrhyhthmias. By far the most useful technique is echocardiography, which allows an objective assessment of the severity of the disease. Haemodynamically significant regurgitation usually results in volume overload and the extent of volume overload can be estimated from the echocardiogram. In addition, Doppler echocardiography can be used to estimate the size of the regurgitant jet.

Diastolic murmurs

Functional diastolic murmurs

Functional diastolic murmurs are less common than functional systolic murmurs (10–15% of all horses), and are most often detected in young fit horses. However, they can be found in horses of any age.

Early diastolic murmurs occur between S2 and S3, are high pitched and musical in character (sometimes called a 'two-year-old squeak'), and are best heard over or just ventral to the heart base on the left or right side of the chest. Their intensity varies from grade 1–3/6, and can vary at different heart rates, often being greatest at slightly elevated rates of 40–60 bpm. There is no evidence that they are associated with valve pathology.

Diastolic murmurs due to valvular disease

Holodiastolic murmurs are relatively common in older horses and are nearly always associated with *aortic valve regurgitation*. Mild pulmonary regurgitation is fairly common but is usually not audible. These murmurs are decrescendo, often musical, with a variable pitch and a buzzing, cooing or rumbling character. The murmur of aortic regurgitation can be very loud (up to 6/6), even in horses without significant volume overload, and the intensity of the murmur is therefore a poor guide to significance. A useful clinical guide can be the arterial pulse quality, which may become short but strong (water-hammer) in horses with moderate or severe aortic regurgitation. The most objective means of assessment is echocardiography. Most horses with aortic regurgitation are retired from athletic use for reasons other than heart disease, but in some cases poor exercise tolerance or even CHF can develop; particularly if mitral regurgitation is also present.

Presystolic murmurs

Presystolic murmurs (ie. late diastolic) may be difficult to differentiate from S4, are low pitched and rumbling or grating in character. There is no evidence that they are of any clinical significance.

III. Arrhythmias

Supraventricular arrhythmias

Second degree atrioventricular block

Second degree AV block (2°AVB, a 'blocked', 'dropped' or 'missed' beat) is the most common arrhythmia in horses. Around 20% of horses have this arrhythmia at rest, which is caused by high vagal tone. It is usually present at low heart rates and is abolished by increased sympathetic tone and decreased parasympathetic tone (e.g. excitement or exercise). Occasionally, 2°AVB is found during heart rate slowing following exercise. There is no evidence that 2°AVB in resting horses has any pathological effect. It is of no clinical importance unless it is very frequent and persists when there is a demand for increased cardiac output.

Diagnosis

On auscultation the underlying rhythm is regular, but periodic pauses of twice the usual diastolic interval are present resulting in a characteristic arrhythmia. During these long pauses, an atrial contraction sound (S4) is usually heard. Often, the S4–S1 interval gradually increases prior to the blocked beat (Wenckebach phenomenon). The block often comes after every 4th or 5th sinus beat, giving rise to the expression of a 'regularly irregular rhythm'.

ECG shows periodic P waves which are not followed by a QRS complex or T wave (Fig. 9.5). In Mobitz type 1 block (Wenckebach phenomenon) there is a gradual prolongation of the P–R interval before the blocked beat. In Mobitz type 2 block, the P–R interval is constant, but some impulses are not conducted.

Sinus arrhythmia

Sinus arrhythmia is a vagally mediated arrhythmia which may be present at low heart rates, but is most commonly detected after submaximal exercise during heart rate slowing. If detected at rest, it is usually abolished by increased sympathetic tone (e.g. excitement or exercise). After exercise, sinus rhythm usually returns once the heart rate returns to normal. It is regarded as a normal physiological arrhythmia related to high vagal tone; certainly there is no evidence that it is correlated with significant cardiac disease.

Diagnosis

On auscultation the rhythm has phases during which the heart rate increases and slows, which may give the impression of irregularity, but there is usually an underlying cyclical regularity. The phases may be associated with respiration, particularly deep sighs.

ECG shows a phasic variation in the R–R interval. Occasionally 2°AVB is also present.

Sinoatrial block/arrest

Sinoatrial block/arrest (sinus block) is a vagally mediated arrhythmia which is usually abolished by increased sympathetic tone. There is no evidence that it is correlated with significant cardiac disease; however, little information has been thoroughly documented.

Diagnosis

On auscultation there are long diastolic pauses during which the sinus node fails to discharge. Consequently, there is no atrial contraction and these pauses are silent (c.f. 2°AVB: see above). The rhythm may be regular or irregular.

ECG reveals pauses that are double or more

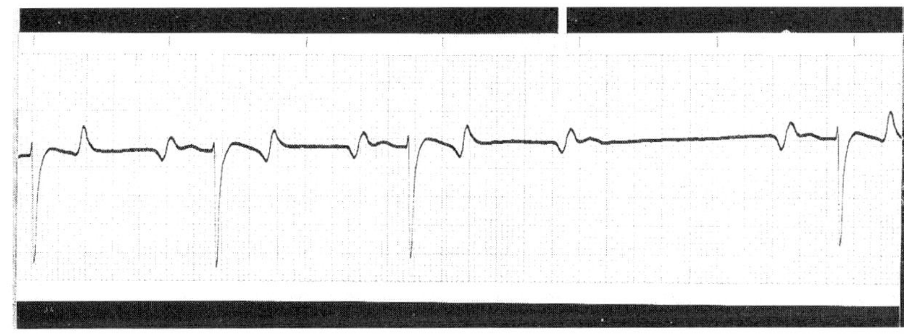

Figure 9.5   Second degree atrioventricular block (2°AVB). An ECG recorded from a 4-year-old Thoroughbred with no clinical signs of heart disease, but a periodically irregular cardiac rhythm. An isolated P wave without subsequent QRS complex is shown by the arrow. On auscultation an isolated S4 (A) heart sound could be heard during the pause between the ventricular contractions.

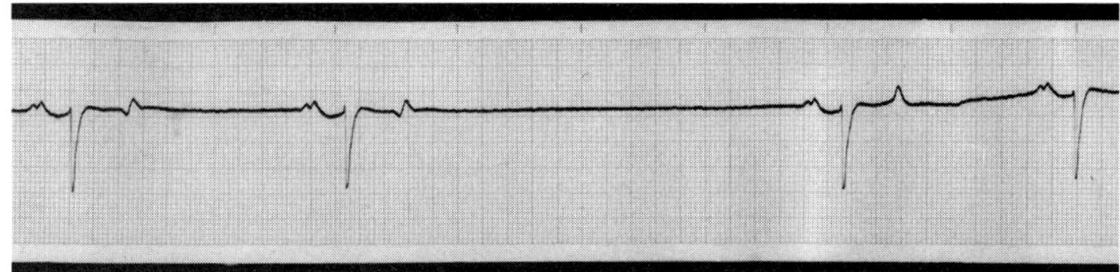

Figure 9.6   Sinoatrial block. An ECG recorded from a 6-year-old Thoroughbred with no clinical signs of heart disease, but a variable cardiac rhythm. The R–R interval between the second and third QRS complexes is approximately twice that of the interval between the first and second and the third and fourth QRS complexes. On auscultation no S4 (A) heart sound could be heard during the pause between the ventricular contractions.

than double the normal R–R interval (Fig. 9.6). The rhythm may be regular or irregular.

Third degree atrioventricular block

Third degree AV block (3°AVB, complete heart block) is present when sinus impulses cannot pass through the AV node, so that tissues distal to this point (junctional or ventricular) have to take up the role of pacemaker. The block is rare and always pathological.

Diagnosis

On auscultation there will be a slow, regular rhythm (a 'junctional' or 'ventricular escape' rhythm). Atrial contraction sounds (S4) may be heard, but these have no fixed relationship to S1 and S2.

The ECG trace will show regular QRS complexes, which may be normal in configuration (junctional or supraventricular) or abnormal (ventricular) in configuration. P waves are also present but have no relationship to the QRS complexes.

Atrial premature complexes (APCs)

APCs result from abnormal impulse formation in the atrial myocardium. Isolated APCs can be an incidental finding. However, frequent APCs can be a sign of myocardial disease, electrolyte imbalance, toxaemia, septicaemia, hypoxia or chronic AV valvular disease. APCs, or the cardiac disease associated with them, may result in poor racing performance. In some instances APCs are thought to be associated with previous episodes of respiratory disease. If APCs are detected, further investigation to establish the underlying cause is indicated.

Diagnosis

On auscultation, APCs can be recognized by the short diastolic interval, usually without a compensatory pause (c.f. ventricular premature complexes). This means that there is an early beat followed by a normal diastolic interval prior to the subsequent S1. Depending on the degree of prematurity, S1 and S2 vary in intensity. Further diagnostic options include exercising ECG (radiotelemetry), 24 hour recordings, echocardiography, haematology, a routine serum biochemistry profile and viral serology.

As the name implies, APCs occur early causing a shortened P–P and R–R interval on ECG. They originate outside the SA node (they are ectopic), and may be of a different configuration from the normal P wave (Fig. 9.7). If APCs are sufficiently early, or at high heart rates, they may be lost in the preceding T wave or QRS complex. They often reset the SA node so that the subsequent P wave follows after a normal P–P interval.

APCs and tachycardia

Atrial tachycardias have a rapid rate and usually a regular rhythm owing to multiple APCs. They may be paroxysmal (short lasting) or sustained. The P waves are often buried in the previous T wave and are difficult to

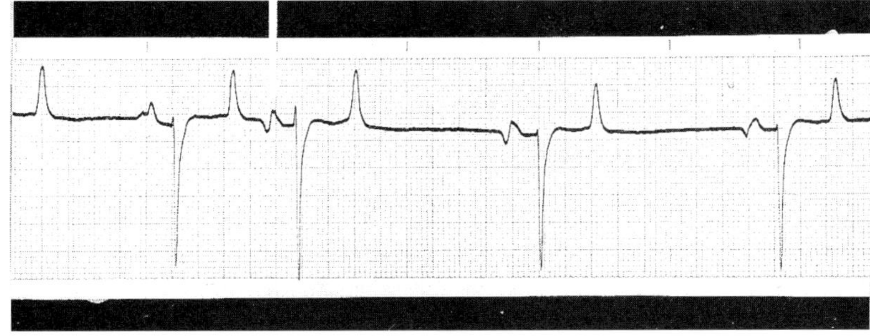

Figure 9.7 An atrial premature complex. The second P wave and QRS complex are much closer to the preceding complex than in subsequent beats. The configuration of the P waves varies. The second P wave (arrow) is an atrial premature complex. On auscultation there was a premature beat followed by a return to the usual S1–S2 interval, without a compensatory pause.

identify. The QRS complexes are normal. If 2°AV block is also present, the rhythm can be fast and irregular.

Atrial fibrillation

Atrial fibrillation (AF) is the most common arrhythmia affecting performance in the horse. It is important for clinicians to recognize AF, in particular to distinguish it from 2°AV block, because long pauses can occur in both arrhythmias. Presenting signs include poor performance, epistaxis, ataxia and tachypnoea. In a significant number of cases, particularly in non-athletic horses, AF is an incidental finding.

AF is commonly found in horses without underlying cardiac disease because the large atria can support the persistence of the arrhythmia once it is set up. AF also occurs in animals with dilation of the atria owing to valvular heart disease (especially mitral regurgitation), and those with frequent APCs. Very seldom is AF found in animals under 15 hands (150 cm) in height.

Those horses without severe underlying heart disease can be successfully converted to sinus rhythm by the oral administration of quinidine sulphate. Once treated, these horses usually return to previous performance levels. However, animals with underlying heart disease are less likely to be successfully treated, and in those horses with an elevated heart rate

(> 60 bpm), or signs of CHF, the drug can be fatal — *treatment with quinidine is contraindicated in these patients.*

Diagnosis

Auscultation reveals an irregular heart rhythm. The heart rate may be normal, slow or elevated (in contrast to the dog where AF is almost always accompanied by a tachycardia). There may be long pauses of up to 8 seconds, sometimes followed by flurries of beats. Sometimes these flurries will come in a cyclical fashion. The S1 and S2 sounds will vary in intensity owing to the variable position of the mitral valve at the beginning of systole. The characteristic finding is the absence of S4. When a long pause is heard, it is important to try to identify S4, because if S4 is present then the cause of the arrhythmia is not AF. In contrast, when 2°AV block is present, S4 is likely to be heard during the pause. In this instance the pauses are usually multiples of the normal R–R interval and the arrhythmia has a regularly irregular predictable nature. It may be helpful to use one's foot as a metronome to get used to the underlying rhythm. *There is no underlying rhythm in AF, the rhythm is irregularly irregular.*

ECG will show that no P waves are present in any lead owing to the absence of any coordinated atrial activity. Fibrillation (f) waves are usually seen in horses, except at high heart rates. The R–R interval is irregular

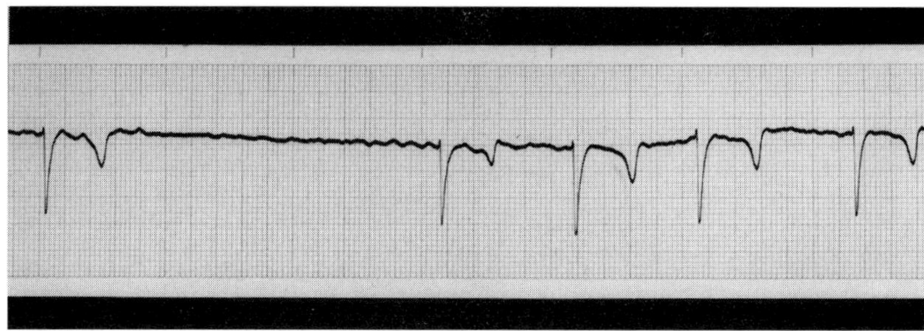

Figure 9.8 Atrial fibrillation. An ECG recorded from an 8-year-old hunter with signs of exercise intolerance and a resting heart rate of approximately 40 beats per minute. The rhythm is completely irregular, and there are no P waves. On auscultation the chaotic rhythm was easily appreciated and there were no S4 (A) heart sounds.

(Fig. 9.8). The QRS complexes may vary slightly, but grossly different QRS complexes may in fact be ventricular premature complexes (see below).

Paroxysmal atrial fibrillation

In some animals AF occurs for a short time before sinus rhythm returns, without treatment. This usually occurs during exercise, and sinus rhythm is re-established within 24 hours. The condition can result in a significant reduction in performance during exercise. It can be difficult to establish the diagnosis in these cases because the paroxysm has often ceased by the time that a veterinary examination is performed. Radiotelemetry is a very useful aid in these cases. Animals that experience repeated bouts of paroxysmal AF may have atrial disease, e.g. as a result of a previous viral infection. Electrolyte imbalance has also been implicated.

Ventricular arrhythmias

Ventricular premature complexes (VPCs)

VPCs are caused by abnormal impulse formation in the ventricular myocardium. The presence of an occasional, isolated VPC is not necessarily abnormal. If no other abnormalities are detected, the abnormal beat may be of no significance. However, if the VPCs are frequent, or a tachycardia or signs of CHF are present, strict rest is indicated. The prognosis is poor unless the underlying disease can be reversed. In many cases the prevalence of VPCs falls between these two extremes and the significance can be highly variable. As a rule, these horses should not be ridden until a thorough investigation directed at detecting underlying heart disease, and treatment aimed at reversing any such disease, have been performed.

Diagnosis

Auscultation will reveal an early beat followed by a longer than normal diastolic pause. The S1 intensity may be greater than normal, and S2 may be relatively quiet depending on the duration of diastole. Echocardiography and clinical pathology (routine haematology and biochemistry, including electrolyte levels) are useful. Radiotelemetry and 24 hour Holter ECG recordings are valuable to document the frequency of the arrhythmia and the effects of exercise.

On ECG, VPCs are early and therefore disturb the R–R interval, resulting in an irregular rhythm. They are ectopic and therefore do not follow the normal conduction pathways, resulting in a different QRS complex from those of sinus origin (Fig. 9.9). However, in horses the duration of the QRS interval may or may not exceed the normal range (> 0.14 sec), so this is not a reliable means of identifying VPCs. If sinus beats are present it is possible to recognize a VPC from its different configuration and amplitude. However, it is more difficult to recognize some VPCs if

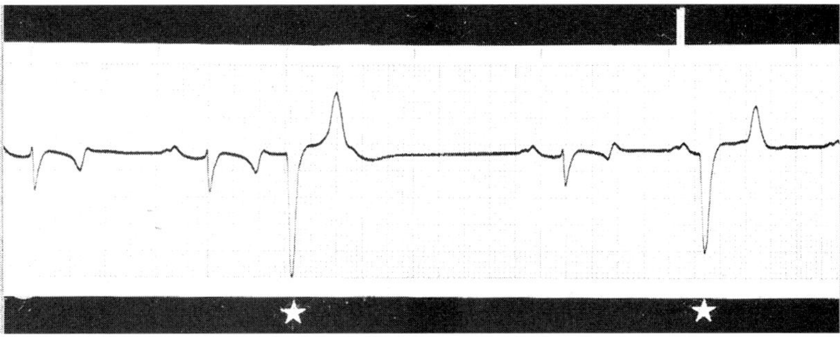

Figure 9.9   Ventricular premature complexes. Bizarre large QRS complexes are seen (stars), which are not preceded by conducted P waves. The first of these can be seen to be followed by a prolonged pause (compensatory pause). More of the strip needs to be seen to assess the frequency of the VPCs and the underlying rhythm, but in this example a P wave may be buried in the T wave following the first VPC, and the P wave preceding the second VPC is too close to it to have been conducted (arrow). On auscultation there was a premature beat with a loud S1 and rather quiet S2, followed by a pause longer than the usual S1–S1 interval.

there is a persistent ventricular tachycardia, in which case there are no sinus beats for comparison. If different QRS abnormalities are present the condition is described as multiform in origin. Usually this indicates more widespread myocardial disease and a less favourable prognosis. The T wave is also widened and of opposite polarity to the QRS complex. The ectopic beat is almost always followed by a full compensatory pause, but it can be found between two normal QRS complexes not disrupting the R–R interval, in which case it is called an interpolated beat.

Ventricular tachycardia

'V. tach.' is defined as four or more VPCs in succession. It may be paroxysmal or sustained. There is nearly always serious underlying cardiac or systemic disease present.

Diagnosis
Auscultation will demonstrate a rapid rhythm which is regular during the periods of ventricular tachycardia, but which may appear irregular if there are short paroxysms interspersed with normal sinus rhythm. P waves may be seen on ECG or hidden by the abnormal QRS complexes. Fusion beats or capture beats may be seen.

Ventricular fibrillation

Ventricular fibrillation (VF) is usually a terminal event in which there are no organized ventricular depolarizations or contraction. The horse collapses and no pulse is palpable. VF is associated with increased myocardial irritability which is usually caused by severe systemic or cardiac disease.

Diagnosis
No clear heart sounds are detected on auscultation and the ECG shows irregular baseline undulations with no QRS complexes, P or T waves.

IV. **Other heart diseases**

Congestive heart failure

Congestive heart failure (CHF) is relatively uncommon in horses. The most common cause is valvular disease, particularly mitral regurgitation. CHF is seldom reversible, except in some cases of myocardial or pericardial disease. Occasionally, towards the end of pregnancy, mares will show signs of CHF, which resolves after the birth of the foal.

Most horses with CHF show marked exercise intolerance. Signs can be divided into those resulting from left-sided or right-sided failure. However, this is a gross over-simplification. In addition, most horses with left-sided disease, such as mitral regurgitation, eventually develop right-sided CHF.

In acute left-sided CHF, the predominant clinical signs are due to the development of pulmonary oedema. Hyperpnoea, tachypnoea and dyspnoea may be observed. Some horses cough but this sign is not as marked as in some other species. In right-sided CHF, the first signs to develop are distension of the jugular veins, and dependent oedema, which usually forms a plaque along the ventral abdomen. Filling of the sheath and distal limbs may be seen. Diarrhoea (due to intestinal oedema) and weight loss may be observed in severe cases.

Auscultatory findings should enable the primary cause of the CHF to be identified, and arrhythmias which complicate the condition may also be detected. Electrocardiography and echocardiography are helpful to define the cause further, assess its severity, and guide prognosis and treatment where appropriate.

Horses with CHF have a poor prognosis unless the underlying cause can be reversed, but this is seldom possible. Horses with mild CHF may be stabilized on treatment so that they can be used as breeding animals or kept as pets, but they are unsuitable for riding purposes. Sudden death may occur, usually when the pulmonary artery ruptures owing to pulmonary hypertension.

Congenital lesions in the growing/adult animal

Congenital heart defects are relatively uncommon in horses compared with other domestic species. Although they may result in foetal or neonatal death, most are not identified until the animal fails to thrive as a youngster, has poor athletic performance when first put into work, or when a murmur is detected at a routine examination. Not infrequently, the congenital lesion is not identified until well into adult life.

Ventricular septal defect

By far the most common congenital lesion in horses, particularly in growing and adult horses, is a ventricular septal defect (VSD). Other defects usually present earlier in life, while VSDs vary in severity and can even be asymptomatic. VSDs result in loud systolic murmurs and usually there is a precordial thrill. Clinical signs associated with a VSD depend upon its size; small defects allow only a limited amount of blood to shunt from the left to right ventricle. Performance can be normal, particularly in non-performance horses. Other horses may have reduced performance, tachycardia, or signs of CHF. Some horses do well until, later in life, they develop aortic regurgitation due to deformation of the aortic ring, which is close to the site of most VSDs.

Diagnosis

Definitive diagnosis requires the use of echocardiography, angiography, or catheterization. Echocardiography is the most accurate of these, provides the best guide to severity and is non-invasive. Because VSDs can have limited effects on exercise tolerance, animals in which this lesion is suspected should not be condemned unless clinical signs are severe or echocardiography demonstrates significant haemodynamic abnormalities.

Using two-dimensional echocardiography, the location of the VSD can be identified and its size measured (Fig. 9.4). In adult Thoroughbreds, VSDs under 2.5 cm in diameter are unlikely to prevent all but the highest level of performance. Doppler echocardiography can be used to measure the velocity of blood flow through the defect and from this information the pressure gradient across the defect, and hence the absolute right ventricular pressure, can be estimated. Right ventricular systolic pressure greater than 60 mm Hg is likely to be associated with clinical signs of poor performance (left ventricular systolic pressure is nearly always in the region of 120 mmHg).

Myocardial disease

Myocardial disease is poorly defined in the horse. Clinical signs vary from poor athletic performance to sudden death, but severe myocardial disease is much less common in horses than in small animals. However, arrhythmias are an important cause of poor athletic performance and may be related to low grade myocardial disease.

Myocarditis is an inflammatory process which is thought to occur in some horses in association with respiratory viral infection. However, this association is anecdotal. Horses with poor athletic performance following a respiratory infection benefit from cardiac investigation, but it must be considered that the reduced exercise tolerance may be due to other post-viral effects. Echocardiography should be used to assess myocardial contractility. A fractional shortening of less than 26% is likely to indicate reduced myocardial performance. Radiotelemetric and 24 hour Holter monitor ECG recordings may show evidence of intermittent arrhythmias such as supraventricular premature beats or tachycardia.

Where signs of CHF develop in horses without loud cardiac murmurs, myocardial or pericardial disease must be suspected. Heart sounds may be quiet and the apical impulse and pulse quality may be weak. A variable murmur may be detected and arrhythmias, especially VPCs, are common.

Severe myocardial disease can be toxic or idiopathic in origin. Monensin toxicity is the most common cause of severe myocardial disease, so that dietary information is helpful.

Clinical pathology may be of value in some cases. Serum cardiac muscle isoenzymes of lactate dehydrogenase (LDH) have been reported to be an indicator of myocardial injury; however, there is little evidence for this at present. Animals with severe disease such as monensin toxicity may appear to have high cardiac isoenzymes, but the true origin may be from skeletal muscle damage. However, the fact that the serum muscle enzyme, creatine phosphokinase (CPK), is elevated in the acute stages of monensin toxicity is diagnostically useful. Haematology and viral serology may provide evidence of viral infection, but clinical signs of myocarditis may develop some weeks after infection when these indicators are even less reliable than in the acute phase.

Bacterial endocarditis

Bacterial endocarditis is a very uncommon condition which carries a grave prognosis if it is not diagnosed early and treated aggressively. It is slightly more common in foals and aged horses, but is sufficiently rare that it is difficult to give a predilection group. The aortic and mitral valves are the most frequently affected.

The predominant clinical signs are usually malaise and weight loss. Fever is often identified. A murmur typical of incompetence of the affected valve may be heard and in a significant proportion of cases ventricular premature beats are present. The source of the infection is seldom identified.

Diagnosis

Clinical pathology is usually extremely helpful, revealing evidence of an acute inflammatory process. A neutrophilia may or may not be present, but hyperfibrinogenaemia is usually very marked, with values in the region of 8–12 g/l being not uncommon. Blood culture can be helpful; several samples should be taken into large quantities of blood for aerobic and anaerobic culture (see 'Blood culture' in Chapter 8: 'Blood disorders'). Unfortunately, cultures are often negative, but antimicrobial sensitivity should be performed if cultures are obtained because a wide variety of organisms may be involved and treatment needs to be specific and long term. Even with a successful bacteriological cure, clinical signs of valvular disease may persist.

When clinicopathological tests are suggestive of a severe inflammatory process, echocardiography is indicated in order to pinpoint the location of the infection. An echocardiogram in horses with endocarditis usually shows a large, vegetative, echogenic lesion on the affected valve. The chordae tendineae may also be affected. Large degenerative nodules are uncommon in horses so that any detected in a patient with suspicious clinical signs is likely to confirm the presence of endocarditis. If there is any uncertainty, it is worth repeating the echocardiogram in a few days. Echocardiography is also useful for assessing the severity of valvular regurgitation. If volume overload is severe, treatment may not be warranted.

Pericarditis

Pericardial disease is very uncommon in horses, but may be recognized rather more frequently in future, now that the use of echocardiography is more widespread.

The development of clinical signs depends on whether diastolic filling of the heart is normal. Filling can be limited by the pericardial sac if it becomes fibrosed (constrictive pericarditis), or if it fills with a significant effusion. If the effusion forms rapidly or is substantial, it may compress the right atrium and limit venous return (tamponade). Presenting signs may be malaise, poor athletic performance or CHF. If the pericardium becomes associated with a pleuropneumonia, respiratory signs will also be present.

Auscultation may reveal muffled heart sounds. If there is a small amount of fluid present, a pericardial 'friction rub' may be detected. This may have one to three components, and has a quality similar to a creaking door. Unlike a pleural rub it is synchronous with the cardiac cycle.

Diagnosis

Identification of a pericardial effusion is best made using echocardiography, when an anechoic area is seen between the echogenic pericardium and the myocardium. Layers or fronds of fibrin on the pericardium or epicardium, or echogenic specks in the effusion, may be seen if there is a bacterial aetiology. If tamponade is present, the right atrium will have a concave outer surface. However, echocardiographic diagnosis of constrictive pericarditis is difficult. The pericardium may appear thickened and the pattern of filling is altered, with a step in the M-mode contour of the ventricular wall and valve motion at mid-diastole.

Appropriate clinicopathological tests are haematology with plasma fibrinogen estimation to identify an inflammatory process. Cytology and culture of the effusion can be helpful in identifying the aetiology of the disease.

Pericardiocentesis

Pericardiocentesis is required to relieve tamponade and may be helpful in obtaining pericardial fluid for cytology and culture. The procedure is not without risk owing to the sensitivity of the epicardium, which can result in arrhythmias when stimulated. Monitoring the ECG and placing an intravenous catheter prior to pericardiocentesis is therefore advisable.

Blind insertion of a catheter is possible in the 5th or 6th intercostal space on the left or right side of the chest, just dorsal to the mid-way point between the elbow and the shoulder level. A long 10–14 gauge catheter, through which a fine polythene tube such as a dog urinary catheter can be threaded, is inserted after infiltration of the skin and intercostal muscle with local anaesthetic. The procedure is best performed by judging the position to insert the catheter using ultrasound guidance.

V. **Vascular diseases**

The association of vasculitis with systemic disease is considered under 'Vascular diseases' in Chapter 8: 'Blood disorders'. The diagnosis and evaluation of much larger vascular lesions is possible by the use of ultrasonography and is considered here.

Ultrasonography of peripheral vasculature

Ultrasonography is a useful technique for evaluation of vascular diseases. Two-dimensional imaging using a linear array or a sector scanner can be used to identify gross lesions. Doppler equipment can be used to investigate blood flow within a vessel, but this facility is generally restricted to specialist centres. These techniques can be useful in investigating a number of clinical situations:

- Aortic or iliac thromboembolism
- Arterio-venous fistulae
- Venous thrombosis
- Identification of moving fluid
- Major vessel rupture

Aortic or iliac thromboembolism

Thromboembolism of the terminal aorta or iliac arteries is an uncommon cause of hind-limb pain and weakness which is exacerbated by exercise. The thrombus may be palpable on rectal examination, although on occasion thrombosis has been diagnosed using ultrasound where no abnormalities were detected by palpation.

A 5 or 7.5 MHz transducer scanner is suitable. For most examinations performed per rectum a linear array transducer is used, but some sector scanners are designed to be suitable for rectal use. Many practices will have equipment designed for examination of the reproductive tract which is equally suitable for this investigation. The thrombus is of mixed echogenicity, with areas of marked hyperechogenicity, particularly in chronic cases in which fibrous tissue has been laid down. Up to 80% of the lumen of the aorta has been shown to be occluded in some cases. The examination should also include the internal and external iliac arteries. The prognosis for athletic use in animals with this condition is poor.

Arterio-venous fistulae

Peripheral arterio-venous fistulae are rare but have been identified by ultrasonography in some animals. The clinical significance of these lesions depends on their size and location. They may be congenital, acquired or iatrogenic. An example of the latter is fistula formation between the jugular vein and carotid artery as a result of poor catheterization technique. Doppler ultrasonography can be used to measure blood flow through the fistula.

Venous thrombosis

Ultrasound is a useful technique to detect the build-up of a thrombus within a vein. A good example is identifying thrombus formation around a jugular catheter, which may prompt the removal of the catheter before complete occlusion of the vessel occurs. Ultrasound can also be used to investigate swelling around veins and identify thrombophlebitis.

For the investigation of superficial vessels, a high frequency transducer such as a 7.5 MHz probe is useful, and a stand-off may be required. Both sector scanners and linear array transducers can be used, but linear array transducers may be more difficult to manipulate in confined areas such as the thoracic inlet.

Identification of moving fluid

In some investigations of soft tissue structures, areas will be identified that are filled with material of a homogeneous density, usually hypoechoic in nature, and the observer will be uncertain whether this structure is a vessel or some other fluid-filled structure. In these situations, pulsation of the structure may lead to its identification as an artery. In some instances echogenic particles will be seen to be moving within the vessel lumen.

Once again, the most useful technique for investigating flow in a vessel is Doppler ultrasound. Not only can the contents of a vessel be confirmed to be moving, but measurements of the velocity of flow and the diameter of the vessel will allow calculation of the volume of blood which is flowing through the vessel.

Major vessel rupture

One of the most common causes of sudden death is rupture of a major artery. By definition, it is therefore difficult for any investigative technique other than post-mortem to be useful in these cases. However, in some horses death is not immediate and investigation may identify the source of haemorrhage in collapsed animals.

The pulmonary vessels are commonly involved. This usually manifests as a profuse bilateral nasal haemorrhage. Occasionally, a vessel ruptures into the pleural space and the presence of a bloody effusion may be identified by thoracic radiography, ultrasonography and thoracocentesis. However, ultrasonography is the most useful of these techniques and thoracocentesis should be avoided if possible. Ultrasonography has the advantage that it can provide information on the type of fluid present, its extent, and the underlying pulmonary disease.

The major pulmonary vessel is the pulmonary artery. This may rupture as a sequel to CHF. Echocardiography may show hypoechoic regions around the base of the artery, a hyperdynamic heart, and abnormal motion of the pulmonary valve in those cases which do not die immediately.

Aortic vessel rupture is a potential cause of sudden death and is not diagnosed ante-mortem. Rupture of a mesenteric artery may be associated with acute colic. In such cases abdominocentesis may reveal frank blood. Fractures of long bones are sometimes associated with haemorrhage from major arteries and in the case of pelvic fractures the blood loss may result in death. In these instances ultrasonography may show the fracture and an associated haematoma. A 3.5–5 MHz linear array or sector-scanning transducer is ideal and can be used transcutaneously or per rectum.

Further reading

Holmes JR (1990) Electrocardiography in the diagnosis of common cardiac arrhythmias in the horse. *Equine Veterinary Education* **2**: 24–27.

McGladdery AJ and Marr CM (1990) Echocardiography for the practitioner. *Equine Veterinary Education* **2**: 11–14.

Long KJ (1992) Two-dimensional and M-mode echocardiography. *Equine Veterinary Education* **4**: 303–310.

Long KJ, Bonagura JD and Darke PGG (1992) Standardised imaging technique for guided M-mode and Doppler echocardiography in the horse. *Equine Veterinary Journal* **24**: 226–235.

Patteson MW (1992) The right electrocardiograph for you? *In Practice* (supplement to the Veterinary Record) **14**: 16–17.

Reef VB (1990) Echocardiographic examination in the horse: The basics. *Compendium of Continuing Education for the Practicing Veterinarian* **12**: 1312–1319.

Robertson SA (1990) Practical use of ECG in the horse. *In Practice* (supplement to the Veterinary Record) **12**: 59–67.

10 Lymphatic diseases

I. Practical techniques

Lymphadenopathy

Lymph node enlargement is the result of reactive hyperplasia, infection, or neoplastic invasion, and is usually incidental to other clinical signs.

In healthy horses, the palpable superficial lymph nodes are usually small and include the submandibular and precrural nodes. Deeper lymph nodes which become palpable as a result of enlargement include retropharyngeal, prescapular, thoracic inlet, supramammary and inguinal nodes.

Lymph node swellings may obstruct dependent lymphatic drainage and cause oedema, as in sporadic lymphangitis, 'strangles' (*Streptococcus equi* infection) and tumours of the lymphosarcoma complex. As space occupying lesions, swollen lymph nodes may obstruct the pharynx, oesophagus, trachea, bronchi or intestinal tract, depending upon their location.

Although neoplastic infiltration may be the result of metastasis from tumours in adjacent tissues, the most common tumour causing lymphadenopathy in horses is lymphoid in origin, i.e. lymphosarcoma (lymphoma).

If the associated clinical signs are inconclusive, biopsy is required to differentiate between inflammatory enlargement (lymphadenitis) and neoplastic infiltration.

Lymph node biopsy

A reasonable sized, representative sample of the node is essential for adequate histopathological examination.

Lymph node excision is ideal for diagnostic pathology, but impractical in the horse.

Fine needle aspiration and smear preparation seldom provides diagnostic information. The sample is small, unlikely to be representative of the lesion and may produce a 'false negative'. An exception is lymph node abscessation.

The best option is incisional biopsy, in which a wedge section is excised under local anaesthesia coupled, if necessary, with sedation. This relatively large sample retains better morphology than a needle core biopsy and improves the chance of a definitive diagnosis.

Wedge section biopsy technique

A wedge section biopsy is most easily collected from a superficial lymph node that can be adequately immobilized against the overlying skin. The local anatomy of the area of lymph drainage should be considered carefully to avoid inadvertent damage to adjacent structures.

- Depending on the site, an area some 10–15 cm square is clipped and surgically prepared over the node. Local anaesthesia is produced by subcutaneous injection of lignocaine along a line following the proposed site of the skin incision. The remainder of the technique must be performed under strict surgical asepsis.
- Ideally the lymph node is immobilized between the fingers and thumb of one hand, leaving the other to make the skin incision. Once the initial incision has been made, the lymph node is maintained in a fixed position against the skin opening. A deep elliptical incision is then made through the capsule of the node and this is continued in a convergent direction into the body of the node. This is most easily performed using a No. 15 scalpel. The wedge section is grasped with tissue forceps and gently withdrawn, while scissors are used to cut any remaining tissue connections.
- In most instances the section is then divided into halves. One half is submitted for bacterial culture and the other is put into formol-saline for histopathology.
- Prior to closure the source of any significant haemorrhage should be identified and ligated. The cut edges of the node are then apposed with a horizontal mattress suture using an absorbable material. Similar material can be used to close the sub-

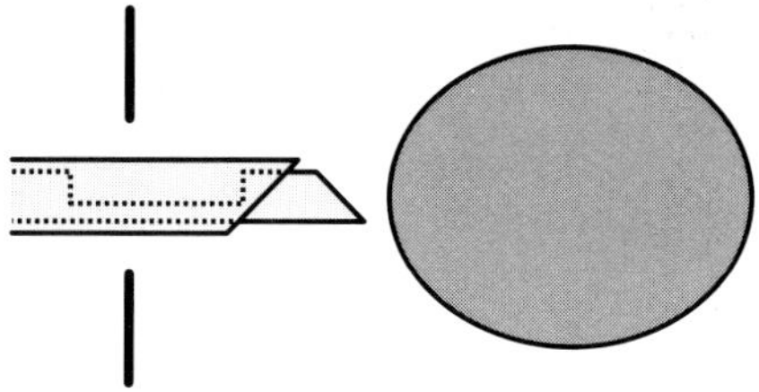

The closed needle is inserted through a skin incision.

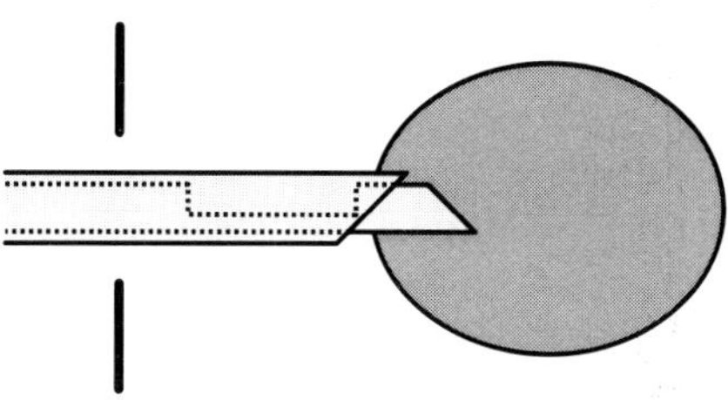

The tip is positioned within the edge of the node.

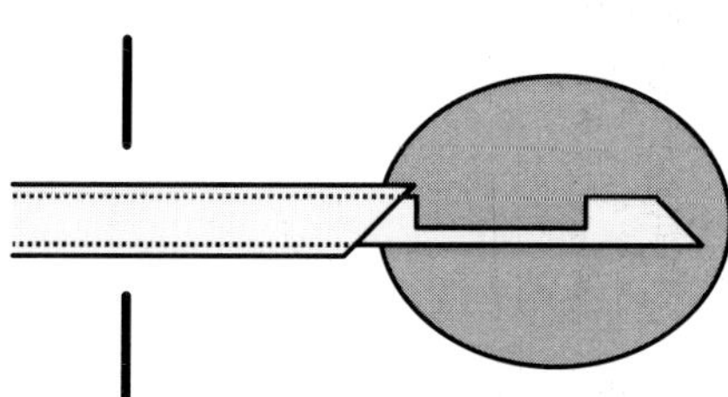

The obturator is advanced.

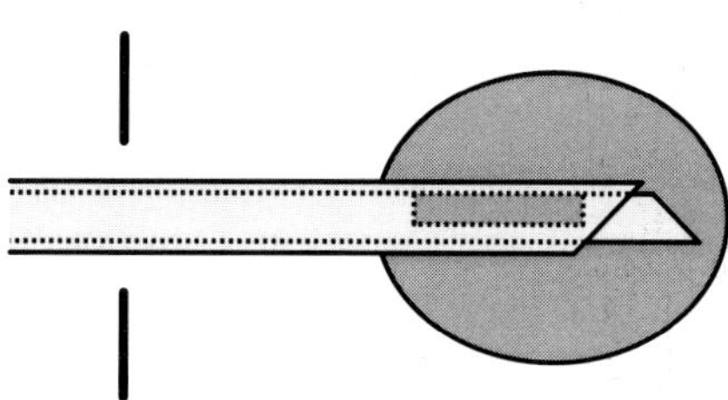

The cannula is advanced to cut the specimen.

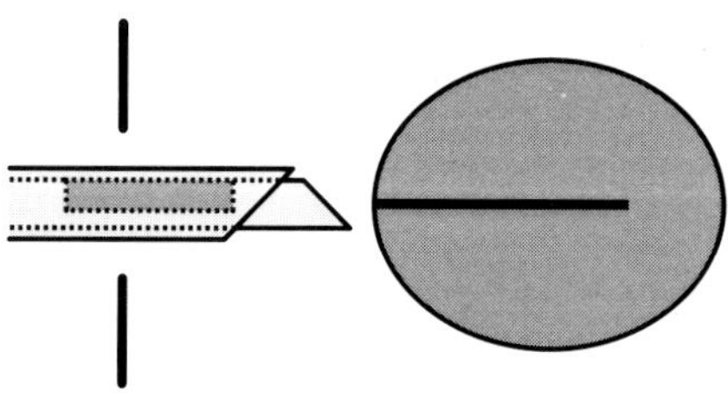

The whole is withdrawn.

Figure 10.1 Technique for needle core biopsy of a lymph node using the 'Tru-Cut' instrument.

cutaneous tissues in a simple continuous pattern. The skin incision is then closed with non-absorbable material in a simple interrupted pattern. Local swelling is usually minimal following the procedure and resolves in 5–7 days.

Comments

- Complications of wedge section biopsy are infrequent, but more common than with the needle technique (see below). The most common complications are local haemorrhage and/or a failure of first intention healing. These risks are reduced by careful attention to good surgical technique during the course of the procedure.

- Poor healing is likely following the incision of a neoplastic mass.

- As with all invasive techniques, the patient's tetanus status should be ascertained.

Needle core biopsy technique

Because of the potential problems associated with healing, a pragmatic alternative to wedge section is needle core biopsy. A core biopsy may be obtained using the 'Tru-Cut' needle (Baxter Healthcare Corporation, California). The 'Tru-Cut' is a 14 gauge punch needle designed for sampling superficial and subcutaneous tissue masses. Its design enables a tissue plug to be trapped and excised within the outer casing of the needle (Fig. 10.1). The technique is as follows:

- A representative lymph node is chosen, ideally one that is superficial and can be held immobile against the overlying skin. An area of skin over the node is clipped and prepared as for the wedge biopsy. A small volume (1–2 ml) of local anaesthetic is infiltrated subcutaneously at the site of needle entry. This allows a small stab incision to be made through the skin with a scalpel. Core biopsy needles are not designed to penetrate the skin and a prior stab incision is always necessary.

- The needle, in the closed position, is then inserted through the skin incision and positioned so that the tip is just entering the lymph node (Fig. 10.1). Where possible, the entry of the needle should be along the direction of the long axis of the node.

- The obturator alone is then advanced into the lymph node allowing tissue to insinuate into its specimen notch. The cannula is advanced in a secondary action to cut the tissue core. Both obturator and cannula are then withdrawn in the closed position. It is not usually necessary to suture the stab incision.

- The sample is retrieved from the needle by advancing the obturator to reveal the specimen notch. It can then be teased into formol-saline using a sterile disposable needle. Providing the biopsy needle is kept sterile, several samples may be collected. However, it is usually preferable to collect a second sample from a different site within the node.

II. **Investigating specific diseases**

Lymphangitis

Sporadic lymphangitis

Sporadic lymphangitis is a common lymphatic obstruction of uncertain aetiology which usually affects one or other of the hind limbs and is traditionally blamed on a protein-rich diet fed during a rest period. However, an infectious aetiology cannot be discounted. Inflammation of the lymphatic tracts and associated regional lymph nodes leads to lymph stasis and, at the extreme, a thickening of the whole limb.

Diagnosis is by recognition of the clinical signs. The earliest change is an acute lameness, but swelling of the limb quickly follows and may be sufficiently severe to cause serum ooze over taut skin surfaces. Secondary infection with the development of cellulitis is possible. Early recognition and treatment of the acute case to resolve oedema formation is extremely important. If oedema persists for more than 7 days, severe fibrosis can develop in the interstitial spaces resulting in permanent swelling and reduced function. This chronic disfigurement is usually refractory to all treatments. There is a tendency for the condition to recur.

Infectious causes of lymphangitis

Inflammation of lymphatic vessels and regional lymph nodes in association with local infection is common. Infections that cause primary lymphangitis are relatively uncommon and usually involve the limbs, producing local swelling and oedema. In contrast to sporadic lymphangitis, these conditions are contagious and involve identifiable bacterial or fungal agents. *Ulcerative lymphangitis* is the most common of these conditions and may be associated with wound infection in conditions of poor hygiene. Transmission is by direct contact (grooming kit), but biting flies are possible vectors. The result is multiple foci of nodular abscessation along lymphatic tracts which erupt to discharge a greenish pus. A number of bacterial causes are implicated including *Corynebacterium pseudotuberculosis*, *Pseudomonas aeruginosa*, and staphylococcal and streptococcal species. Diagnosis is based on culture.

The clinician should be aware of two other forms of infectious lymphangitis which, although very rare, are still notifiable in the UK and other parts of the world. *Cutaneous glanders* or 'farcy' is the cutaneous form of a debilitating pneumonic disease caused by *Pseudomonas mallei*. It has been eradicated from most of Western Europe and is now confined to parts of Asia. Lymphatic infection is associated with the development of nodules which discharge a 'honey-like' pus. Diagnosis is based on culture and serum antibody assay. In the UK an intradermal hypersensitivity test would be undertaken by the Ministry of Agriculture, Fisheries and Food using an antigen extract of the bacterium ('Mallein test'). *Epizootic lymphangitis* is caused by a yeast-like fungus, *Histoplasma farciminosum*, which gains access to superficial wounds to produce skin nodules from which a thick creamy pus erupts. The disease is now of limited occurrence world-wide, being found in parts of the African and Asian continents. The clinical presentation is similar to the cutaneous form of glanders, from which it can be distinguished by smear cytology and/or Mallein test.

Lymphosarcoma in horses

Lymphosarcoma is the commonest tumour of the equine haematopoietic system and probably the commonest internal tumour of horses. It tends to occur in middle-aged and older horses, but cases are commonly recorded in yearlings and young horses. There is no predisposition of breed or sex.

The site of tumour development and the associated range of presenting signs can be grouped conveniently into one of four categories:

- Abdominal lymphosarcoma — probably the commonest form
- Thoracic lymphosarcoma
- Multicentric lymphosarcoma
- Cutaneous lymphosarcoma — probably the least common form

However, individuals often present tumour foci and clinical signs which overlap these divisions, resulting in a wide variety of clinical presentations. In all cases there is weight loss and a common non-specific finding is intermittent fever which is probably associated with tumour necrosis.

A definitive antemortem diagnosis of lymphosarcoma is obtained by demonstrating neoplastic lymphocytes in the peripheral blood, bone marrow, pleural or peritoneal fluids, or in a biopsy sample of a lymph node or tumour mass. Most usually a diagnosis is obtained from the histology of a tumour mass. Otherwise, the clinical pathology of lymphosarcoma tends to be non-specific.

The techniques employed to narrow down the differential diagnoses of the presenting clinical signs are outlined below. They are described in detail elsewhere in this book under the appropriate organ systems.

Abdominal lymphosarcoma

Abdominal lymphosarcoma (alimentary form) is characterized by the development of discrete (focal) or diffuse lesions. Occasionally, both conditions occur together.

Discrete lesions

Sites of lymphocyte infiltration include the intestinal wall, abdominal lymph nodes, mesentery, omentum and possibly the spleen. Such lesions can achieve considerable size before causing clinical signs. In general, clinical signs are associated with external pressure on the gut (causing acute colic), or focal invasion of the gut wall itself (causing recurrent colics). Ventral oedema may occur.

Diagnosis

- A palpable, solid mass (or masses) at rectal examination is suspicious.
- Abdominocentesis may provide diagnostic exfoliative cytology, but this is rarely the case with lymphosarcoma.
- Clinical pathology is likely to provide non-specific information (see later).
- Laparotomy demonstrates the mass(es) and the extent of gross infiltration.

Diffuse lesions

Extensive infiltration of the intestinal mucosa/submucosa with lymphocytes causes destruction of the villous architecture. Local lymph nodes are also likely to be involved. The result is malabsorption and the presenting signs depend upon which part of the gut is involved.

Infiltration of the small intestine is always associated with a loss of weight despite an adequate food intake. However, the appetite is often variable. Ventral oedema may be present and occasionally there are signs of chronic low grade pain such as teeth grinding or repetitive yawning. Faecal consistency is normal.

Infiltration of the large intestine (or large intestine plus small intestine) produces the same signs as above, but with chronic diarrhoea.

Diagnosis

- In a serum biochemistry profile, hypoalbuminaemia is usual (protein-losing enteropathy) and in the circumstances indicates the need for an oral glucose tolerance test (see 'Tests of intestinal malabsortion' in Chapter 2:'Alimentary diseases'). The serum alkaline phosphatase may be raised (see later).
- The oral glucose tolerance test will usually indicate malabsorption if the small intestine is involved.
- In cases of diarrhoea, a rectal biopsy may demonstrate lymphocyte infiltration of the large intestine.
- Abdominocentesis is indicated, but rarely provides diagnostic exfoliative cytology.
- Intestinal biopsies obtained by laparotomy will provide diagnostic histopathology.

Comment

- At laparotomy or post-mortem examination, diffuse lymphocytic infiltration of the intestinal tract is usually not appreciable. There is often no palpable thickening of tissues and a definitive diagnosis always requires histopathology. However, both diffuse and discrete lesions can occur together.

Thoracic lymphosarcoma

Thoracic lymphosarcoma (mediastinal form) is characterized by space-occupying lesions within the thorax owing to the development of thymic/mediastinal tumours with associated

11 Fluid, electrolyte and acid–base balance

The purpose of this chapter is to address the diagnostic assessment of fluid, electrolyte and acid–base balance in various disease states of the adult horse.

In the text that follows it is necessary to consider fluid, electrolyte and acid–base balance separately, but the clinician must never lose sight of their mutual interdependence. There is a dynamic relationship between these parameters; a change in one will induce changes in the others. Because of this the assessment of changes that have been caused by disease must be monitored throughout the period of corrective treatment; a treatment aimed at correcting one parameter will certainly have an effect on the others. Although it is outside the scope of this book to describe treatments in detail, the required action will be indicated by the interpretation of clinical findings.

The first section of this chapter deals with fluid balance and its assessment. However, quite apart from the volume of fluid which is needed to correct an imbalance, the required composition of that fluid must be determined by assessment of blood electrolyte concentrations, acid–base considerations and the plasma protein status. These parameters are considered individually in the subsequent sections and their application to common conditions are summarized in the final section on 'Common conditions affecting fluid and electrolyte balance'.

Fluid balance

Some 60% of an adult horse's body weight consists of water, which is distributed between the intracellular fluid (ICF) and extracellular fluid (ECF) compartments. Water moves freely between these compartments to maintain the osmotic equilibrium, but at any one time its relative distribution is governed by the prevailing concentrations of solutes on each side. A decrease in the volume of either compartment changes its osmotic forces, which results in a redistribution of water between the two sides until the osmotic equilibrium is resumed. The osmolality of the ICF is maintained for the most part by *potassium* and *phosphates*, whereas ECF osmolality is primarily a function of *sodium* and *chloride* ions.

In health, the ICF contains approximately two-thirds of the total body water. In a 500 kg horse, this amounts to some 200 litres of fluid. The ECF contains about one-third of total body water which in a 500 kg horse amounts to some 100 litres. Disturbances in the water balance result from either:

- A reduced intake associated with deprivation, dysphagia or other disease
- An increased loss associated with diarrhoea, high intestinal obstruction or excessive sweating
- A combination of these factors

Assessment of fluid balance

An acute loss of fluid from the ECF will increase its osmolality and water is transferred from the ICF. When the loss exceeds 5% of total body water, the result becomes clinically detectable as dehydration. Depending upon the clinical circumstances, dehydration will be accompanied by electrolyte and acid–base disturbances and, in the case of gut catastrophes, endotoxaemia.

Clinical signs associated with dehydration

The collective clinical signs can provide a diagnostic guide to the extent of fluid loss and its effect upon the circulation. Key features are as follows:

- Increases in the heart and pulse rates are indicative of hypovolaemia and/or endotoxaemia.
- Changes in pulse pressure reflect the integrity of the peripheral circulation. If the pulse is weak or absent and the capillary refill time prolonged, hypovolaemia and/or endotoxaemia are indicated.

- Changes in the capillary refill time (CRT) reflect the integrity of the peripheral circulation. Refill times in excess of 2 seconds indicate poor perfusion and circulatory compromise.
- Dryness of the oral mucous membranes indicates dehydration.
- A decrease in jugular distensibility when the vein is raised indicates a fall in venous pressure.
- A decrease in skin elasticity is consistent with dehydration. However, this is a very subjective test in horses. A fold pulled up at the point of the shoulder is probably more reliable than the skin of the neck region.
- Coldness of the extremities and a decreased rectal temperature indicate developing shock.
- A decrease in urine production accompanies renal hypoperfusion, but can be difficult to assess.
- Changes in body weight are a sensitive indicator of sudden alterations in fluid balance during the course of illness and/or treatment. An increase or decrease of 1 kg represents a gain or loss of approximately 1 litre of fluid. Unfortunately, suitably accurate weighing facilities are rarely available in practice.

The collective clinical information will not provide an accurate measure of the per cent dehydration of body weight, but it allows a subjective assessment of mild, moderate or severe dehydration. All signs are accentuated in acute dehydration and at their extreme indicate the development of hypovolaemic shock. The following observations are offered as a guide:

- Mild but detectable changes in the clinical signs reflect mild losses of 5–7% of total body water.
- A thready pulse, extended CRT (3–4 seconds) and reduced skin elasticity suggest moderate losses of 8–10%.
- Dry mucous membranes, prolonged CRT (4–5 seconds), weak or undetectable pulse and a marked decrease in skin elasticity indicate severe losses of 10% or greater.

Clinical pathology

In addition to clinical observations, simple blood parameters can be used to indicate the severity of dehydration. However, where facilities are available they are best used in a serial manner to follow the course of dehydration over a critical period.

Packed cell volume (PCV). A blood sample taken into anticoagulant (EDTA or heparin) is suitable for PCV estimation, but the technique has potential drawbacks. Excitement of the patient at collection may introduce error as a result of splenic contraction. Alternatively, an anaemic animal that has become dehydrated may show a PCV which is within a normal range. However, in all cases serial measurements should reveal any progressive dehydration. In general terms a PCV > 45% indicates a reduction in the ECF volume and a loss of sodium.

Total plasma protein (TPP) estimation. A heparinized blood sample is suitable for total plasma protein estimation, which may be undertaken in the field using a refractometer. However, concurrent protein loss can produce a spuriously low result. Thus a patient suffering a protein-losing enteropathy as well as dehydration may show a total plasma protein which is within the normal range. In addition, chronic infection can raise the plasma fibrinogen and globulin concentrations so that the total plasma protein will be raised, even in the absence of dehydration. However, as with PCV, serial measurement should reveal any progressive dehydration.

Urea and creatinine concentrations. Most serum or plasma biochemistry parameters, including urea, are raised by acute dehydration. However, significant increases in both urea and creatinine reflect prerenal failure associated with hypovolaemia (i.e. renal hypoperfusion). This condition is usually reversible if fluid therapy is not delayed.

Electrolyte balance

The problem in assessing electrolyte balance is that only the concentration of electrolytes in the plasma portion of the ECF can be determined with ease. ICF electrolyte concentrations can be determined, but the techniques are not usually available to the practitioner. However, knowing the distribution and function of the various electrolytes enables an empiric interpretation of their status from the results of a blood sample. Those of clinical importance in fluid and acid–base balance are *sodium, potassium, chloride* and *bicarbonate*. The first three can be measured in either serum or plasma, but bicarbonate estimation can only be undertaken on a blood sample collected into lithium heparin (see later). Whole blood samples must be separated soon after collection, since any tendency to haemolysis will alter electrolyte concentrations in serum or plasma. Table 11.1 includes typical blood electrolyte ranges for the adult horse.

Table 11.1. Typical blood biochemistry ranges* for the adult horse.

Content	Range
Total protein	60–70 g/l
Albumin	30–40 g/l
Globulin	20–35 g/l
Urea	3.2–5.2 mmol/l
Creatinine	128–188 µmol/l
Sodium	135–145 mmol/l
Potassium	3.3–5.0 mmol/l
Chloride	93–103 mmol/l
Bicarbonate	25–33 mmol/l

*Adapted from data supplied by the Clinical Pathology Diagnostic Service, Department of Clinical Veterinary Science, University of Bristol.

Sodium

Sodium is the major cation within the ECF and is largely responsible for maintaining the compartment's osmotic forces and thereby its fluid volume. However, the laboratory estimation of serum or plasma sodium concentration cannot be interpreted in absolute terms as a blood deficit or excess. This is because its concentration at any one time depends upon fluctuations within the total 'exchangeable' body stores of water, sodium and potassium, which can be transferred between compartments. The relationship of these factors has been defined by the following equation:

$$\text{Serum or plasma Na}^+ \text{ concentration } = \frac{\text{Exchangeable Na}^+ + \text{Exchangeable K}^+}{\text{Total body water}}$$

From this equation it follows that decreases in serum or plasma sodium concentration below the normal range (hyponatraemia) may be due to an excess of total body water, a loss of sodium or potassium, or a combination of these factors. However, increases in serum or plasma sodium concentration above the normal range (hypernatraemia) may be due to a loss of total body water, an excess of sodium or potassium, or a combination of these factors.

Hyponatraemic states (< 135 mmol/l) usually occur in diarrhoeic diseases where massive losses of fluid and electrolyte are followed by oral intake of water and partial replacement of the lost fluid. Hypernatraemic states (> 145 mmol/l) are rare, but can follow acute dehydration or excessive sodium replacement in fluid therapy.

Potassium

Potassium is the major cation of the ICF; only 2% of its total body store is present in the ECF. Consequently, serum or plasma potassium concentrations are of very limited value in estimating total body potassium. Even when the blood concentration is normal or raised, total body potassium stores could be depleted.

It is commonly observed that the serum or plasma concentration of potassium increases during acidosis and decreases in alkalosis. Cells tend to take up hydrogen and release potassium in states of acidosis and the reverse occurs in alkalosis. A knowledge of blood potassium concentration, together with a clinical assessment of the circulatory status, may therefore be used to infer extremes of acid–base balance. However, the situation may be complicated in conditions where there is a net loss of potassium from the circulation.

Decreases in serum or plasma potassium concentration below the normal range (hypokalaemia: < 3.3 mmol/l) are often associated with diarrhoea or, importantly, a decreased food intake. *Large amounts of potassium are excreted by the normal equine kidney, so that deficits soon occur when a horse's feed intake is reduced.* Deficits are readily replaced by the intake of sufficient quantities of hay. Marked hypokalaemia is usually indicative of a severe acid–base imbalance (alkalosis). If the blood potassium concentration is *less than* 3.3 mmol/l, or the horse is unable to eat, then supplementation must be considered.

Increases above the normal range (hyperkalaemia: > 5 mmol/l) are unusual in the horse unless associated with severe acidosis, haemolysis or, rarely, impaired renal function. Spurious hyperkalaemia in blood samples may follow spoilage associated with haemolysis or leakage of potassium out of red cells. It is for this reason that prompt separation of serum or plasma from blood cells is important when sampling. If possible, hyperkalaemia should be confirmed by a second sample. For obvious reasons, whole blood samples are unsatisfactory if laboratory processing is delayed.

Chloride and bicarbonate

Chloride and bicarbonate are the major anions of the ECF and demonstrate an inverse relationship. Since chloride is largely located in the ECF, changes in its serum or plasma concentration tend to reflect changes in its whole-body status. A decrease in the serum or plasma concentration of chloride below normal range (hypochloraemia: < 93 mmol/l) is usually the result of an increased loss to the gastrointestinal tract (diarrhoea or high obstruction) or, alternatively, a massive loss in sweating.

The role of bicarbonate is to act as a buffering system and its plasma concentration therefore reflects the horse's acid–base status. Marked decreases in bicarbonate accompany moderate to severe acidotic states. In a state of metabolic acidosis there is a decrease in plasma bicarbonate and an increase in serum or plasma chloride concentration. In metabolic alkalosis the reverse is true.

Calculation of fluid and electrolyte losses

In many instances a polyionic fluid such as lactated Ringer's solution is given empirically to correct fluid loss and the effect is subsequently monitored using clinical and clinicopathological parameters. However, as the following example shows, it is possible to make a crude though revealing calculation of fluid and electrolyte deficits based upon clinical examination and simple clinicopathological data.

Clinical example

The example is a 500 kg horse with severe diarrhoea. Clinical examination reveals a raised heart rate (60–80 bpm), a thready pulse, a prolonged CRT (3–4 secs) and reduced skin elasticity. These findings suggest modest dehydration (8–10%). Clinical pathology reveals a PCV in excess of 45% and low plasma concentrations of sodium (130 mmol/l) and potassium (3.0 mmol/l). From this assessment the animal is clearly dehydrated and there is a loss of electrolytes to the bowel. Above all, the sodium deficit needs to be corrected, which in the first instance should stabilize the ECF volume. *The correction of sodium and volume deficits are the major concerns when considering fluid and electrolyte therapy.*

Once the percent clinical dehydration has been assessed, the magnitude of the required fluid volume for replacement can be estimated as follows:

Approximate fluid deficit (litres) =
Supposed clinical dehydration (%) x
Body weight (kg)

In this example the magnitude of fluid requirement is therefore:

8–10% of 500 litres = 40–50 litres

Using these figures and the given clinico-pathological data, it is then possible to estimate the sodium and potassium deficits. For this we make two assumptions: (1) that the horse's plasma sodium concentration in health is the mean of the laboratory's normal range (135 to 145 = 140 mmol/l), and (2) that the horse's total body water prior to dehydration was 60% of its body weight, i.e. 300 litres.

Since the plasma concentration of sodium has the following relationships (see above under: 'Electrolyte balance'):

$$\text{Plasma Na}^+ = \frac{\text{Exchangeable Na}^+ + \text{Exchangeable K}^+}{\text{Total body water}}$$

Then *before* dehydration the sum of exchangeable Na^+ and K^+ is derived from:

Plasma Na^+ x Total body water =
Exchangeable Na^+ + Exchangeable K^+

This, by substitution of the given figures becomes:

140 x 300 = 42 000 mmol

But *after* dehydration the sum of the Exchangeable Na^+ and K^+ is reduced because the plasma Na^+ concentration is low (130 mmol/l) and there is a fluid deficit of 40–50 litres as follows:

130 x (300 – 50) to 130 x (300 – 40) =
32 500 to 33 800 mmol

The deficit of Na^+ + K^+ therefore becomes:

[42 000 – 33 800 mmol] to [42 000 –
32 500 mmol] = 8200 to 9500 mmol

In diarrhoea, some 70% of the Na^+ + K^+ loss is sodium. In consequence:

The Na^+ deficit = [8200 x 0.7] to [9500 x
0.7] = 5740 to 6650 mmol

and by subtraction:

The K+ deficit = 2460 to 2850 mmol

In summary, this crude assessment of the patient's requirement indicates:

A total body water deficit of 40–50 litres
A Na^+ deficit of 5740–6650 mmol
A K^+ deficit of 2460–2850 mmol

By selecting 40–50 litres of a polyionic solution

the sodium deficit would almost be corrected. Polyionic solutions approximate in ionic composition and concentration to plasma and in such solutions the sodium content is usually of the order of 130–140 mmol/l. However, the potassium deficit would remain far short of replacement. This is not a problem if the horse is eating or oral supplementation with potassium chloride is permissible. Nevertheless, if fluid therapy is repeated over several days in the absence of oral supplementation, substantial potassium deficits can result.

NB This calculation provides a rough idea of the immediate replacement volume. However, after replacement is achieved there will be a continuing maintenance requirement of 50–100 ml fluid per kg per day, which the patient may or not be able to sustain for itself.

Acid–base balance

Disturbances of acid–base balance may be due to an increased production, or a decreased excretion, of acids or bases. A number of mechanisms can cause these disturbances. The accumulations of organic or inorganic acids and bases in the body produce states of metabolic acidosis or metabolic alkalosis. These acid–base imbalances often accompany conditions for which fluid therapy is indicated. Corrective fluid therapy will usually redress the acid–base balance by diluting out acid or base excesses and improving tissue perfusion. *In consequence, specific correction of acid–base imbalance is often unnecessary and on occasion can even be harmful.*

Metabolic acidosis is the most common acid–base disorder in horses. It occurs most frequently in association with obstructive gastrointestinal disease and diarrhoea. Much more rarely, it is associated with renal failure. The underlying causes of acidosis in these situations are either increased base loss and/or reduced peripheral perfusion causing a switch from aerobic to predominantly anaerobic metabolism in tissues, with a consequent build up of lactate. The physiological response is an increase in the respiratory rate (to blow off CO_2) which may be seen among the clinical signs. Metabolic acidosis usually causes few adverse effects.

Metabolic alkalosis is uncommon in horses but is usually associated with a depletion of serum or plasma chloride concentration. Alkalosis may occur transiently with hypochloraemia in the early stages of diarrhoea or high intestinal obstruction.

Changes in blood pH can also follow changes in respiratory ventilation. Hypoventilation produces respiratory acidosis due to an increasing partial pressure of CO_2 in the blood. Repiratory acidosis occurs during general anaesthesia in the horse in association with a central depression of respiration and an increase in the partial pressure of CO_2 in the blood. With due care it is of little consequence. In contrast, hyperventilation produces respiratory alkalosis due to a decreasing partial pressure of CO_2 which is 'blown off'. Respiratory alkalosis may follow hyperventilation associated with exercise.

Assessment of acid–base balance

Although blood gas and pH measurements provide the only accurate guide to acid–base status, plasma bicarbonate estimations are acceptable for most clinical situations. Plasma bicarbonate concentrations are most commonly estimated from the total CO_2 in plasma, of which 95% is considered to be bicarbonate. However, delays in determining total CO_2 concentration can cause spuriously low values and to avoid this, venous blood samples must be collected anaerobically into heparinized syringes and processed as soon as possible. Unfortunately, the close proximity of sophisticated equipment is required for these analyses and this is not usually the case in practice. In practical terms, however, the need to correct a metabolic acidosis by specific bicarbonate therapy is rare — unless the plasma concentration falls below 15 mmol/l.

The decision to administer sodium bicarbonate solution requires caution since it may cause persistent metabolic alkalosis with respiratory depression, hypernatraemia (by supplementing excess sodium), hypokalaemia, and a net hyperosmolality. However, in the exceptional cases where plasma bicarbonate falls below 15 mmol/l, supplementary bicarbonate should be given because many of the body's metabolic processes cannot function below a pH of 7.

At specialist centres, estimations of the quantity of bicarbonate required to restore a deficit are usually related to replacement of the deficit in extracellular fluid. Since the lower range of normal plasma bicarbonate concentration is usually some 25 mmol/l, a *base deficit* (i.e. bicarbonate deficit) is calculated by subtracting the patient's plasma bicarbonate concentration (mmol/l) from 25 mmol/l and substituting in the following equation to derive the bicarbonate requirement:

HCO_3^- requirement (mmol/l) = 0.3 ×
Body weight (kg) × Base deficit (mmol/l)

This equation allows calculation of the bicarbonate deficit in extracellular fluid, which is presumed to be some 30% (0.3) of body weight. To continue the earlier example of the 500 kg horse with severe diarrhoea (see above under: 'Calculation of fluid and electrolyte losses'), if its plasma bicarbonate concentration was found to be very low, say 12 mmol/l, then its base deficit would be 25 − 12 = 13 mmol/l. By substituting in the above equation, its bicarbonate requirement would be 0.3 × 500 × 13 = 1950 mmol.

Since 1 g of $NaHCO_3$ yields 12 mmol HCO_3^-, the horse's requirement is $^{1950}/_{12}$ = 163 g, which can be given intravenously as a 5% solution over 30–45 minutes. It is standard practice to replace half the calculated deficit so that overcorrection is avoided. Further blood samples should be taken during treatment to monitor bicarbonate concentrations.

Plasma protein status

An identifiable drop in total plasma protein (TPP) concentration over time indicates protein loss during a disease process. In horses this is most usually associated with a protein-losing enteropathy in which there is a net albumin loss. Whole plasma replacement is indicated where continued protein losses are occurring, or where continued fluid therapy has resulted in the dilution of plasma proteins to a concentration below 40 g/l — in these cases subcutaneous oedema is likely to follow the drop in plasma osmotic pressure.

Assessment of the plasma protein requirement

The plasma volume of a horse is approximately 5% of its body weight and the normal range of TPP is approximately 60–70 g/l. Assuming a mean TPP of 65 g/l, a horse with a plasma concentration reduced to 40 g/l has a deficit of some 25 g/l.

From these suppositions, a 500 kg horse would have a plasma volume of 25 litre (5% of 500) and its total protein deficit would be 25 g/l × 25 = 625 g. If a suitable donor has a TPP of 70 g/l, then the volume of plasma required to replace 625 g protein is $^{625}/_{70}$ = 8.9 litres. In practice, half this volume would probably suffice.

In ideal circumstances, donor plasma should be compatible with the recipient's red cells. Unfortunately, routine cross-matching only demonstrates plasma agglutinins (i.e. the positive test end-point is agglutination), whereas many equine erythrocyte alloantibodies act as haemolysins and do not show on routine tests. Compatibility testing is therefore a sophisticated *in vitro* procedure which is limited to specialist laboratories and is impractical in the field. In general terms, however, the risks associated with an initial plasma transfusion are minimal in horses, particularly if the donor is genetically similar to the recipient.

Common conditions affecting fluid and electrolyte balance

Examples of the common conditions of the adult horse which require investigation and treatment for fluid and electrolyte imbalance are given below.

Reduced water intake

Any disease process associated with reduced water and food intake will inevitably produce signs of progressive dehydration. In these circumstances the loss of Na^+ from the ECF is low, but K^+ deficits soon develop if the food intake is reduced.

Clinical assessment: clinical signs of dehydration will not develop until after 2–3 days of deprivation.

Clinical pathology: in the early stages clinical pathology will be unremarkable, but after 2–3 days there will be modest increases in PCV, TPP and serum or plasma Na^+, K^+ and Cl^-.

Requirement: within one or two days of the onset of deprivation, oral fluids are sufficient to meet the daily requirement. After 3 days the patient will have developed more severe dehydration, which must be treated initially with an intravenous polyionic replacement fluid, followed by oral maintenance fluid (50–100 ml/kg/day).

Comments on oral and maintenance fluids

- Fluid administration by stomach tube is generally advocated in cases of mild dehydration, but only when intestinal absorption is not compromised by ileus, obstruction or severe gastroenteritis.
- Depending on the size of horse, 4–10 litres can be given at frequent intervals during the day (per 2–3 hours if necessary).
- Oral fluid formulations should be isotonic or hypotonic. Hypertonic fluid given orally to a hypovolaemic horse will cause a net movement of fluid into the gut lumen.
- If maintenance with an intravenous fluid is required over several days, continued use of a polyionic replacement fluid will lead to the high sodium load being excreted, together with water, thus defeating the object of rehydration. Where there has been more water than electrolyte loss (as in water deprivation or inappetance), water is the main requirement and the use of 5% dextrose provides an isotonic source of electrolyte-free fluid. However, flow rates for 5% dextrose in water should not be greater than 1–2 l/hour, otherwise the renal threshold is exceeded and osmotic diuresis follows.
- In an inappetant horse the potassium requirement increases daily. Oral supplementation is beneficial in these circumstances and may be given as 50 g (equivalent to 675 mmol of potassium) per 500 kg in several litres of water by nasogastric tube, 2–3 times daily.

Colic

Fluid, electrolyte and acid–base disturbances are associated with those acute colics in which fluid is sequestered in the gut lumen and/or there is associated strangulation. Examples include all forms of high obstruction, and displacement with torsion of the large intestine.

Clinical assessment: the clinical signs of colic will be coupled with signs of hypovolaemia.

Clinical pathology: the PCV and TPP are raised, indicating dehydration, but serum or plasma Na^+, K^+ and Cl^- may register normal. If plasma bicarbonate estimations are possible, these will be seen to be low in cases of severe circulatory disturbance (metabolic acidosis).

Requirements: intravenous polyionic replacement fluid, with or without a plasma volume expander to counter shock. If bicarbonate estimations are possible, isotonic $NaHCO_3$ may be indicated.

Comments on replacement fluids

- Polyionic solutions are the replacement fluids of choice since their composition closely resembles that of the ECF. This type of solution is largely confined to the extracellular space and provides expansion of the plasma volume.
- The rate of administration in adults should be 3–5 l/hour, but where there are signs of hypovolaemic shock, a more rapid infusion of fluid is required to increase intravascular pressure (10–12 l/hour). However, it should be remembered that fluids delivered this quickly tend to be excreted rapidly before

redistribution to other fluid compartments can occur.

- As well as providing a source of bicarbonate precursor, such as lactate, polyionic solutions will frequently improve peripheral perfusion and produce a marked reduction in acid–base abnormalities. For this reason, specific bicarbonate treatment may not be indicated in colic or shock. If facilities for acid–base determinations are not available, $NaHCO_3$ should be used with caution and limited to 1–2 mmol/kg body weight.

- Normal saline (0.9%) is not appropriate for administration in most clinical circumstances because both the sodium and chloride concentrations are considerably higher than those found in horse plasma. Saline can induce hypokalaemia (by dilution of existing blood K^+), hyperchloraemia (by excess supplementation of Cl^-) and metabolic acidosis (by promoting hyperchloraemia and diluting out blood bicarbonate). In addition, it lacks the bicarbonate precursors that are often added to proprietary polyionic fluids.

Diarrhoea

The extent of fluid and electrolyte losses and the development of acidosis depend upon the severity of the enteric lesion and whether or not the patient continues to drink during the illness.

Clinical signs: clinical signs of dehydration will be minimal in mild cases, but signs of toxaemia and dehydration will accompany severe diarrhoea.

Clinical pathology: mild cases in which the patient is not systemically ill and continues to drink will hardly affect clinicopathological parameters. In severe cases the PCV will increase as a result of dehydration and the serum or plasma electrolytes will be depressed due to enteric loss. There may be an associated loss of albumin to the gut, so that the TPP may not markedly increase with dehydration. If plasma bicarbonate estimations are possible, these will be low in severe cases.

Requirements: in mild cases, oral fluids may be sufficient. At most, intravenous polyionic fluids would be required for replacement, followed by oral fluids for maintenance. Severe cases require intravenous polyionic infusions for replacement and possibly plasma volume expanders to counter shock. When plasma protein concentrations are low, donor plasma can be used as a volume expander. If plasma bicarbonate estimations are possible, isotonic $NaHCO_3$ may be indicated.

NB The large potassium deficits which can accompany diarrhoea cannot be replaced by intravenous infusion. If clinical circumstances permit, oral supplementation of potassium is preferable (see above under: 'Comments on oral and maintenance fluids').

Exertional dehydration

Endurance exertion over relatively short distances is unlikely to be associated with clinical signs of dehydration. Exertion over long distances in which there is also profuse sweating may produce clinicopathological evidence of dehydration with falls in Na^+ and especially K^+ and Cl^-.

Requirements: mild cases simply require oral fluids. More extreme cases require intravenous polyionic replacement fluid.

NB On occasion, hypocalcaemia is also associated with long distance exertion and results in an increase in neuromuscular irritability (see Chapter 5: 'Endocrine diseases').

Further reading

Vaala WE, Johnston JK, Marr CM and Orsini JA (1995) Intensive care. In: *The Equine Manual* pp. 737–755. London: W.B. Saunders.

12 Respiratory diseases

I. Practical techniques: upper respiratory tract

Diseases of the upper and lower respiratory tracts are common in horses. This chapter describes practical techniques for the diagnosis of these conditions using equipment which is available to the practising veterinary surgeon.

Endoscopy

Endoscopy allows direct visualization of many parts of the respiratory tract, and the use of flexible fibreoptic or videoendoscopic equipment has become an essential component in the evaluation of respiratory tract diseases. The parts of the tract that are accessible to examination are determined by the equipment available. Although a narrow 1 or 1.2 m endoscope will permit examination of most parts of the upper respiratory tract in adult horses, it is unlikely to have sufficient length to allow examination of the bronchial tree — an instrument of 2 m or longer (such as a human colonoscope) is needed for bronchoscopy. Fine paediatric endoscopes may be required for foals. Adequate disinfection of the instrument between horses is essential to prevent cross-infection by pathogens.

Technique

The horse is restrained as necessary. A nose twitch is usually sufficient, and this helps stabilize the head. Chemical sedation is sometimes required, but this should be avoided where functional assessment of the larynx or palatal arch is needed. It is helpful to have three people to perform the examination: one holds the horse and twitch; one stabilizes the endoscope at the nostril, and one has charge of the controls. For routine examinations, the endoscope is introduced through one nostril and passed along the ventral nasal meatus.

The regions of the tract that can be examined can be conveniently divided into seven areas:

- Nasal chambers
- Nasopharynx
- Auditory tube diverticula (guttural pouches)
- Palatal arch
- Epiglottis
- Larynx
- Trachea and bronchi.

Nasal chambers

The ventral nasal meatus and ventral concha (Fig.12.1) are examined as the endoscope is advanced to the nasopharynx. However, detailed examination of these areas is more easily performed as the instrument is slowly withdrawn towards the nose. As the endoscope is retracted within the nasopharynx to the choana, dorsal deviation of the tip will allow

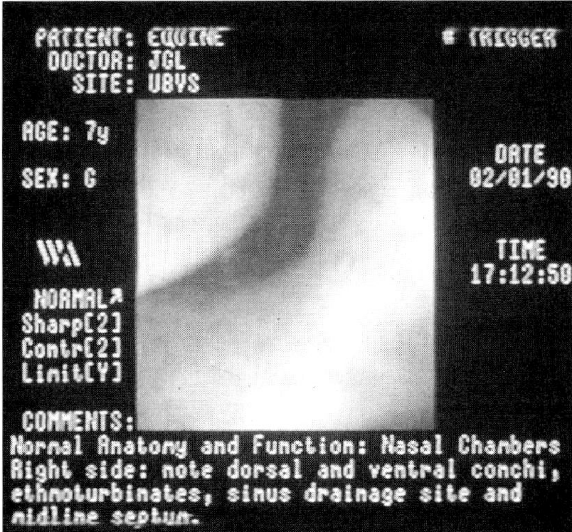

Figure 12.1 Endoscopic view of the ventral nasal meatus and ventral concha.

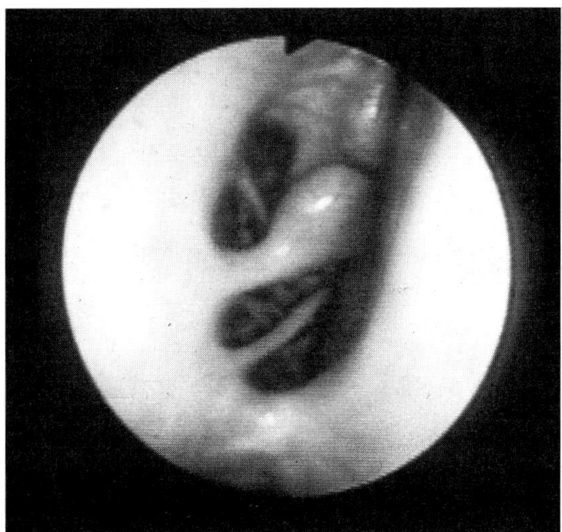

Figure 12.2 Endoscopic view of the ethmoidal labyrinth and great ethmoturbinate.

examination of the ethmoidal labyrinth and great ethmoturbinate (Fig.12.2). The naso-maxillary opening of the paranasal sinuses opens into the lateral wall of the middle meatus in this region. Although this opening cannot be examined directly, discharges originating within the sinuses may be seen streaming into the nasal cavity here. Progressive *ethmoidal haematomas* commonly occur in the region of the ethmoidal labyrinth, and appear as a grey/green mass protruding rostrally into the middle nasal meatus.

The middle nasal meatus can also be examined from the nares, but it is narrower than the ventral meatus, and is easily traumatized if the endoscope is forced along it. The conchal surfaces should be examined for fungal plaques, ulcers, masses, etc. Paranasal sinus disease may result in distension of the conchi and narrowing of the meati. Nasal septal disease (deviation, cysts, thickening, etc.) may be observed.

Nasopharynx

The walls of the nasopharynx and pharyngeal recess commonly show *hyperplastic lymphoid nodules* in young horses up to 5 years of age (Fig. 12.3). This is considered to be a normal finding, but it can result in adventitious respiratory noises if excessive.

Pharyngeal paralysis is an important cause of dysphagia and nasal return of food. Endoscopically this appears as sagging of the pharyngeal walls, persistent dorsal displacement of the soft palate and dissemination of food debris/saliva within the nasopharynx.

Guttural pouches

Examination of the guttural pouches is possible by introducing the endoscope from the ventral nasal meatus into the nasopharynx, and passing it in a dorsal direction under the cartilaginous flap of the auditory tube (Fig. 12.4). A flexible wire leader, passed down the biopsy channel of the instrument, is passed under the flap first, and used to elevate the flap by rotation of the endoscope, thus allowing entry of the endoscope itself into the auditory tube. A rotating movement as the endoscope is advanced facilitates this entry. The endoscope is then advanced into the pouch. Each pouch is divided into medial and lateral compartments by the stylohyoid bone. The medial pouch (Fig. 12.5) is larger than the lateral pouch, and coursing along its caudolateral wall are several important structures including the internal carotid artery, the cranial cervical ganglion, the

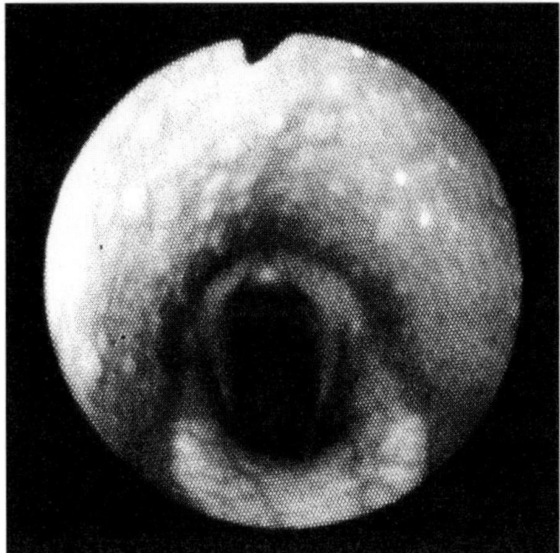

Figure 12.3 Endoscopic view of the nasopharyngeal wall of a young adult horse showing hyperplasia of the lymphoid follicles.

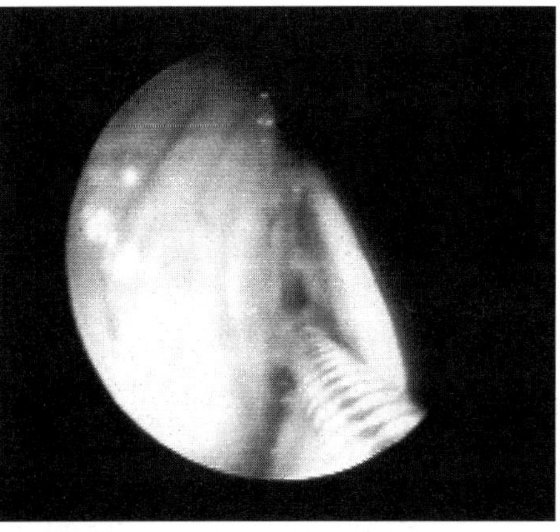

Figure 12.4 Endoscopy of the guttural pouch. A lead wire is passed underneath the cartilaginous flap of the auditory tube to aid subsequent passage of the endoscope into the tube.

vagus, the glossopharyngeal, hypoglossal, spinal accessory and sympathetic nerves.

Palatal arch

The soft palate is a continuous sheet which forms the floor of the nasopharynx. Its free (caudal) border normally lies beneath the epiglottis (Fig. 12.6) and is therefore obscured from view unless it becomes displaced dorsally during swallowing (Fig. 12.7). Congenital

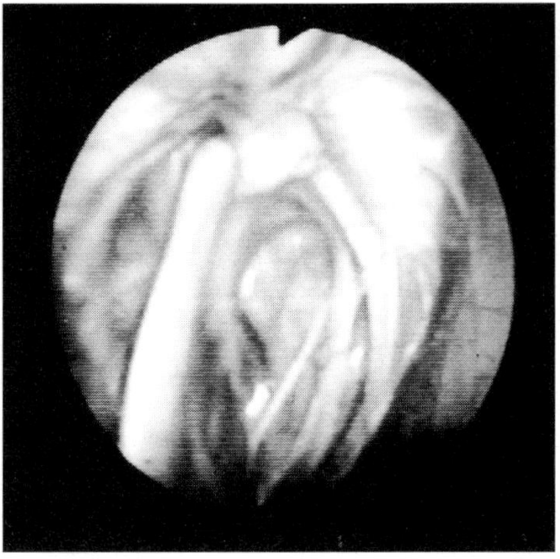

Figure 12.5 Endoscopic view of the medial compartment of the guttural pouch.

lesions of the soft palate are a cause of nasal reflux of milk in foals. They are readily diagnosed endoscopically — the defect allows direct visualization of the oral cavity from the nasopharynx.

Laryngopalatal dislocation

Laryngopalatal dislocation (dorsal displacement of the soft palate) involves movement of the free caudal edge of the palate dorsal to the epiglottis. In performance horses this condition results in exercise intolerance associated with an adventitious respiratory noise (gurgling). The condition is usually intermittent and cannot be diagnosed at rest. At a specialist centre, endoscopy during exercise on a high-speed treadmill may allow an accurate diagnosis. Horses twitched for endoscopy often displace the soft palate initially, but it usually returns to its normal position after swallowing. Frequent displacement of the palate or many unsuccessful swallowing attempts to correct it at rest are suspicious of laryngopalatal dislocation, but not diagnostic. Similarly, billowing and displacement of the soft palate during nostril occlusion, with difficulty of replacement, are also suspicious.

Pharyngeal cysts

Pharyngeal cysts are most commonly located in the subepiglottic tissue, and they are usually visible by endoscopy, but occasionally cysts

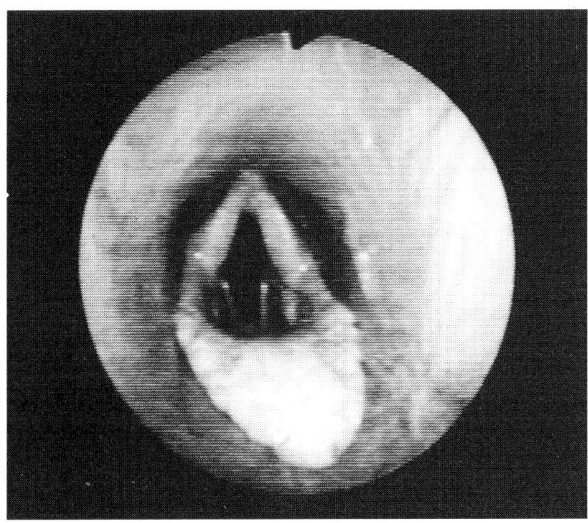

Figure 12.6 Endoscopic view of the soft palate. The caudal border lies beneath and is obscured by the epiglottis. The epiglottis has a serrated edge and fine vessels are visible on its dorsal surface.

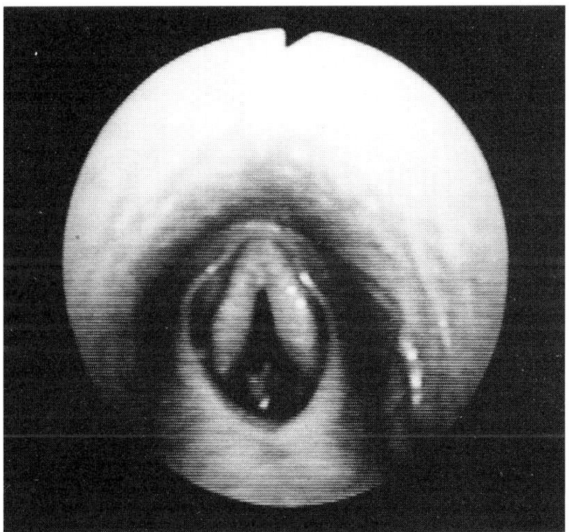

Figure 12.7 Endoscopic view of the soft palate in its dorsally displaced position. The caudal border is visible, since it has become displaced above the epiglottis.

may be obscured by the caudal margin of the soft palate.

Epiglottis

The epiglottis is a leaf-like structure that projects rostrodorsally from the base of the larynx. The edge is serrated, and the dorsal surface possesses fine arcuate blood vessels (Fig. 12.6). *Epiglottic entrapment* involves the dorsal reflection of subepiglottic tissue and arytenoepiglottic folds over the epiglottis, thus obscuring its apex, lateral margins and dorsal surface. Endoscopically, the outline of the epiglottis is visible, but the serrated edges and dorsal vessels are obscured by the entrapping tissue. Hypoplasia of the epiglottis resulting in reduced length, width and thickness of the epiglottis can be assessed subjectively by endoscopy, but requires radiography to confirm the diagnosis. The condition predisposes to epiglottic entrapment and laryngopalatal subluxation.

Larynx

The larynx is viewed from the nasopharynx, but the eccentric position of the endoscope invariably produces a degree of perceived asymmetry of the rima glottidis. If uncertainty about the significance of slight asymmetry exists, the procedure should be performed via each nostril in turn.

In most normal horses, an endoscope can be introduced into the larynx and trachea without inducing a severe cough response. However, in horses affected by lower airway disease, the cough reflex may be very sensitive and paroxysmal coughing occurs. In these cases, the topical application of diluted lignocaine solution (50:50 sprayed over the larynx via a catheter passed down the biopsy channel) will abolish this response.

Trachea and bronchi

The trachea (Fig. 12.8) can be examined in its entirety if a sufficiently long endoscope is used (>1.8 m). Strictures of the tracheal lumen (congenital, iatrogenic or traumatic) can be observed, although radiography may yield more useful information. Discharges often accumulate at the thoracic inlet, and their nature (mucus, purulent material, blood) can be assessed and samples obtained by aspiration (see below). A haemorrhagic discharge observed after exercise is suggestive of *exercise-induced pulmonary haemorrhage.*

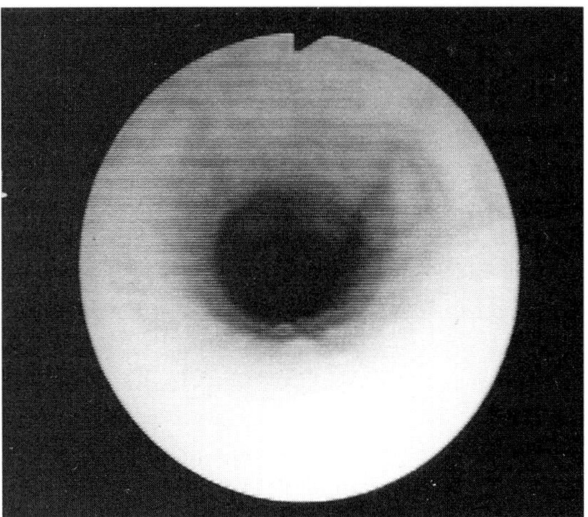

Figure 12.8   Endoscopic view of the trachea.

Foreign bodies such as brambles may lodge in the distal trachea/main bronchi and are an uncommon cause of chronic coughing — they can usually be identified and retrieved by endoscopy.

The bronchial tree can be examined as far as the length and diameter of the endoscope permits. The carina (Fig. 12.9) normally presents as a sharp angle at the junction of the right and left principal bronchi. Thickening of the angle (owing to mucosal oedema and inflammation) and hyperaemia may be seen in chronic lower airway diseases. A unilateral

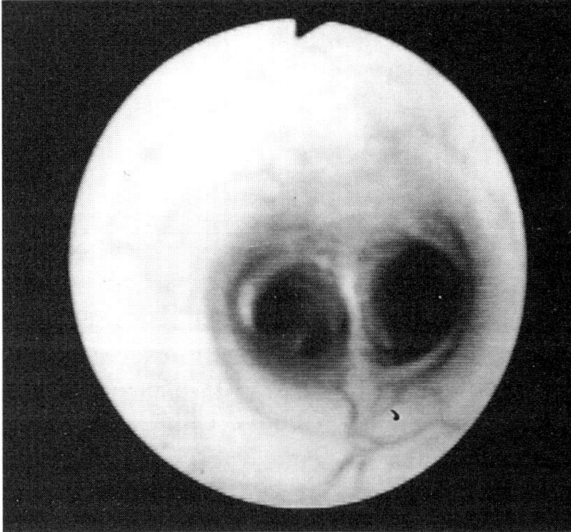

Figure 12.9   Endoscopic view of the carina and tracheal bifurcation.

purulent discharge draining from only one principal bronchus indicates a focal lung lesion on that side (e.g. focal pneumonia, pulmonary abscess or foreign body). Passage of the endoscope down the bronchial tree may induce significant coughing which renders the examination difficult. This reaction can be reduced by repeated infusions of small volumes of dilute lignocaine solution as the endoscope is advanced. The bronchial walls can be assessed for thickening, inflammation and collapse. Intraluminal masses are rarely diagnosed in the horse.

Examination of the paranasal sinuses

Percussion

The horse has five paired paranasal sinuses: frontal; sphenopalatine; ethmoidal; superior maxillary and inferior maxillary. Of these, the frontal and maxillary sinuses are the most important sites of disease. Percussion can be helpful in detecting fluid or space-occupying lesions, or in demonstrating pain in the region of the sinus. The fingers of one hand are tapped sharply over the bone overlying the sinus (Fig. 12.10). Changes in resonance will be more easily appreciated if the mouth is opened at the same time (e.g. by placing a finger in the interdental space). Comparison of resonance or pain reaction are made on both sides of the face. The topographical anatomy and areas of percussion of the frontal and maxillary sinuses are shown in Figures 12.11 and 12.12.

Endoscopy

The paranasal sinuses are interconnected and open into the middle meatus via the nasomaxillary ostium. This opening cannot be visualized directly but drainage of discharges from the opening into the nasal cavity may be observed by examining the caudal aspect of the middle nasal meatus (see endoscopy section above under: 'Nasal chambers'). Deformation of the nasal meati may occur in chronic sinus

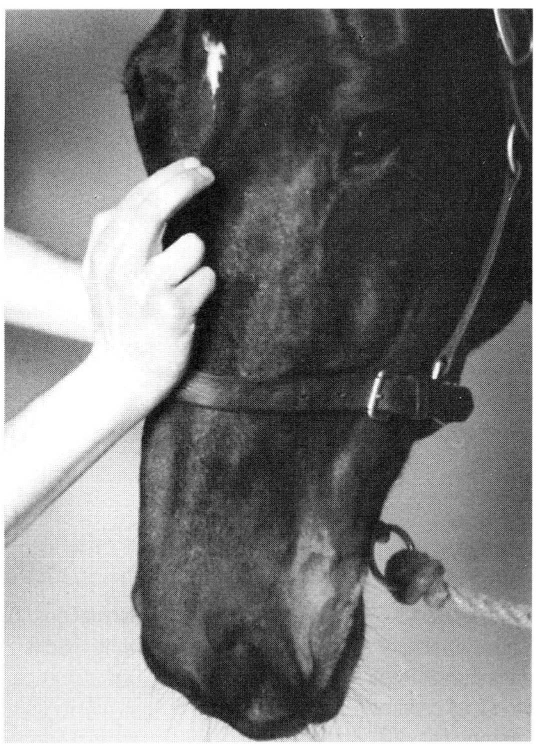

Figure 12.10   Percussion of the paranasal sinuses. The fingers of one hand are tapped sharply onto the bone overlying the sinus.

disease owing to expansion of the sinus cavities.

Sinus centesis

This allows the collection of fluid samples for cytology and culture. The precise site for centesis may be determined by clinical and radiographic features, but in cases of generalized sinus disease the sites shown in Figure 12.13 are satisfactory. The procedure is performed in the standing, sedated horse as follows:

- The site is clipped and prepared for aseptic surgery, and the skin is infiltrated with local anaesthetic. A 0.5 to 1.0 cm incision is made through the skin and subcutaneous tissues.
- A 2 mm Steinmann pin attached to a Jacob's chuck is used to drill a hole through the bone (Fig. 12.14). It may be necessary to displace the levator labii superioris muscle dorsally from the rostral maxillary site. In

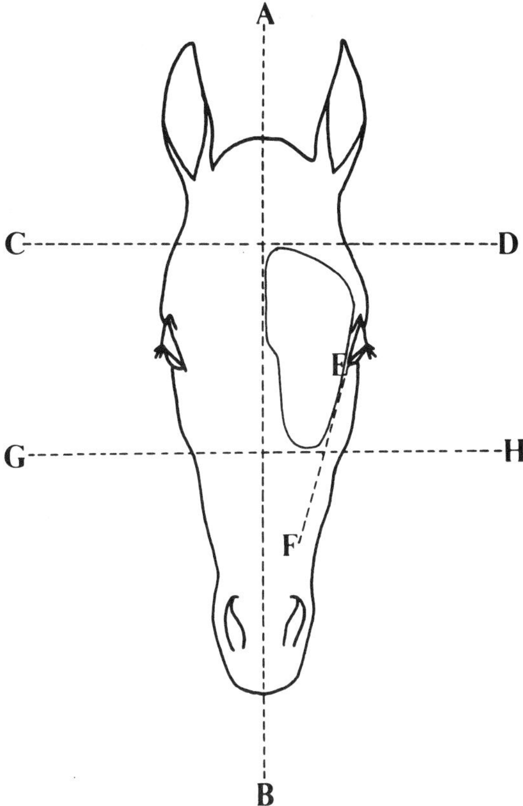

Figure 12.11   Topographical anatomy of the left frontal sinus. The left and right sinuses are separated by a bony septum in the midline of the head (A–B). The caudal margin of the frontal sinus is rostral to the temporomandibular joint at a line drawn through the middle of the zygomatic arches (C–D). The lateral margin is a line drawn from the medial canthus of the eye to the nasomaxillary notch (E–F). The rostral extent of the sinus lies on a line drawn between the midpoints of the medial canthus to the nasomaxillary notch on each side (G–H).

many horses with chronic paranasal sinus disease the overlying bone is sufficiently thinned to allow access into the sinus with a 16 gauge needle and there is no need for a prior drill hole.
- Fluid can be collected via a needle or polythene tubing (Fig. 12.15). Lavage with sterile saline may be helpful if the fluid content of the sinus is inaccessible or highly viscous.
- The centesis site is left to heal by second intention.

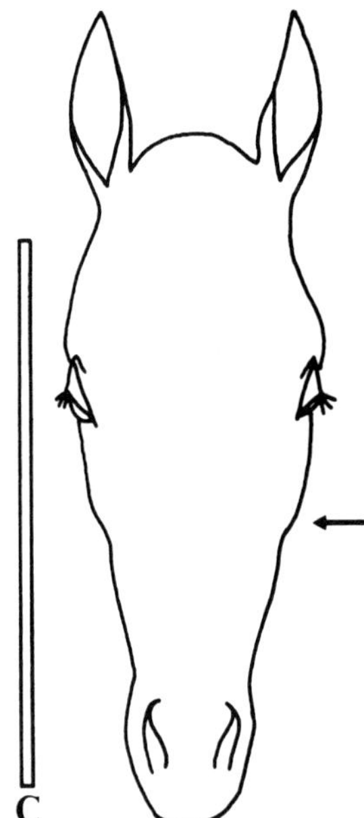

Figure 12.16   Lateral radiography of the paranasal sinuses and nasal cavity. The cassette (C) is placed alongside the head and the horizontal X-ray beam centred at the rostral limit of the facial crest.

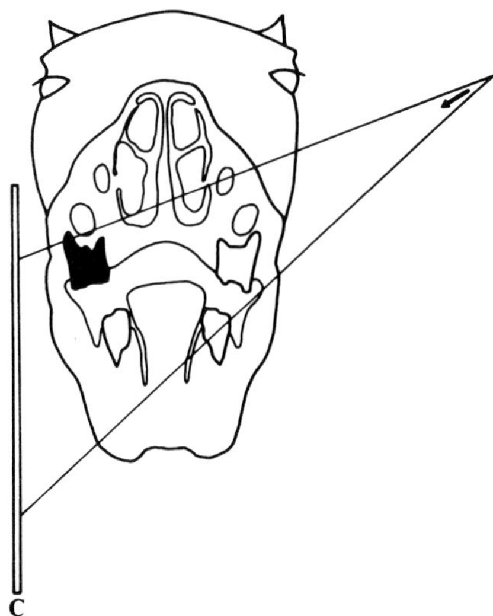

Figure 12.17   Thirty degree oblique radiography to demonstrate the roots of the maxillary cheek teeth. Cross section through the head at the level of the rostral end of the facial crest. The cassette (C) is placed on the affected side, and the X-ray beam angled down from the contralateral side. The maxillary cheek teeth and roots of the affected side (shaded) will be highlighted on the film away from the other teeth.

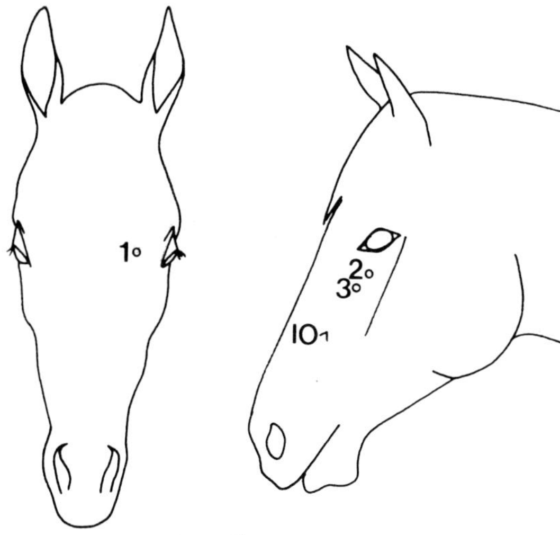

Figure 12.18   Recommended portal locations for endoscopic examination of the paranasal sinuses. (1) Frontal sinus: 60% of the distance laterally from the midline to the medial canthus, and 0.5 cm caudal to the medial canthus. (2) Caudal maxillary sinus: 2 cm rostral and 2 cm ventral to the medial canthus. (3) Rostral maxillary sinus: halfway between the rostral end of the facial crest to the level of the medial canthus, and 1 cm ventral to a line joining the infraorbital foramen (IO) and the medial canthus.

Comments

- The trephine hole will heal rapidly by granulation and second intention healing, and requires minimal aftercare other than daily cleaning with dilute antiseptic solution.

- If the trephine hole is to be used for daily medication or flushing, the opening should be plugged with a rolled plug of sterile gauze to delay healing (Fig. 12.24).

Examination of the guttural pouches

Endoscopy

Evidence of possible guttural pouch disease may be apparent by routine endoscopic examination of the pharynx (see above under: 'Endoscopy'). The following observations might be suggestive of guttural pouch disease:

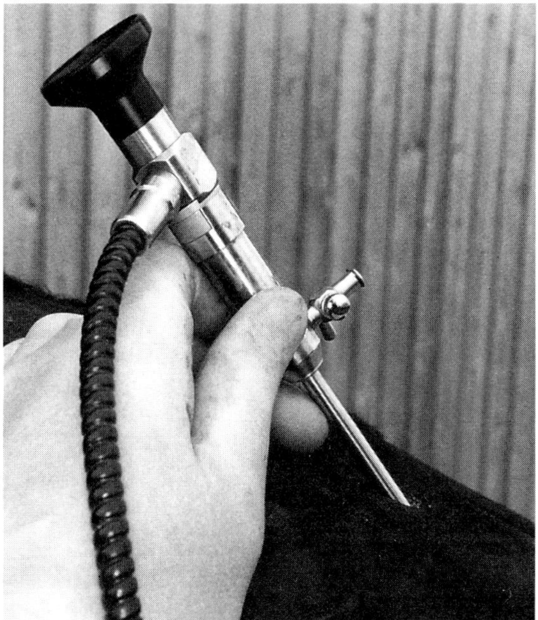

Figure 12.19 Direct sinus endoscopy. A rigid arthroscope has been introduced into the frontal sinus via a small trephine hole.

- Blood or pus draining from the opening of one or both auditory tubes into the pharynx
- Pharyngeal paralysis
- Laryngeal hemiplegia
- Collapse of the pharyngeal roof

Guttural pouch mycosis may be confirmed by the identification of a mycotic plaque within the pouch. In most cases, the mycosis affects the dorso-medial wall of the pouch over the internal carotid artery. Extreme care must be exercised when examining horses with potential guttural pouch mycosis, especially those with a history or evidence of haemorrhage. The presence of free blood/haematoma within the pouch hinders the examination, and care must be taken to ensure that the endoscope does not dislodge a blood clot over the artery that could initiate further haemorrhage. The degree of neurological dysfunction (pharyngeal paralysis; laryngeal hemiplegia) should be assessed prior to undertaking treatment of mycotic disease.

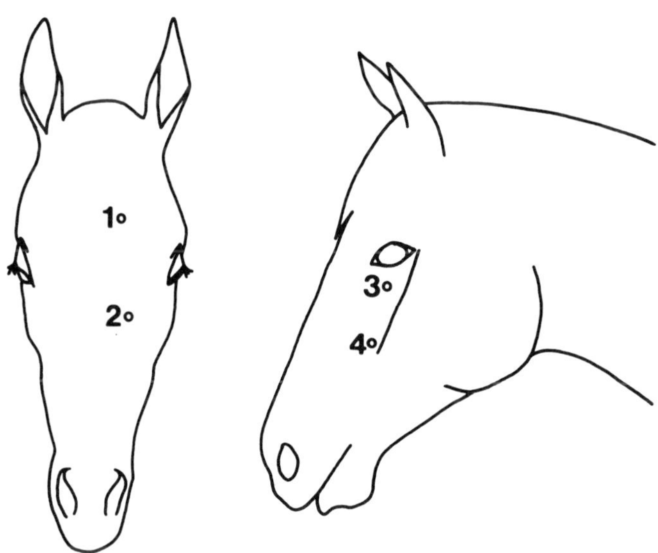

Figure 12.20 Routine sites for sinus trephination. (1) Frontal sinus (frontal portion): 4 cm from the midline on a line joining the supraorbital processes. (2) Frontal sinus (turbinate portion): 5 cm from the midline at a level 3–4 cm caudal to the rostral end of the facial crest. (3) Caudal maxillary sinus: 2.5–3 cm dorsal to the facial crest, and 2.5–3 cm rostral to the medial canthus; as far into the angle formed between the rim of the bony orbit and the facial crest as possible. (4) Rostral maxillary sinus: 2.5 cm caudal and 3.5 cm dorsal to a point at the rostral limit of the facial crest. NB in young horses this opening will be adjacent to the cheek teeth and there will be minimal access to the sinus.

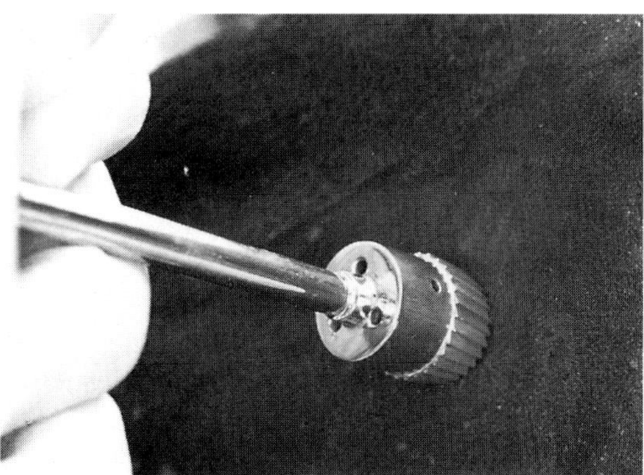

Figure 12.21 Trephination (caudal maxillary sinus). The trephine is pressed against the skin to mark the site of the skin incision.

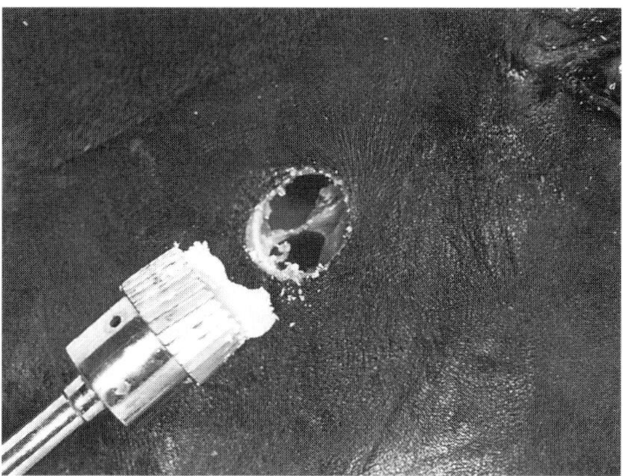

Figure 12.23 Trephination. The trephine is used to create a window in the bone, allowing entry into the sinus cavity.

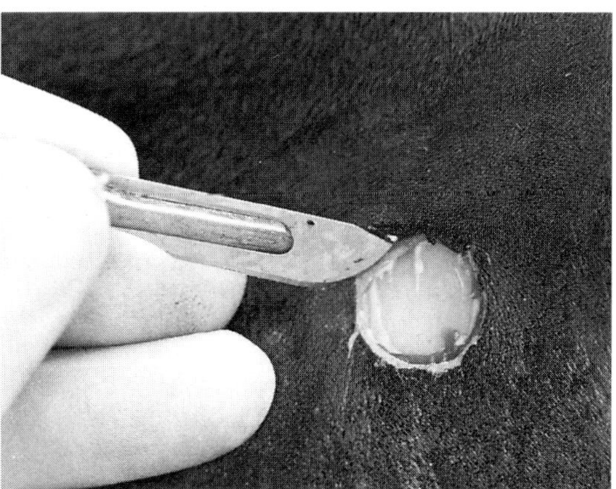

Figure 12.22 Trephination. The skin, subcutaneous tissue and fascia are excised to reveal the surface of the bone.

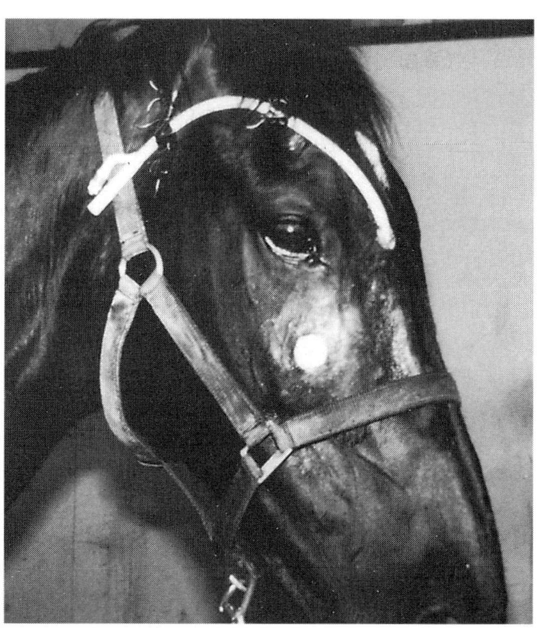

Figure 12.24 Trephine hole into the rostral maxillary sinus plugged with sterile cotton gauze to prevent too rapid healing. A Foley catheter is secured in the frontal sinus via another trephine hole to permit medication/flushing.

Endoscopy can provide limited information about conditions such as tympany, empyema and chondroids. Although these diseases may be confirmed by endoscopy, other techniques, especially radiography, will supply more useful information. Diverticulitis is recognized as a generalized inflammation of the walls of the pouches, and may be associated with neuropathies such as pharyngeal and laryngeal paralysis.

Catheterization

A catheter can be passed into the guttural pouch either blindly or under endoscopic guidance to allow the collection of samples for cytology and culture.

If a catheter is to be inserted blindly, the distance from the nostril to the opening of the auditory tube (which corresponds to the level of the lateral canthus of the eye) should be marked on the catheter. The catheter should be stiffened by threading it over a wire guide which has a 30 degree curve at the distal 2 cm level. The catheter is passed along the ventral nasal meatus until the mark reaches the nose. The curved end is turned laterally and the catheter advanced under the flap-like opening of the auditory tube. This is facilitated if the catheter is advanced as the horse swallows. Entry into the auditory tube is recognized by a lack of resistance as the catheter is advanced into the pouch.

Radiography

Air within the guttural pouches provides a good, natural radiographic contrast agent which makes radiography a useful clinical technique in the assessment of guttural pouch disease. Standing lateral views are taken in the same manner as for the paranasal sinuses (see above). The medial and lateral compartments of the pouches can be identified. Fluid lines may be seen in cases of empyema or haemorrhage. Chondroids can also be identified. Compression by retropharyngeal masses causes distortion of the outlines of the pouches. Abnormally large air-filled pouches are seen in cases of guttural pouch tympany.

Examination of the larynx

Palpation

The index fingers of each hand are pushed under the tendon of the sternocephalicus muscle on either side of the neck, and the cranial dorsal larynx in the region of the muscular process is palpated. In advanced cases of idiopathic laryngeal hemiplegia, atrophy of the dorsal cricoarytenoid muscle on the left side makes the muscular process more prominent.

Arytenoid depression test

The first and second fingers of both hands are located over the muscular processes of the arytenoids, which are then depressed. In horses with laryngeal hemiplegia, this results in a stridorous respiratory noise. The test is best performed shortly after exercise. Vibration of the left arytenoid cartilage may also be detected at this time in horses with left laryngeal hemiplegia.

Slap test

This test is used to assess the adductor function of the arytenoids. The response can be evaluated either by palpating the muscular process or by visualizing the larynx by endoscopy. An assistant gently slaps the horse on one side of the thorax; this results in a reflex movement or flicking of the contralateral muscular process resulting in adduction of the corniculate process and vocal cord. In a horse with left laryngeal hemiplegia, the flicking of the left muscular process in response to slapping the right thorax is diminished or absent. In normal horses, the response of both arytenoids is symmetrical. The test should be performed while the horse is breathing quietly and during expiration.

Endoscopy

Endoscopy is used to view the larynx and to evaluate the range of movement of the arytenoid cartilages. The procedure may need to be performed at rest and after exercise. Examination during exercise on a treadmill may be particularly helpful in subtle cases of laryngeal hemiplegia.

The larynx is viewed by passing the endoscope along the ventral meatus in the usual way. The visible parts of the larynx are assessed for gross abnormalities of structure (e.g. arytenoid chondritis) and evidence of previous surgical interference (e.g. absence of one or both laryngeal ventricles). The paralaryngeal structures (epiglottis, palatine arch and pharyngeal walls) are also evaluated.

The symmetry of the glottis and positions of the corniculate processes and vocal cords are examined at rest. In cases of laryngeal hemiplegia where the paralysis is complete, the affected arytenoid cartilage shows little or no movement and is displaced (along with the vocal cord) to the midline (Figs. 12.25 and 12.26). The opening to the laryngeal ventricle on the affected side is more obvious.

The depth of respiration and degree of arytenoid abduction during expiration can be increased by temporary occlusion of the nostrils or the injection of a respiratory stimulant (e.g. doxapram hydrochloride). Observation of arytenoid adduction following stimulation of swallowing (e.g. by flushing water through the endoscope) is also useful. Asynchronous abduction of the arytenoids is not in its own right regarded as abnormal, provided that both arytenoid cartilages can abduct maximally. However, a deficient, exaggerated or biphasic arytenoid abduction is abnormal.

Comment

- In horses with mild degrees of laryngeal hemiplegia, abnormalities of arytenoid abduction may be difficult to detect at rest. These horses should be reassessed immediately after strenuous exercise or, at specialist centres, during exercise on a high speed treadmill. During or immediately after

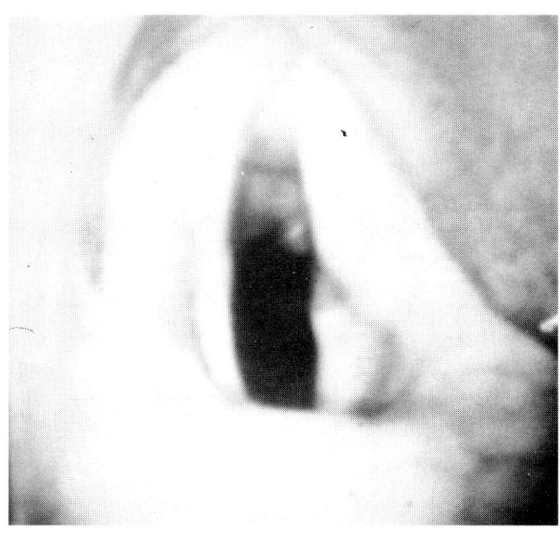

Figure 12.26 Endoscopic view of larynx with left laryngeal hemiplegia. The left arytenoid cartilage and vocal cord are displaced towards the midline.

exercise a normal horse will have a symmetrically dilated larynx with both arytenoids at maximal abduction. In horses with laryngeal hemiplegia, the larynx will appear asymmetric, with incomplete abduction on the affected side.

Radiography

Standing lateral radiographs of the pharynx and larynx can provide useful additional information about the condition of the larynx and surrounding structures. The absence of one or both laryngeal ventricles indicates previous surgery (laryngeal ventriculectomy). Radiographic examination of the larynx prior to laryngeal prosthesis surgery may be helpful in identifying osseous metaplasia of the cartilages that might complicate the surgery. Dorsal displacement of the soft palate, sub-epiglottic cysts, epiglottic entrapment and rostral displacement of the palato-pharyngeal arch may all be diagnosed radiographically. In addition, epiglottic size and conformation can be assessed.

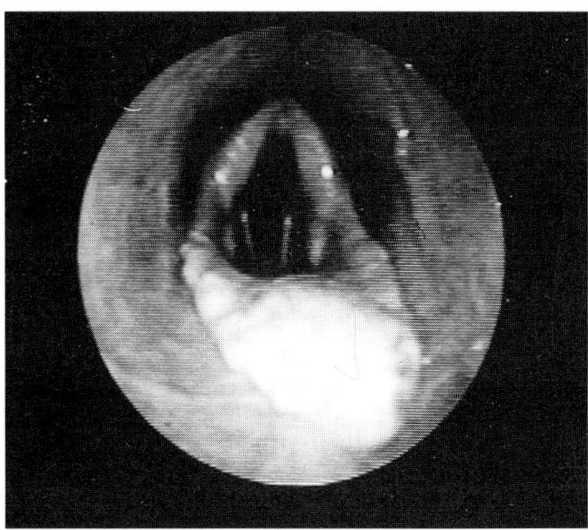

Figure 12.25 Endoscopic view of the normal resting larynx.

II. Practical techniques: lower respiratory tract

Auscultation

Auscultation of the trachea and chest should be performed in a quiet environment. Air movement sounds in the trachea are clear and well-defined with inspiratory sounds being similar to expiratory sounds. Referred sounds from both the upper and lower airways may be heard at the trachea. Gurgling/bubbling sounds can be heard over the distal cervical trachea of horses that have large amounts of lower airway secretions. The secretions tend to pool in the trachea in this region.

Lung sounds audible over the chest will vary depending on the body condition of the horse and the depth of breathing. Lung sounds may be difficult to appreciate in fat horses, whereas in thin horses many more sounds can be heard. Respiratory sounds can be accentuated by increasing the depth of breathing using a re-breathing bag (Fig. 12.27). A large reservoir bag, such as a plastic bin liner, is placed over the nostrils and the resulting accumulation of carbon dioxide in the air stimulates the depth of breathing. The bag can be left in place for a variable period depending on the response of the horse. Horses with chronic obstructive pulmonary disease (COPD) or pneumonia may cough paroxysmally when the bag is used, which limits its usefulness. Care should be taken when using the technique in horses with painful pleural conditions.

The normal caudal lung border runs in a gently curving line from the 18th rib, with the following landmarks (Fig. 12.28):

- 17th intercostal space — border level with the tuber coxae
- 13th intercostal space — border level with the mid thorax
- 11th intercostal space — border level with the point of shoulder; then curving down to the elbow

Airflow sounds in the chest are normally slightly louder on the right side than the left and inspiratory sounds are slightly louder than expiratory sounds. The sounds are most readily heard over the area of the carina where the large airways divide but air sounds at the lung periphery may be difficult to detect in normal horses. Comparisons should always be made between the left and right sides.

Intestinal sounds are commonly heard on

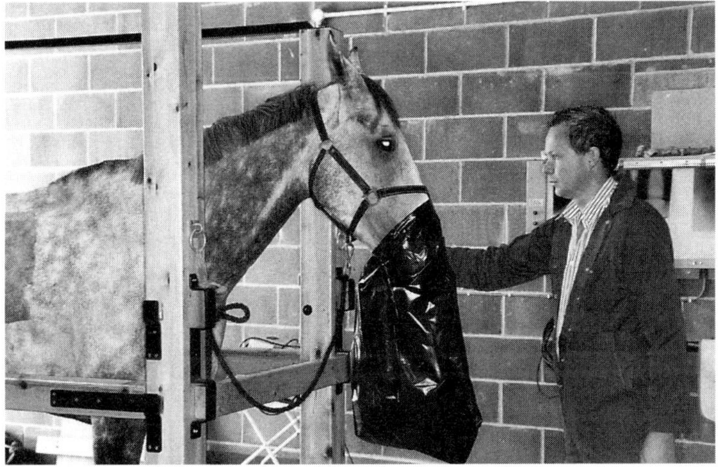

Figure 12.27   Use of a re-breathing bag. A reservoir bag is placed over the horse's nostrils and the horse allowed to breathe several times into and out of the bag until the depth of respiration is sufficiently increased.

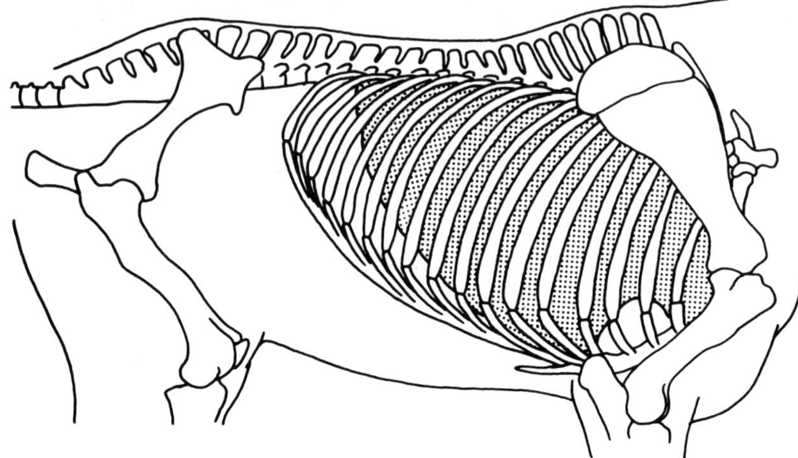

Figure 12.28
Topographical anatomy showing the relationship between the caudal border of the lung and the intercostal spaces.

thoracic auscultation which may mimic abnormal respiratory sounds, such as pleural rubbing sounds. True respiratory sounds will occur at the same phase of respiration with every breath, whereas intestinal sounds are random. It is therefore essential to watch the respiratory rhythm as the lungs are auscultated.

Abnormalities of normal airflow sounds

These include the following:

- A generalized increase in the intensity of sounds, e.g. mild COPD.
- The expiratory sounds are louder than inspiratory sounds, e.g. consolidation or pleural effusion (owing to increased transmission of large airway sounds).
- A localized or unilateral absence or decrease in the intensity of sounds, e.g. pulmonary or pleural abscess, pleural effusion.
- An abrupt change from soft to harsh sounds, e.g. effusion or consolidation.
- A bilateral absence of sounds in the ventral chest, e.g. bilateral pleural effusion (often accompanied by the radiation of heart sounds over a larger than normal area).
- The complete absence of sounds in the dorsal chest (uni or bilateral), e.g. pneumothorax.

Adventitious sounds

Adventitious airflow sounds are abnormal lung sounds which include crackles ('rales') and wheezes ('rhonchi').

Fine crackles are described as 'velcro-like' and tend to occur mainly during late inspiration — they can be heard in COPD and pulmonary oedema/congestive heart failure. Coarse crackles are popping sounds that occur during inspiration or expiration, and are commonly heard in COPD.

Wheezes are musical notes of varying pitch and duration. They occur in obstructive airway diseases, including COPD and bronchopneumonia, and may arise during inspiration or expiration.

Pleural friction (rubbing) sounds may be heard in pleuritis cases, although the sounds are lost when a significant effusion is present. These are usually fine crackling, crunching or creaking sounds that are heard mainly at end inspiration/early expiration.

Percussion of the chest

Percussion of the chest is particularly useful for the detection of pleural pain and effusions. The technique may be performed using a plexor and pleximeter, or with the fingers. When using the fingers, the first two fingers of one hand serve as a pleximeter (placed in an intercostal space), and the first two fingers of the other hand serve as a plexor to sharply tap the fingers of the first hand (Fig. 12.29). The area of percussion is similar to the area of auscultation, remembering that there is an area of cardiac dullness (larger on the left than the right) in the ventral thorax. The entire chest on both sides should be percussed working in parallel lines from dorsal to ventral and anterior to posterior. Normal lung tissue will sound resonant and hollow, whereas solid tissue or fluid will sound dull and flat.

Comment

- Pain on percussion is common in pleuritis cases, especially before large quantities of effusion have accumulated.

Aspiration of tracheal fluid

Transtracheal aspiration

This technique allows the aseptic collection of samples from the lower respiratory tract that are suitable for cytology and bacterial culture. The procedure is performed in the standing horse using restraint (twitch or sedation) as necessary. The procedure must be performed under aseptic conditions and sterile gloves should be worn by the operator. A small area over the middle to lower trachea is clipped and prepared aseptically. The technique is then as follows:

- A bleb of local anaesthetic is injected under the skin in the midline, and a small stab incision is made with a scalpel blade (Fig. 12.30).
- The trachea is grasped by one hand to stabilize it, and the tracheal lumen is entered by pushing a 12 to 14 gauge needle or catheter (directed downwards) through the skin incision and between two tracheal rings (Fig. 12.31). NB Care should be taken to avoid penetrating a cartilage ring or damaging the opposite wall of the trachea, and the bevel of the catheter/needle should face downwards. Once the tracheal lumen is entered, air may be heard passing in and out of the catheter/needle as the horse breathes.
- A 5 or 6 French gauge sterile dog urinary catheter is then passed through the catheter/ needle and threaded down the trachea until the end is at the level of the thoracic inlet (Figs 12.32 and 12.33).
- 30 to 50 ml of sterile saline (without any bacteriostatic agents) are injected through the catheter and immediately aspirated. Only a small proportion of the delivered fluid is likely to be retrieved. The position of

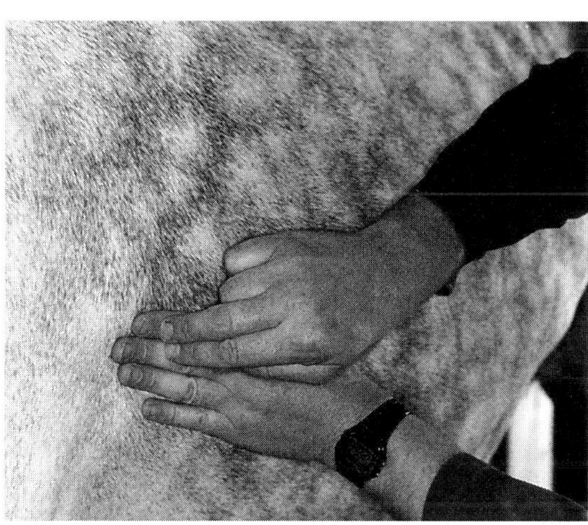

Figure 12.29   Chest percussion using the fingers of one hand to sharply tap the fingers of the other hand pressed against the chest wall.

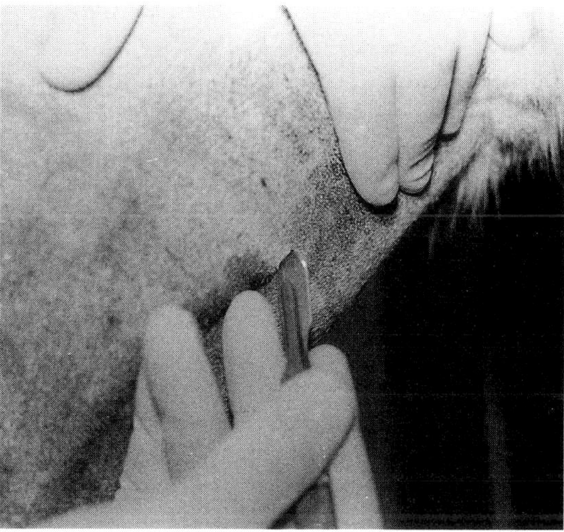

Figure 12.30   Transtracheal aspiration. A small stab incision is made through the skin in the midline over a bleb of local anaesthetic.

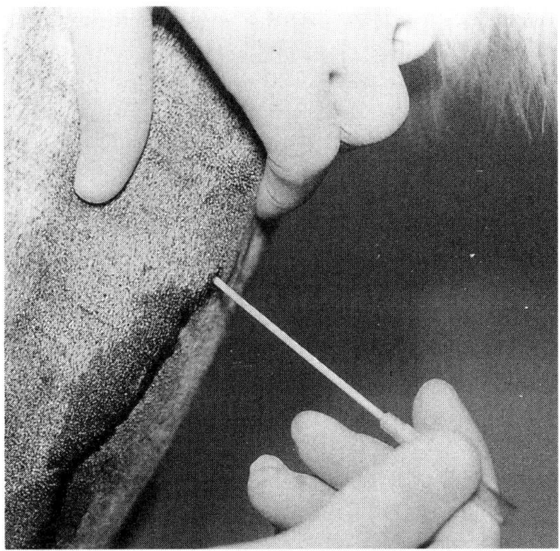

Figure 12.31   Transtracheal aspiration. A 12 gauge over-the-needle catheter is pushed between two tracheal rings into the tracheal lumen.

the urinary catheter may need to be adjusted several times, or the flushing/aspiration repeated until a satisfactory volume of fluid is recovered.

On completion of aspiration, the urinary catheter is removed, followed by the introducer catheter. However, if a needle is used as an

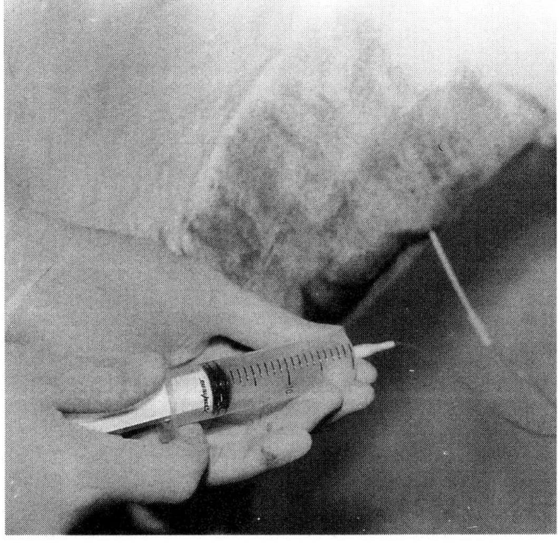

Figure 12.32   Transtracheal aspiration. A sterile dog urinary catheter is threaded into the tracheal lumen and lavage/aspiration performed with sterile saline.

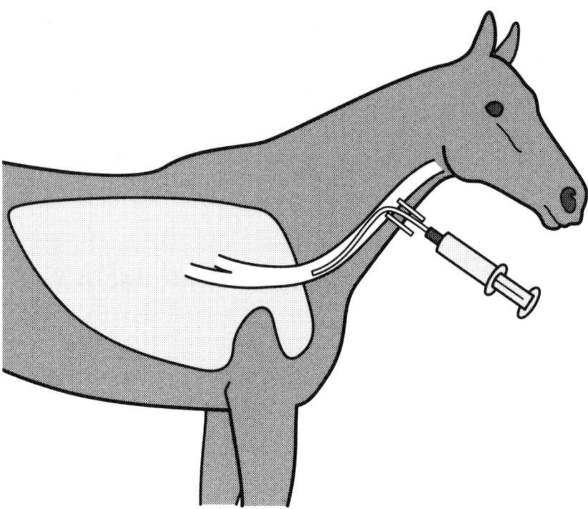

Figure 12.33   Diagram illustrating transtracheal aspiration. The catheter is passed until the distal tip is at the level of the thoracic inlet.

introducer, it should be removed with the urinary catheter to prevent it from cutting off the catheter tip within the trachea.

An alternative to the catheter, or needle and urinary catheter, is a commercially available 16 gauge through-the-needle catheter with 58 cm tubing. If this system is used, local anaesthesia and a stab incision are generally unnecessary.

Complications of transtracheal aspiration

The clinician should be aware of the potential complications of this technique:

- Damage to the tracheal cartilage, with resultant chronic infection.
- Breaking of the catheter within the trachea. Most horses will cough up the damaged catheter within 30 minutes without long-term sequelae.
- Breaking of the catheter in a subcutaneous site as a result of initial misplacement of the catheter/needle. The catheter must be removed surgically in these cases.
- Local infection/cellulitis at the site of tracheal puncture owing to contamination of the site by bacteria from the lower airways. In this instance hot fomentations, surgical drainage and appropriate antibiotic

therapy will be necessary. Routine prophylactic antibiotics given systemically or injected locally may prevent this complication, and should always be used if malodourous or frankly purulent material is aspirated.

Endoscopic tracheal aspiration

This procedure allows the collection of tracheal aspirate samples suitable for cytology. It relies on the availability of a sufficiently long endoscope (usually 2 m) to reach the distal cervical trachea.

A flexible endoscope is passed in the usual way via the nares into the trachea. When the tip has reached the distal trachea, a catheter is passed down the biopsy channel until it protrudes from the end. Thirty ml of sterile saline are injected through the catheter, which forms a pool at the thoracic inlet. The catheter tip is positioned into this pool and the sample is aspirated. Only a small proportion of the delivered fluid is likely to be retrieved.

Comment

- Samples collected in this way are suitable for cytology, but unsuitable for bacteriological culture since the endoscope is unavoidably contaminated by bacteria residing in the upper respiratory tract. Guarded aspiration catheters are available that will reduce the risk of contamination of samples obtained in this way.

Bronchoalveolar lavage (BAL)

This technique samples fluid and cells from the alveoli and distal airways. BAL is undertaken in the standing, sedated horse and may be performed using an endoscope or a 'blind' technique.

Cytology of BAL fluid provides a more accurate reflection of the state of the small airways and alveoli than that of tracheal aspirates. BAL is ideally suited to the assessment of diffuse lower airway and alveolar

diseases. When performed blindly, the segment of lung being lavaged is unknown, and the technique should, therefore, not be used in focal lung diseases. Endoscopy permits more accurate placement of the lavage tube, but the precise location can still be difficult to assess.

Endoscopic technique

A 2 m (or longer) endoscope is passed in the usual way to the carina and then into a mainstem bronchus. It is advanced down the bronchial tree until it wedges in an airway (usually about a fourth generation bronchus if an endoscope with an external diameter of 8 mm is being used). Lavage is performed via a catheter passed down the biopsy channel. NB Coughing can be severe as the endoscope passes down the bronchial tree, but this can be reduced by infusing a small volume of dilute lignocaine solution at each bronchial division.

The volume and type of fluid used for BAL is a matter of personal preference. Most clinicians use sterile saline, infused in 50 ml aliquots to a total volume of about 300 ml. The retrieval rate for this fluid varies, but is usually in the region of 75%.

Blind technique

Commercially available BAL tubes or homemade tubes fashioned for the purpose (Fig. 12.34) can be used when the technique is performed blind. The tube is passed in the same way as the endoscope until it lodges in a bronchus, at which point the lavage is carried out as above (Fig. 12.35).

Thoracic radiography

Thoracic radiographs can be helpful in the diagnosis and monitoring of chest diseases in foals (especially pneumonia), and some lung diseases (especially interstitial disease, pneumonia, neoplasia, etc.) and pleural diseases (effusions) in the adult. Rare earth intensifying screens and high speed radiographic film are necessary. The cassette should not be hand-

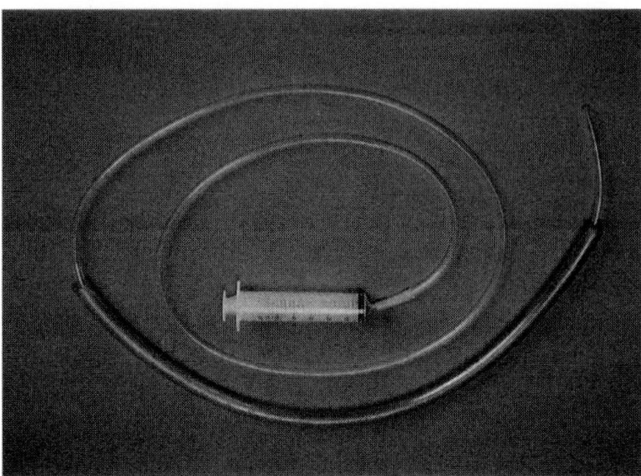

Figure 12.34   BAL tube consisting of a stomach tube (external diameter 12 mm) through which a smaller tube (external diameter 5 mm) is threaded. The small tube is lodged in a small bronchus, and the lavage/aspiration performed.

held, and can be suspended in a bag hanging from a drip stand. An air gap of approximately 25 cm between the patient and the film eliminates the need to use a grid. The horse must be standing perfectly still when the radiograph is taken, and sedation should be used if necessary.

In the foal, both lateral and ventrodorsal or dorsoventral projections can be used, and the entire chest may be covered by a single 35 x 43

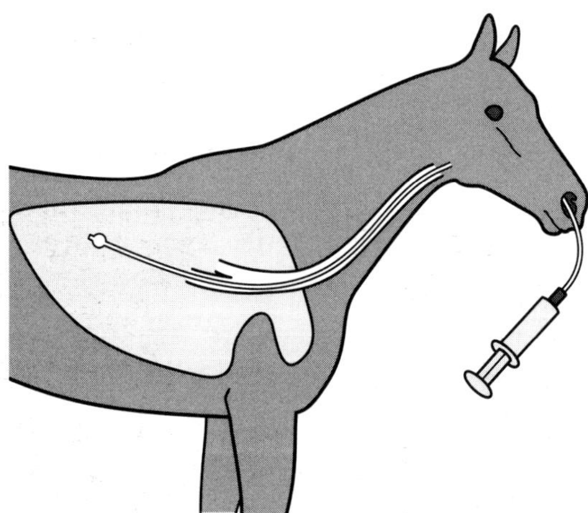

Figure 12.35   Diagram illustrating BAL performed with a balloon-tipped catheter. The catheter is passed via the nose, larynx and trachea into the bronchial tree. It is lodged in a small bronchus, and the balloon is inflated prior to performing lavage.

cm film. In the adult horse only lateral views are possible, and four overlapping views are often necessary to cover the entire thorax. A focus-film distance of 2 m is ideal, but if low power mobile or portable generators are used the distance may need to be reduced to 1 m in order to keep the exposure times short enough to avoid motion artefacts.

Good quality radiographs of a field which encompasses the caudodorsal lung area are possible using low output generators. This view enables detailed evaluation of peripheral lung tissue and third generation pulmonary vessels. Radiographic examination of other lung fields requires the use of powerful generators at specialist centres. See 'Further reading'.

Lung biopsy

Lung biopsy is indicated in diffuse pulmonary diseases of unknown aetiology such as disseminated nodular or widespread interstitial diseases. Solitary lung masses identified by radiography, ultrasonography or endoscopy can also be investigated by biopsy.

Parenchymal lung biopsies may be obtained either by a percutaneous route using a biopsy needle, or by a trans-bronchial technique via endoscopy using a grasping biopsy wire. Both techniques are performed in the standing horse.

Percutaneous technique

A 'Tru-Cut' biopsy needle (Baxter Healthcare Corporation, California) is suitable for the percutaneous technique. The selected site on the chest wall is clipped and prepared aseptically. In diffuse lung diseases the 7th or 8th intercostal space (left or right), approximately 8 cm above the level of the elbow joint, is recommended. The technique is as follows:

- The skin, intercostal muscles and pleura are infiltrated with local anaesthetic, and a 5 mm stab incision is made through the skin.
- The biopsy instrument is introduced through the intercostal space, avoiding the vessels and nerves that run along the caudal margins of the ribs (Fig. 12.36). The

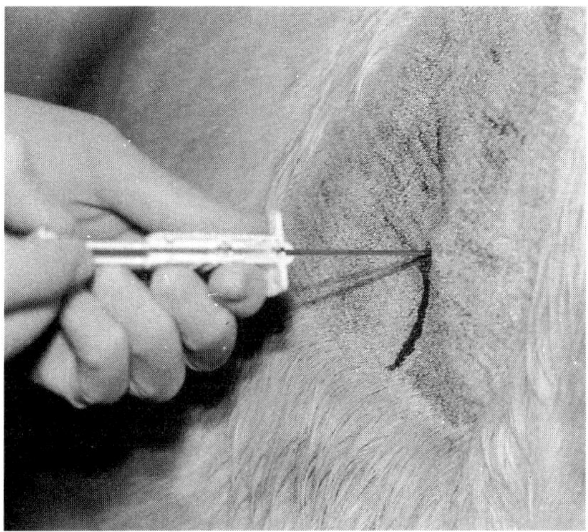

Figure 12.36   Percutaneous lung biopsy using a 'Tru-cut' biopsy needle.

needle can often be felt to 'pop' through the pleura.

- The needle is then inserted about 2 cm into the lung tissue, and the biopsy taken. Two or three biopsies are usually taken.
- The skin is sutured as necessary.

Comment

- Complications are rare with this technique, but could include haemorrhage and pneumothorax. Transient epistaxis or haemoptysis is sometimes observed following biopsy.

Trans-bronchial technique

An endoscope is passed in the same way as for BAL (above) until it lodges in a bronchus. The biopsy wire (jaws closed) is pushed down a small airway until resistance is met. The jaws are opened and the wire is advanced as far as possible prior to closing the jaws and retrieving the sample. Four to six repeat samples are usually taken. Biopsies of bronchial wall or endobronchial masses can also be obtained by this method.

Comment

- Samples obtained by the trans-bronchial route tend to have crushing artefacts that

may render histological interpretation difficult.

Ultrasonography of the chest

Ultrasonography is ideally suited to the investigation of pleural diseases, especially pleural effusions, where the technique can provide some clues as to the nature of the fluid (i.e. transudate or exudate), as well as the presence of adhesions and loculations. Consolidated lung, pulmonary abscesses and pulmonary masses may also be imaged if these lesions are adjacent to the pleural surface. Ultrasound waves are not transmitted through aerated lung (Fig. 12.37), so the technique is of little value in airway disease or focal lung diseases where the diseased area lies deep to the lung surface.

Either linear array or sector scanners can be used. A 5 MHz transducer is generally satisfactory — this produces an optimal image quality in the 5–10 cm depth range. In horses with large pleural effusions, a 3.5 MHz or lower frequency transducer may be necessary. The area to be scanned should be clipped, cleansed and washed in spirit to degrease the surface. An acoustic coupling gel is then applied to the skin. The intrathoracic structures are imaged by placing the probe in the intercostal spaces and scanning both sides of the chest in a systematic fashion (Fig. 12.38).

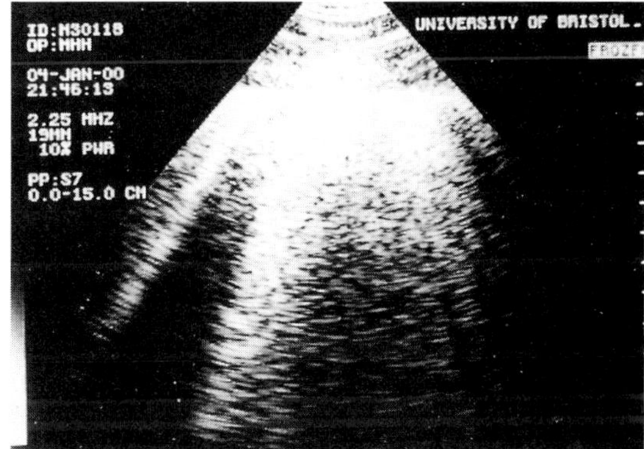

Figure 12.37   Ultrasonographic appearance of normal lung.

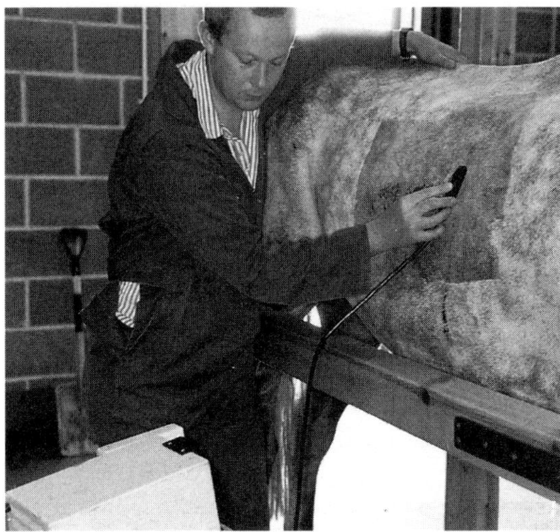

Figure 12.38 Ultrasonographic examination of the thorax using a 5 MHz linear array rectal probe.

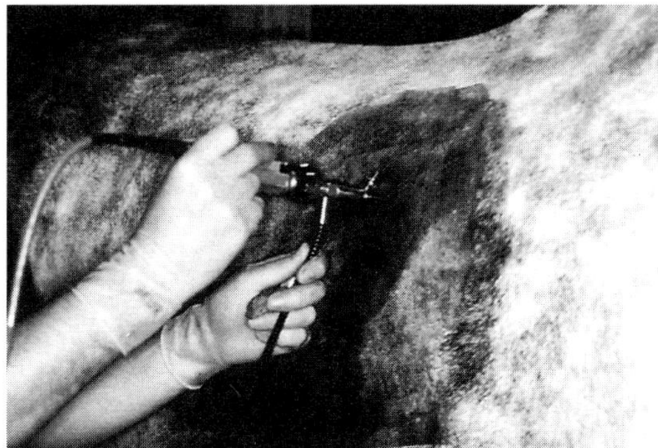

Figure 12.39 Pleuroscopy using a rigid arthroscope. A unilateral pneumothorax is created as soon as the chest cavity is entered, which provides space to allow the intrathoracic structures to be examined.

The normal anatomical boundaries of the lung (as described earlier in the section on 'Auscultation') are important landmarks.

Pleuroscopy

Direct endoscopic examination of the pleural cavity is occasionally helpful in some neoplastic diseases affecting the pleural surfaces. It may also be helpful in aiding biopsy of pleural masses. Either rigid endoscopes (such as arthroscopes or laparoscopes) or flexible endoscopes may be used. The technique is as follows:

- The horse should be sedated as necessary.
- An area over the dorsal lung at the 10th intercostal space is clipped and prepared aseptically. Local anaesthetic is infiltrated in the skin and down through muscle to the level of the parietal pleura.
- A stab incision is made through the skin and a purse-string suture placed around it. The intercostal tissues are bluntly dissected (avoiding the blood vessels and nerves that run along the caudal margins of the ribs) down to and including the parietal pleura. As the pleural cavity is entered, air will be heard to rush in through the wound — this creates a pneumothorax which allows space

for examination with the endoscope (Fig. 12.39).

- The endoscope is introduced and the pleural cavity examined. The dorsal and middle parts of the thorax can be visualized in this way.
- On completion of the examination, the endoscope is withdrawn, and the purse-string suture tightened to seal the chest wall defect.
- The pneumothorax may be drained by inserting a sterile cannula with an attached three-way tap into the cavity dorsal to the endoscopy portal. Air is repeatedly aspirated through the cannula using a 50 ml syringe.

Comment

- Prophylactic broad-spectrum antibiotic therapy should be administered before and for several days after the procedure.

Thoracocentesis

Thoracocentesis allows sampling of pleural fluid for cytology and culture. Repeated thoracocentesis is also used in the treatment of pleuritis to provide drainage for accumulated effusions.

Thoracocentesis is generally performed in the ventral third of the chest, taking care to avoid damage to the heart. The precise site will vary depending on the distribution and quantity of fluid in each individual horse. When ultrasonography is available, it may be helpful to aid selection of the best site. The technique is as follows:

- The usual site is the 6th–7th intercostal spaces on the right, or the 8th–9th intercostal spaces on the left.
- A large area should be clipped and prepared aseptically. *Care should be taken to avoid the lateral thoracic vein which runs subcutaneously over the ventral part of the chest wall.*
- Local anaesthetic is infiltrated subcutaneously and into the intercostal muscles down to the level of the parietal pleura.
- A blunt ended cannula (6–7 cm long, 12 or 14 gauge) is suitable for sampling small volumes of fluid. This is introduced through a stab incision in the skin, and pushed down through the intercostal muscles (avoiding the vessels and nerves which run along the caudal margin of the ribs) until it enters the pleural cavity. This can be appreciated by a palpable decrease in resistance.
- If fluid is not present in the cavity, air will be drawn into the chest once the pleura is penetrated, so a device such as a three-way tap is essential to seal the end of the cannula.
- If fluid is present, it will usually drain from the cannula under gravity, and samples can be collected for bacteriology (into aerobic and anaerobic blood culture bottles) and cytology (into EDTA).
- Following completion of the procedure, the cannula is withdrawn; there is usually no need to suture the skin.

Comment

- If large volumes of fluid are to be drained in addition to sampling, wider bore sterile cannulas can be used (such as metal bitch urinary catheters or human thoracic drainage cannulas: Fig. 12.40). It is usually necessary to suture the skin after the use of these larger cannulas.

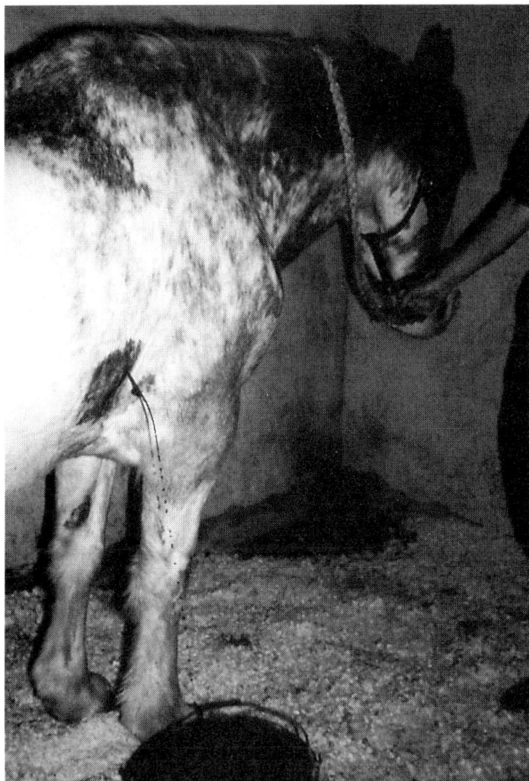

Figure 12.40   Thoracocentesis. Drainage of a large volume of pleural fluid using a metal bitch urinary catheter.

Arterial blood collection

In the adult horse, arterial blood samples for blood gas analysis are usually collected from either the common carotid artery or the facial artery.

Carotid artery

The carotid artery is punctured on the right side of the neck in the region of the lower third as follows:

- The artery is palpated as a cord-like structure deep to the jugular vein.
- The area is prepared aseptically, and a 2 inch x 19G (51 x 1.0 mm) needle is pushed into the vessel which is stabilized with the fingers of one hand. When the artery is penetrated, blood will squirt out under pressure. Several

attempts may be required to penetrate the artery. Alternatively, placement of the needle using ultrasound guidance may help.

- Blood is collected into a 2 or 5 ml syringe which has been previously filled with a small volume of sodium heparin solution (1000 iu/ml) to eliminate any air space. All air bubbles are expelled from the syringe which is then sealed with a cap.

- Following removal of the needle from the artery, firm finger pressure is applied for several minutes to prevent haematoma formation.

Facial artery

The facial artery can be sampled at a site just lateral to the lateral canthus of the eye. The area is prepared aseptically, and the artery is stabilized with the fingers of one hand. The vessel is punctured with a 1 inch x 23G (25 x 0.65 mm) needle, and the sample collected as described above.

Comment

- Arterial samples should be analysed immediately, or alternatively they can be stored in ice for up to 6 hours.

Nasopharyngeal swabbing

Nasal and pharyngeal swabs can be used for the isolation of respiratory viruses and bacteria. The viruses of clinical importance are:

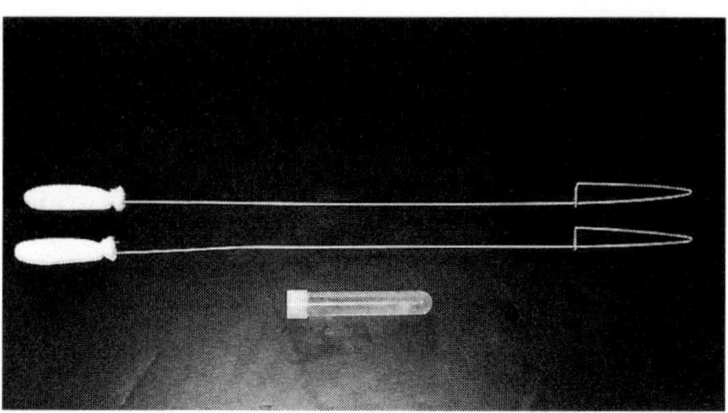

Figure 12.41 Gauze nasopharyngeal swabs suitable for collection of samples for virus isolation.

equine herpesvirus — types 1 and 4 (EHV-1 and EHV-4); equine influenza, and equine viral arteritis (EVA). Lesser clinical signifi-cance is attached to equine adenovirus and equine rhinovirus.

Successful isolation of these viruses depends upon sample collection at the correct time (early in the course of infection), the use of suitable viral transport medium, and rapid transport to the laboratory. Large gauze swabs are the most suitable (Fig. 12.41). These are inserted through the nares and passed along the ventral nasal meatus to the nasopharynx. The swab should be rotated and left in the nasopharynx for several minutes before it is withdrawn and then placed immediately into viral transport medium containing antibiotics. The swab is detached using wire cutters. Samples should be sent to the laboratory on ice or in a cool transport container as soon as possible.

III. **Clinical pathology**

Cytology of tracheal aspirates and BAL fluid

Preparation

Tracheal aspirate samples may be sufficiently cellular to allow a smear to be made immediately after collection onto a glass slide, which is fixed or air-dried, and stained.

BAL fluid and less cellular tracheal aspirate samples should be centrifuged in conical tubes (1500 x g for 10 minutes), and the sediment used to prepare a smear. Alternatively, a smear may be prepared using a cytocentrifuge. Smears should be made as rapidly as possible, since cellular changes occur within hours after collection. If immediate processing is not possible, the cells can be fixed by adding an equal volume of 40–50 % ethanol.

Suitable stains for cytology include Wright's stain, Wright's–Giemsa stain, May–Grunwald Giemsa stain, Sano Trichome and Papanicolaou stains.

Samples from confirmed or suspected pneumonia cases can be Gram-stained to give an early indication of the nature of the infection. A Ziehl–Nielson stain may be helpful to indicate mycobacterial infection.

Total nucleated cell counts can be useful in BAL samples, and are performed using a Neubauer haemocytometer. Cell counts obtained with Coulter counters are unreliable.

Interpretation

Tracheal aspirates

Tracheal aspirates from normal horses contain mainly ciliated columnar epithelial cells and alveolar macrophages. Macrophages may be seen to contain phagocytosed material such as fungal spores and degenerate cells. Haemosiderin granules are commonly seen in the macrophages of Thoroughbred horses in race training — this is a normal finding and may not indicate clinically significant exercise-induced pulmonary haemorrhage. Varying numbers of neutrophils are found in normal horses, which may account for up to 40% of the total cells present. Other cells that may be found include goblet cells, squamous epithelial cells, eosinophils, lymphocytes, basophils and mast cells.

Inflammatory diseases such as COPD and bronchopneumonia usually result in large numbers of neutrophils (which may comprise 95–98% of the total cells) and increased amounts of mucus in tracheal aspirates. Curschmann's spirals (casts of inspissated mucous plugs from small airways) are also seen in chronic lower airway disease.

High numbers of eosinophils are seen in horses with lungworm (*Dictyocaulus arnfieldi*) infection. Larvae may also be recovered in tracheal washes in these cases.

BAL samples

BAL samples from normal horses contain mainly macrophages and lymphocytes (approximately 40–50% of each). Neutrophils normally account for less than 5%. Other cells include mast cells, epithelial cells and eosinophils. Horses with COPD tend to show an increase in neutrophils. Animals with pneumonia show large numbers of neutrophils with toxic changes (provided that a diseased segment of lung has been sampled).

Pleural fluid analysis

Normal fluid

Normal horses have a small volume (up to 8 ml) of pleural fluid that can be retrieved by thoracocentesis. The fluid is clear, watery and pale straw coloured. The total nucleated cell count is normally less than 4×10^9/l, the total protein less than 3 g/dl and the specific gravity about 1.015. Neutrophils predominate (approximately 70%) with smaller numbers of large mononuclear cells (20%), lymphocytes and eosinophils.

Pleural effusions

Pleural effusions may be classified as transudates, modified transudates, exudates or chylous effusions.

Transudates

Transudates have normal cell counts and protein levels. They may be identified in early neoplastic diseases, congestive heart failure and hypoproteinaemia.

Modified transudates

Modified transudates are transudates with added cells (mesothelial cells, macrophages, neutrophils or neoplastic cells) and/or protein. They tend to appear pink and slightly cloudy. In the horse they are most commonly associated with neoplasia.

Exudates

Exudates have high cell counts (more than 10 x 10^9/l), high protein content (more than 3.0 g/dl) and high specific gravity (1.018). They are usually thick and cloudy, and tend to clot spontaneously. The majority of cells are neutrophils. Exudates are seen in pleuritis (pleuropneumonia) and some neoplastic conditions.

Chylous effusions

Chylous effusions appear milky white; the colour clears when the sample is shaken with ether. They possess high triglyceride concentrations, and a large proportion of the cells are lymphocytes.

Arterial blood gas analysis

Normal values of partial pressures of O_2 (PaO_2) and CO_2 ($PaCO_2$) are 85–100 mm Hg, and 35–45 mm Hg respectively.

Hypoxaemia (PaO_2 <80 mm Hg) occurs in diseases resulting in mismatching of ventilation and perfusion, such as pulmonary oedema, pneumonia and COPD.

Hypoxaemia with hypercapnea ($PaCO_2$ >45 mm Hg) indicates hypoventilation, e.g. severe COPD with airway obstruction.

Viral serology

Serology is the most convenient way of diagnosing viral infections but should be seen as complementary to nasopharyngeal swabbing, rather than as an alternative technique. In most cases, acute and convalescent serum samples (taken early in the infection, and 2–3 weeks later) are required. A four-fold rise in antibody titre is regarded as diagnostic of infection.

Sinus aspirates

Cytology and culture of fluid obtained by centesis can be helpful in differentiating primary sinusitis and sinusitis that is secondary to dental disease. The presence of food material indicates dental disease. Bacterial cultures from primary sinusitis cases generally yield single bacterial species, whereas multiple species are often present in secondary sinusitis cases.

Aspiration of relatively acellular, bright yellow fluid from a sinus is suggestive of a sinus cyst.

Haematology

Haematology provides non-specific information in patients with respiratory disease. The following points are offered as a general guide:

- Erythrocyte parameters will be depressed by most long-term respiratory diseases.
- Total white cell counts are likely to be raised (leucocytosis), largely as a result of neutrophilia, in bacterial respiratory diseases such as 'strangles' *(Streptococcus equi)*, post-viral infections, or pneumonia/pleuropneumonia. Lymphopenia commonly occurs during the acute phase of viral infections, but the effect is often transient and it is not a pathognomonic finding. Monocytosis is usually a feature of chronic inflammatory conditions associated with suppuration, granulomatous reactions or tissue necrosis.
- Plasma fibrinogen concentration is a sensitive indicator of bacterial inflammation. It is a better prognostic indicator than leucocyte parameters when monitoring the course of bacterial respiratory disease.

Chapter appendices

Investigating the causes of nasal discharges and coughing are common problems of differential diagnosis which confront the practitioner. Appendix 12.1 suggests applications of some of the diagnostic techniques covered in this chapter for the investigation of nasal discharges. The nature of the discharge and whether or not it is unilateral or bilateral reflect the type and site of the underlying lesion. Discharges may be variously mucoid, mucopurulent or purulent, and may additionally contain blood or food. Sometimes the discharge may be distinctly malodorous. Unilateral discharges usually indicate lesions associated with the nasal passages or paranasal sinuses. Bilateral discharges suggest a lesion caudal to the nasal septum, but an exception is guttural pouch empyema which often produces a predominantly unilateral discharge. Appendix 12.2 suggests techniques for the investigation of persistent coughing.

Further reading

Chan C and Munroe G (1995) Endoscopic examination of the equine paranasal sinuses. *In Practice* (supplement to the Veterinary Record) **17**: 419–422.

Greet TRC (1992) Differential diagnosis of equine nasal discharge. *Equine Veterinary Education* **4**: 23–25.

Mair TS and Gibbs C (1990) Thoracic radiography in the horse. *In Practice* (supplement to the Veterinary Record) **12**: 8–10.

Mair TS (1994) Differential diagnosis and treatment of acute onset coughing in the horse. *In Practice* (supplement to the Veterinary Record) **16**: 154–162.

Marr C (1993) Thoracic ultrasonography. *Equine Veterinary Education* **5**: 41–46.

McGorum B (1994) Differential diagnosis of chronic coughing in the horse. *In Practice* (supplement to the Veterinary Record) **16**: 55– 60.

Appendix 12.1. Some applications of diagnostic techniques for the investigation of nasal discharge.

Discharge	Possible cause	Aids to diagnosis
Mucoid/mucopurulent	Respiratory virus	Viral isolation; serology
	Bacterial infection	Nasopharyngeal swab
	Paranasal sinus cyst	Endoscopy; radiography
Mucopurulent/purulent	Sinusitis	Percussion; endoscopy; radiography; centesis (culture); direct sinus endoscopy
	Guttural pouch empyema	Endoscopy; catheterization (culture); radiography
	Fungal rhinitis	Endoscopy; biopsy for histopathology/culture
	Lower airway disease	Auscultation; endoscopy; tracheal aspiration/BAL for cytology; thoracic radiography
Discharge with food (dysphagia)	Oesophageal obstruction	Endoscopy; radiography
	Pharyngeal paralysis:	
	– guttural pouch mycosis	Endoscopy
	– trauma of the head and neck	Neurological examination (see Chapter 14)
	– lead poisoning	Lead estimation in: blood; liver/kidney, and top soil
	– botulism	Check clinical signs and feedstuff (see Chapter 14)
	Pharyngeal mass — abscess/neoplasia	Endoscopy; endoscopic biopsy; radiography; culture
	Pharyngeal foreign body	Endoscopy
	Palatal defect	Endoscopy; radiography
	Guttural pouch tympany	Endoscopy; radiography
	Guttural pouch empyema	Endoscopy; catheterization (culture); radiography
	Grass sickness	Check clinical signs; radiography of the oesophagus (megoesophagus and pooling of contrast medium); endoscopy of the oesophagus ('reflux oesophagitis'); post-mortem histopathology of the coeliacomesenteric ganglion
Discharge with dyspnoea	Pharyngeal abscess	Endoscopy; radiography; culture
	Guttural pouch tympany	Endoscopy; radiography
	Guttural pouch empyema	Endoscopy; catheterization (culture); radiography
	COPD	Auscultation; tracheal aspiration/BAL for cytology; thoracic radiography

Appendix 12.1. Some applications of diagnostic techniques for the investigation of nasal discharge *(continued)*.

Discharge	*Possible cause*	*Aids to diagnosis*
	Pulmonary abscess/pneumonia/pleuropneumonia	Auscultation; chest percussion; endoscopy; tracheal aspiration/BAL for cytology and culture; thoracic radiography; ultrasonography (pleural effusion); thoracocentesis for cytology and culture of effusion
Discharge with necrotic smell	Dental disease	Examine mouth; radiography
	Chronic sinusitis	Percussion; endoscopy; radiography; centesis (culture); direct sinus endoscopy
	Fungal rhinitis	Endoscopy; biopsy for histopathology/culture
	Guttural pouch infection	Endoscopy; culture
	Neoplasia	Endoscopy; endoscopic biopsy; radiography
	Gangrenous pneumonia	Auscultation; chest percussion; tracheal aspiration/BAL for cytology and culture; thoracic radiography; ultrasonography (pleural effusion); thoracocentesis for cytology and culture of effusion
	Inhaled foreign body	Endoscopy
Discharge with blood	Nasal tumour	Endoscopy; radiography
	Guttural pouch mycosis	Endoscopy
	Fungal rhinitis	Endoscopy; biopsy for histopathology/culture
	Foreign body	Endoscopy
Epistaxis	Ethmoidal haematoma	Endoscopy; radiography; haematology (anaemia)
	Turbinate necrosis	Endoscopy; culture
	Guttural pouch mycosis	Endoscopy; haematology (anaemia)
	Exercise induced pulmonary haemorrhage	Endoscopy; thoracic radiography; haematology (anaemia)
	Trauma	Radiography

Appendix 12.2. Some applications of diagnostic techniques for the investigation of coughing.

Possible cause	Aids to diagnosis
Acute coughing **Viral infection:** 　　　**EHV-1 and EHV- 4** 　　　**Equine influenza** 　　　**Equine viral arteritis** 　　　**Adenovirus** 　　　**Rhinovirus**	Viral isolation; serology
'Strangles' (*Streptococcus equi*)	Nasopharyngeal swab
Choke and other causes of dysphagia	Endoscopy; radiography; see also Appendix 2.1 in Chapter 2
Acute small airway obstruction in COPD	Auscultation; tracheal aspiration/BAL for cytology; thoracic radiography
EIPH	Endoscopy; thoracic radiography
Pulmonary abscess/pneumonia/pleuropneumonia	Auscultation; chest percussion; tracheal aspiration/ BAL for cytology and culture; thoracic radiography; ultrasonography (pleural effusion); thoracocentesis for cytology and culture of effusion
Inhaled foreign body	Endoscopy
Tracheal collapse	Endoscopy
Chronic coughing **COPD**	Auscultation; tracheal aspiration/BAL for cytology; thoracic radiography
Post-viral airway disease	History of preceding viral respiratory disease; serology indicating recent infection
Lungworm	Tracheal aspiration/BAL for cytology (eosinophilia) and larvae
Pulmonary abscess/pneumonia/ pleuropneumonia	Auscultation; chest percussion; tracheal aspiration/ BAL for cytology and culture; thoracic radiography; ultrasonography (pleural effusion); thoracocentesis for cytology and culture of effusion
Summer pasture associated obstructive pulmonary disease	Auscultation; tracheal aspiration/BAL for cytology; thoracic radiography; change environment
Thoracic neoplasia	Endoscopy; thoracic radiography; ultrasonography (pleural effusion); thoracocentesis for cytology; pleuroscopy

13 Musculoskeletal diseases

I. Lameness examination

Problems associated with the musculoskeletal system of horses are common and usually present as a physical deformity or lameness. The diagnostic approach involves a number of basic steps:

- Defining the problem to be investigated
- Localizing the site(s) of abnormality
- Characterizing the nature of the pathological change

History

Apart from details of breed, age and sex, the essential background information should include:

- The duration of ownership and use (or intended use) of the horse
- Details of recent management including housing, feeding, shoeing and exercise

- Any previous medical problems known to the owner

The owner should be allowed to describe in his/her own way the reasons for presenting the animal and should then be questioned more specifically to try to define the primary complaint. Once this is achieved, further details can be added, particularly in relation to the owner's observations:

- The limb or limbs thought to be affected
- The timing and nature of the onset of signs
- Details of any associated events or incidents
- The progression of signs since their onset
- Any changes in management (or attempts at treatment) as a result of the problem and their effects
- A summary of the current state of the problem

Physical examination

Every effort should be made to examine the entire musculoskeletal system, even in the presence of obvious abnormalities at one site. The examination at rest falls into two stages.

(1) There should be an overall inspection of the horse from all angles, noting particularly:

- General body condition
- Conformation of the body, limbs and feet (see below)
- Posture and weight bearing on the limbs
- Skeletal and soft tissue symmetry
- Any localized swellings or thickenings
- Any evidence of generalized or systemic disease

Conformation is the outward appearance of an animal. Ideal conformation is generally accepted to be that which does not bring excessive force(s) to bear on any individual structure. In consequence, it requires symmetry and alignment of the limbs, leading to straight limb flight and even weight bearing. Deviation from good conformation will result in excessive tensile or compressive forces being concentrated on one part of the limb during weight bearing. Over the course of time, the cumulative effect may be injury or disease.

Deviation from straight limb flight is inefficient and may result in interference with the gait and self-inflicted injury. The dividing line between conformational variation, adopted posture and pathological deformity is poorly defined in many cases.

(2) A detailed evaluation of the individual regions of the limbs should be undertaken by:

- Inspection to reveal deformity, swelling or thickening, skin wounds and muscle wasting
- Palpation to detect heat and pain, well as characterizing the precise location and consistency of any swellings or thickenings
- Manipulation of limb joints to evaluate their range of movement, i.e. detecting restriction, instability, pain or crepitus

All three procedures should involve comparison of the region under examination with the contralateral limb to detect potentially significant asymmetries.

The forelimb

Examination of the foot

Initially, the feet should be inspected with regard to their size, shape, symmetry and balance.

Variations in foot shape may be due to conformation, trimming, shoeing, disease, or lameness. Not infrequently, abnormalities are actually a result of a complex combination of these factors which have distorted foot shape over a prolonged time.

The feet should show symmetry between contralateral limbs and between the medial and lateral halves of each foot. The angle between the dorsal wall of the hoof and the ground should be approximately 45–50 degrees in the forelimbs and slightly more upright (50–55 degrees) in the hindlimbs.

The foot is said to be balanced when its shape and position in relation to the limb are such that weight is equally distributed over it. The angle between the dorsal wall of the hoof and the ground should be the same as that of the pastern. This relationship constitutes the *hoof–pastern axis* (Fig. 13.1). A common abnormality, thought to predispose to foot lameness, is the combination of an overlong toe and a low collapsed heel leading to a 'broken back' hoof–pastern axis . The dorsal wall of the hoof should be parallel to the wall at the heel as viewed from the side of the horse. There should be no rotatory deformity of the foot ('toe in or toe out') and the heels should be of equal height.

The hoof wall, coronary band and solar surface should then be examined in detail.

The hoof wall should be straight and not splayed out toward the bearing surface. The outer surface of the hoof should be smooth. 'Rings' on the hoof wall may result from nutritional variations, previous episodes of systemic disease, or laminitis. The variations of horn growth associated with nutritional change or systemic disease result in rings which emerge parallel to the coronet and each other. In contrast, laminitic rings appear to diverge at the heel and converge at the dorsal wall, reflecting uneven growth from the coronet. The hoof wall should also be carefully examined for cracks and their location, depth and any associated lesions of the coronary band noted.

The coronary band should be palpated, particularly dorsally, for evidence of 'dipping', which may indicate downward displacement of the pedal bone as a result of laminitis.

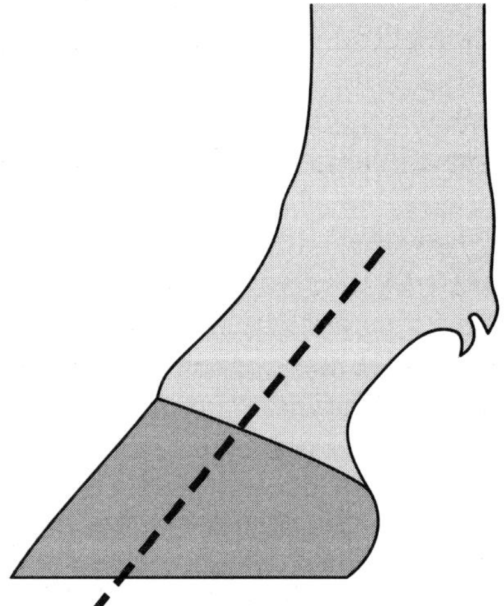

Figure 13.1 The hoof–pastern axis.

Palpation of the coronary band may also reveal local swelling, pain or heat secondary to trauma or infection. The proximal part of the lateral cartilages can be palpated above the coronary band and should be checked at the same time. Distension of the distal interphalangeal joint ('coffin joint') is occasionally palpable just proximal to the coronary band dorsally.

The digital pulse at the fetlock should be palpated in association with examination of the foot to see if it is increased in volume on one or both sides. An increased digital pulse suggests inflammation or laminitis in the foot.

The foot is then picked up and the solar surface examined. The sole should be concave and not flat. In the forelimb, the heel to toe length should equal the width of the bearing surface at its widest point, while the hind foot is generally longer and more pointed. The foot (or shoe) should be inspected for uneven wear and an attempt made to correlate this to limb movement and foot placement during motion. The shoe should be evaluated for type, positioning, nail numbers and their placement.

The frog and solar surface of the foot must then be picked clean of bedding and dirt and the superficial layers of horn pared away with a hoof knife before they can be adequately examined. Initial inspection should check for the presence of foreign bodies embedded in the foot, or other obvious solar injury. The surface is then carefully searched for discolouration which may indicate bruising (usually red/ purple areas), or possible infection (particularly black spots or lines). Careful attention should be paid in this part of examination to the white line, heels and frog, including the sulci as these are common sites of infection.

Palpation of the hoof capsule itself usually requires the mechanical advantage provided by hoof testers, unless the sole is very thin and compressible. The hoof testers are used to apply pressure to all parts of the hoof, including the frog, in a systematic manner — always remembering that they exert pressure at two points. Areas that seem to be painful are checked several times to try to localize the painful focus as accurately as possible and ensure that the response is consistent. Suspect areas should be compared with the equivalent site in the contralateral limb if the significance of the horse's response is in doubt. Percussion of the wall and sole with a light hammer or the hoof testers may also be helpful in determining the presence of foot pain. Consistently painful areas should be explored further with the hoof knife to see if deep infection or bruising are the underlying cause.

The distal interphalangeal joint should be flexed and extended and stressed medially, laterally and in rotation, checking for pain, restriction, instability and crepitus. The same manipulations apply in the examination of all limb joints, although they are less easy to perform on the more proximal joints in the horse.

Examination of the pastern and fetlock

The pastern is checked for thickening around the proximal interphalangeal joint ('pastern joint'), or on its palmar aspect, where lie the superficial and deep digital flexor tendons and the distal sesamoidean ligaments.

The fetlock joint should be inspected and palpated for swelling due to synovial effusion. This usually begins as a fluctuant fluid swelling between the palmar aspect of the distal third metacarpal bone and the branches of the suspensory ligament. More severe effusion may produce a swelling which is apparent on the dorsal aspect of the joint. Articular effusion should be distinguished from distension of the digital sheath which produces a more palmar swelling around the digital flexor tendons at the back of the fetlock, i.e. behind the branches of the suspensory ligament. This is sometimes constricted on the palmar aspect of the proximal sesamoid bones by the annular ligament. The proximal sesamoid bones themselves and the insertions of the branches of the suspensory ligaments are palpated for pain and swelling.

Examination of the metacarpus

The three metacarpal bones are palpated for evidence of pain, heat and swelling; this is particularly relevant to young horses, where dorsal metacarpal periostitis and/or stress fractures (sore shins) and 'splints' are seen most commonly. Palpation of the small metacarpal bones should include their axial (medial), palmar and abaxial (lateral) surfaces as far as possible. Firm cold painless 'splints' in middle-aged and older horses are a common incidental finding which is usually of no significance.

The palmar metacarpal soft tissues are a common source of lameness and should be carefully palpated with the limb bearing weight and then with the foot raised. The individual structures to be checked are the superficial digital flexor tendon, the deep digital flexor tendon, the inferior check ligament and the suspensory ligament:

- Swelling of the superficial digital flexor tendon commonly renders the normally straight palmar surface of the metacarpus convex, i.e. the tendon becomes 'bowed'. Severe swelling makes it impossible to distinguish the deep flexor tendon as a separate structure — however, it is comparatively rare for this tendon to suffer strain injury.
- Inferior check ligament injuries produce a swelling in the proximal and middle thirds of the palmar metacarpus dorsal to the superficial digital flexor tendon and do not usually disturb the straight palmar contour of the region.
- The body and branches of the suspensory ligament are easy to palpate in the mid and distal thirds of the metacarpus. However, the proximal third of the ligament is located between the two small metacarpal bones and is more difficult to assess clinically. Defining the margins of the suspensory ligament using the thumbs is helpful in assessing whether there is any thickening present.

The digital extensor tendons (common digital extensor and lateral digital extensor) should be palpated from their muscular origins above the carpus and followed down the dorsal aspect of the distal limb.

Examination of the carpus

The dorsal aspect of the carpus ('knee') is examined for synovial swellings owing to effusion in the two more mobile carpal joints (the antebrachiocarpal and midcarpal joints), or tenosynovitis of the extensor tendon sheaths (extensor carpi radialis, extensor carpi obliquus, common digital extensor and lateral digital extensor).

Joint flexion allows palpation of the dorsal margins of the carpal joints for capsular thickening and alteration in the underlying bony contours. Separated bone fragments can occasionally be palpated within the antebrachiocarpal or mid-carpal joints when these are flexed.

The palmar aspect of the joint is examined for swelling of the carpal sheath and stability of the accessory carpal bone. In horses with carpal sheath distension, the palmar aspect of the distal radius is palpated with the carpus flexed to detect radial osteochondromas.

Examination of the elbow and shoulder

Effusions or thickenings of the elbow and shoulder joints are not generally palpable, but regional swelling may occur, particularly with traumatic injury or joint infection.

The stability of the olecranon should be specifically checked by manipulation, especially in horses demonstrating a 'dropped' elbow. *Auscultation with a stethoscope over bony prominences during manipulation or movement can be helpful in detecting crepitus associated with proximal limb fractures.*

Muscle wasting as a result of lameness is usually most apparent in the largest muscle masses, i.e. around the shoulder and scapula of the proximal limb, even where the precipitating cause is a foot problem. Rapid and severe wasting of specific muscle groups may accompany lower motor neurone injury,

e.g. following trauma to the suprascapular nerve.

The hindlimb

Examination of the foot, fetlock and metatarsus of the hindlimb is essentially similar to examination of the lower forelimb.

Examination of the hock

A number of different conditions may give rise to swellings around the hock:

- Effusion of the tarsocrural joint ('bog spavin') is usually most apparent on the dorsomedial aspect of the hock, though smaller fluctuant swellings may also be apparent plantarolaterally and plantaromedially.
- Distension of the tarsal sheath ('thoroughpin') produces plantar swellings proximal to the hock on either side of, and slightly cranial to, the Achilles tendon.
- Inflammation of the plantar ligament ('curb') causes thickening on the plantar aspect of the hock centred about 10 cm distal to the point of the hock.
- Degenerative joint disease of the small hock joints ('bone spavin') may produce thickening on the medial aspect of the distal hock, though this is not always detectable.

The Achilles tendon should be examined for thickening indicative of strain injury and the positioning and stability of the superficial digital flexor tendon over the point of the hock should also be checked. Extension of the hock should cause extension of the stifle owing to the action of the reciprocal apparatus. If it can be accomplished independently and results in relaxation of the Achilles tendon, then rupture of the peroneus tertius should be suspected.

Examination of the stifle

Effusion of the femoropatellar joint causes palpable swelling between the three distal patellar ligaments. The collateral ligaments can also be palpated medially and laterally.

In cases of suspected intermittent upward fixation of the patella, attempts can be made to lock the joint by reversing and turning the horse in tight circles. Alternatively, locking may be demonstrated by pushing upwards on the patella while keeping the horse's weight on the affected limb by pulling laterally on the tail.

The demonstration of stifle instability due to ligamentous injury is occasionally possible. The integrity of the medial collateral ligament can be tested by placing the shoulder against the lateral aspect of the stifle and abducting the distal limb while palpating the medial aspect of the femoropatellar joint for abnormal widening.

The author has never convincingly demonstrated instability as a result of cruciate ligament injury in the horse, but a technique has been described. This involves standing behind the horse with arms brought around the suspect limb and the hands clasped together at the proximal end of the tibia. The clinician's knee is placed in close contact with the plantar aspect of the calcaneus and his/her toe placed behind the bulbs of the horse's heel. The tibia is pulled sharply caudally and released to allow it to return cranially while feeling for laxity and crepitation. Clearly the temperament of the horse should always be taken into consideration before determining whether it is safe to attempt such a manoeuvre.

Examination of the pelvis and hip

The hip joint is the most deeply buried of the limb joints and the least amenable to direct physical examination. The correct alignment of its components can be evaluated to some extent by checking that the relationships between the greater trochanter, tuber coxae, tuber sacrale and tuber ischii are symmetrical. Hip problems tend to result in outward rotation of the affected limb.

As in the forelimb, muscle wasting as a consequence of hindlimb lameness is usually most noticeable proximally, particularly over the gluteal region, regardless of the site of the problem. The thigh muscles may also show evidence of a loss of bulk as a consequence of persistent or severe lameness.

The pelvis can be evaluated by a combination of inspection and internal palpation of the bony landmarks by rectal examination. In the case of suspected pelvic fractures, rectal examination while the animal is walked slowly forward or rocked from side to side is often helpful in revealing crepitus and movement of bone fragments. Rectal examination also enables assessment of the central alignment of the sacrum and caudal lumbar vertebrae, along with their overlying muscles, and the presence and character of the pulse in the terminal aorta and iliac arteries.

Iliac or aortoiliac thrombosis is an uncommon occlusive condition of the terminal aorta which is diagnosed by rectal examination. The lesion is associated with ischaemia of one or both hindlimbs and is seen as a lameness or apparent weakness of one or both hindlegs at exercise. In severe cases there may be an acute onset at exercise with severe pain and recumbency. The affected limb(s) feels cold distally and there is reduced pulsation of the common digital artery. When the aortic pulse is detected per rectum and followed caudally with the fingertips, a firm irregular enlargement is felt at the termination of the aorta where it branches into the internal and external iliacs. The enlargement may be unilateral or bilateral (consistent with one or both hindlegs being affected) and of reduced or unappreciable pulse volume. If available, ultrasonography of the terminal aorta and its iliac branches is a more sensitive diagnostic technique than rectal examination.

NB The immediate and much more usual differential for hindlimb pain at exercise is *exertional rhabdomyolysis* (see later under: 'Myopathies').

The back

The equine back is an area where objective physical examination remains difficult. Inspection will reveal asymmetries due to swelling, muscle atrophy and curvature deformities. Palpation may be helpful in assessing the presence of pain and muscle spasm — however, it is often difficult to be certain of the significance of mild or moderate responses in relation to the presenting complaint. Some pointers to a diagnostic approach are given below.

History

Clinical signs associated with chronic back pain are extremely varied, the most consistent being a loss of the horse's performance or ability to jump. This may coincide with a distinct alteration of behaviour or temperament, e.g. uncharacteristic resentment of rugging up, grooming, or picking up of the hindlegs. Unfortunately, there is a tendency amongst owners to seize upon a 'back problem' as a cause of poor performance, which may more correctly be attributed to problems of schooling, horsemanship, or obscure organic disease. A detailed history of the horse's management, its tack, performance and temperament must be considered.

Examination

If possible, the dorsal midline of the back should be viewed from above as the horse is standing square, to check that it is correctly aligned. Some degree of lateral curvature suggests a degree of muscle spasm on one side. The symmetry of the pelvis should be checked from behind and the quarters and back should be inspected for muscle wastage; abnormal findings could be indicative of sacroiliac injury. Where there is damage to the muscle or ligaments of the sacroiliac region, it is usually possible to evoke discomfort by exerting pressure over the tuber coxae and/or over the midline at the lumbar region.

Pinching over the dorsal spinous processes at the withers normally causes 'dipping' of the spine (dorsiflexion), whilst pinching over the sacral region normally causes an extension (ventroflexion). Reluctance to comply, or a rigidity of the spine, may reflect some underlying bony pathology. Similarly, pressure with a blunt point over the dorsal spinous processes, caudal sacrum and flank can be used to stimulate spinal flexion away from the stimulus, enabling assessment of the animal's willingness and ability to carry out this movement.

Firm stroking of the longissimus dorsi with a blunt point normally produces lateral flexion of the thoracic and lumbar spine. Resentment suggests painful muscle involvement, but if it is detected on both sides then it could reflect pain in the vertebral column of the mid-back.

In a straight line walk and trot, back pain can produce a restricted hindlimb action with poor hock flexion and a tendency to drag the toes of one or both hindlimbs. Sharp turning to flex the spine will be resented or appear difficult with clumsy, jerky movements. Backing up is also resented.

Radiography

Radiography of the equine back requires powerful equipment and is associated with considerable radiation scatter. Its use is limited to a few specialist centres.

Haematology and biochemistry

Clinical pathology is generally non-specific, but serves to rule out other causes of reduced performance (e.g. anaemia, intercurrent infection, chronic rhabdomyolysis).

Evaluation of the gait

Observation

Sophisticated technologies are now available in some referral centres for the detailed and objective analysis of the gait of the moving horse, including force plates to quantify ground reaction forces and videographic recording of limb and body movements. However, these have yet to find their way into routine use and the clinician's observation of movement remains the mainstay of gait evaluation. The aims should be to identify:

- The presence or absence of a gait abnormality
- The limb or limbs involved
- The character of any abnormality present
- The degree of abnormality

The gait is usually best evaluated on a hard level surface. Ideally this should be done in a safe enclosed area, free of distractions and dangers such as traffic and other horses. The horse should be restrained with a headcollar or bridle and bit, and allowed 30–50 cm of headrope to permit sufficient freedom of head movement.

Abnormalities of gait are usually most apparent when the horse is moving at the walk and slow trot. Variations in foot placement and limb movement, e.g. shortening of one phase of the stride in one limb, are generally easiest to appreciate at the walk when limb movement is slower. The abnormalities in head and hind-quarter movement resulting from pain during weight bearing are usually most apparent at the slow trot. The horse should be observed moving in a straight line at an even pace from in front, from both sides, and behind.

Lunging the horse in tight circles is a helpful way of demonstrating more clearly lamenesses that are subtle or inapparent when the horse is moving in a straight line. If circumstances do not permit such an examina-tion, trotting the horse around sharp corners may accentuate lameness in a similar though more transient way.

Horses with forelimb lameness owing to pain on weight bearing shift the distribution of weight from the affected limb across to the contralateral forelimb and back to the hindlimbs. This is achieved, at least in part, by raising the head and neck as the lame forelimb takes weight, the head being lowered again as the sound forelimb strikes the ground. This downward nodding of the head as the sound forelimb strikes the ground is generally the easiest abnormality of movement to appreciate and allows identification of the lame (or lamer) forelimb. The sound limb may also be heard to strike the ground with greater force, particularly if the horse is shod.

With hindlimb lameness the gluteal region on the affected side will rise and fall through a greater range of motion than that of the sound limb. This is often most easily appreciated as a 'hiking up' of the gluteal region on the affected side during weight bearing on that limb.

Several abnormalities of limb movement may also be appreciable in the lame horse:

- *Alteration in the relative lengths of phases of the stride*. The cranial phase of the stride is that part which occurs in front of the footprint of the contralateral limb, while the caudal phase occurs behind it. If the animal is moving in a straight line the overall stride length in a pair of contralateral limbs must be symmetrical, therefore a reduced cranial phase must always be accompanied by an increased caudal phase. Overall reductions in stride length frequently accompany bilateral orthopaedic conditions leading to a 'pottery' or restricted gait
- *Alteration in the arc of foot flight*. Lowering of the arc or foot flight may occur as a compensation to reduce impact when the foot lands, or to reduce limb flexion during protraction. If severe it may lead to dragging of the toes. Exaggerated elevation of a foot owing to hyperflexion of the limb joints is occasionally seen, e.g. in 'string-halt'.
- *Variations in the path of foot flight and in foot placement*. These may occur for similar reasons to those outlined for alterations in the arc of foot flight (above). The foot may be swung medially or laterally during protraction of the limb. The foot may land asymmetrically, contacting the ground first at the toe, heel or on one or other side.

There is tremendous variation in the pattern of foot flight between different horses, some of which can be related to breed and conformation. Bilateral and symmetrical deviations from the ideal, which are unassociated with other evidence of lameness, may not be of clinical significance, e.g. some horses seem to drag the hind toes regularly during protraction without experiencing other evidence of hindlimb dysfunction.

Records of lameness evaluation should contain some assessment of the severity of the problem. This should be recognized as an essentially subjective exercise as spontaneous variations may occur with time, exercise, and ground surface. Nevertheless, it can be helpful in communicating findings to other clinicians and when re-evaluating cases. A variety of scoring systems are employed, e.g. 0 to 5, or 1/10th to 10/10ths lame, with higher scores representing more severe grades of lameness.

Provocative tests

Provocative tests may be used for three basic reasons:

(1)   To demonstrate occult lameness in a horse that appears 'sound' on initial gait evaluation
(2)   To exacerbate a mild lameness
(3)   As an aid to localization of the abnormality causing the lameness

A variety of manoeuvres are employed of which the most common are *flexion tests*. A flexion test is performed by holding the joint under consideration in a firmly flexed position for a time — usually about a minute. Once the limb is released, the horse is observed during immediate movement, usually at the trot, to note any change in gait compared with that seen before undertaking the test. Limitations to the technique include the following:

- It is often difficult to flex a single joint in isolation, particularly in the hindlimb, with a resulting lack in specificity of the response.
- The response is not necessarily consistent; the same test performed on several different occasions within a single examination may yield varying results.
- There are not hard and fast criteria for determining what constitutes a 'positive' response.
- Both false positive and false negative results may be obtained. Flexion of an abnormal joint may not noticeably influence the gait and, conversely, flexion of a normal joint may produce some degree of lameness when the horse is trotted off, particularly if a severe degree of flexion is maintained for a prolonged period of time.

To reduce these problems it is important to standardize the technique employed and apply caution to the interpretation of results.

Standardization of the flexion test

- Always flex joints for the same period of time; one minute is generally considered a satisfactory period.
- Fully flex the joint concerned and hold it in this position with firm pressure. Standardizing the force employed is obviously more difficult than standardizing the time, but it should at least be consistent for each examination performed on one individual.
- Explain to the handler that the horse must be trotted away as soon as the limb is put down and at the same speed as it was moving when the gait was initially evaluated.
- The horse should be trotted away for at least 20–30 m, turned and trotted back again, past the observer, so that the degree and persistence of any response can be fully evaluated.
- Ensure that the response to any individual flexion test has fully subsided before proceeding to perform other similar tests on other joints or limbs.
- Perform equivalent tests on the contralateral limb to allow comparison of the response.
- If possible, repeat positive tests to check that the result is consistent.

Interpretation of flexion tests

It is impossible to lay down incontrovertible rules regarding what constitutes a positive response to a flexion test. It should be interpreted in the light of other information about the horse and it is wise to avoid using it as the sole basis for a firm diagnosis.

In general terms the more severe, persistent and consistent the response to a test, the more likely the result is to be significant. The extent of the response therefore influences the weight given to it in the final analysis of the results of a lameness investigation. It is important to remember that several joints will be flexed when performing a flexion test and that a positive response may therefore be due to a lesion in one of a number of locations. Trying to eliminate the response to a flexion test by using local analgesia can be helpful in localizing a source of lameness. However, it does presuppose that the response to flexion is not going to diminish spontaneously with time and repetition.

Extension tests

Extension tests can be performed in a similar manner. The most commonly employed involves extension of the distal limb joints by standing the horse with the toe of the suspect limb elevated on a small wooden wedge and the contralateral limb raised for one minute, followed by trotting the horse off.

Pressure tests

The effect of pressure on a particular area can also be evaluated, e.g. digital pressure on a suspect splint lesion, or frog pressure applied by standing the horse with the frog on the handle of a shoeing hammer. The limitations outlined for flexion tests apply equally to these other provocative tests.

II. Local analgesia

General considerations in local analgesia

'Nerve blocking' is time consuming, invasive, sometimes hazardous and reliant on subjective evaluation of gait for its interpretation. Despite these disadvantages, in many lame horses it remains the only way to answer the question: 'where does it hurt?'

Local anaesthetic solutions can be used in a variety of ways to localize the source of pain responsible for lameness. The technique depends on accurate placement of the anaesthetic solution into or around the structure to be anaesthetized, followed by evaluation of its effect on gait.

The results of local analgesia are most easily and reliably interpreted when the horse is showing an adequate and consistent degree of lameness in the first instance. Interpretation is more difficult and less reliable if the initial lameness is very slight or inconsistent. Techniques for accentuating the degree of lameness, e.g. lunging the horse in tight circles on hard ground, have been described previously. In the case of chronic low grade lameness, it may be helpful to try to exacerbate the problem by exercising the horse for a few days to make the lameness more apparent, prior to the use of local analgesia.

Conversely, caution should be exercised with the use of local analgesia in acute lameness if there is a possibility that the cause may be an injury which could be exacerbated by the abolition of pain under local anaesthesia. An example would be an animal with an undisplaced fracture where the fracture line may extend and displace with the increased weight bearing promoted by relieving the associated pain. Initial radiographic and/or scintigraphic examination (see later) may be prudent in such cases.

Local anaesthetics may be used for:

- Perineural infiltration around specific nerves to desensitize the regions of the limb supplied by that nerve
- Intrasynovial analgesia of joints, tendon sheaths or bursae

- Local infiltration around suspect superficial lesions.

Perineural analgesia — general considerations

Perineural analgesia in the diagnosis of lameness is confined to the distal limb, i.e. below the elbow and stifle. The peripheral nerves in the distal limb are largely sensory since the muscles supplied by motor nerves are located proximally. In general, blocking of nerve conduction at these more distal levels does not significantly interfere with the horse's ability to move the limb normally.

Materials

A number of different local anaesthetic solutions can be used for perineural analgesia. It has been suggested that mepivacaine and prilocaine cause less inflammatory reaction than lignocaine and they are commonly employed for this reason. *Solutions without adrenaline, corticosteroid, antibiotic or other additivies should be used.*

It is advisable to use fresh bottles of sterile solution for each examination, though not necessarily each block. Fresh sterile needles should be used for each injection site. The needle diameter and the length required varies depending upon the block to be performed; the author's preferences are outlined below. Perineural analgesia should ideally be performed in a clean, quiet, well lit, relatively confined area without bedding (in which displaced or dislodged needles can easily be lost).

Preparation and restraint of the horse

Opinions vary on the necessity for clipping the hair at the site of perineural analgesia. It is undoubtedly possible to clean the site for needle puncture more effectively if the hair is clipped. However, the incidence of infection appears to be low if the hair and underlying skin are simply scrubbed with antiseptic solution and rinsed with spirit prior to injection.

Clipping is recommended in horses with thick coarse hair or 'feather' around the distal limb, as this allows palpation of the appropriate landmarks for injection. A tail bandage is helpful when performing blocks on the hindlimb to keep the the tail hair out of the way. Alternatively, the tail should be held to one side by an assistant.

The degree of restraint necessary will vary depending on the temperament of the horse under examination. The use of a bridle and bit together with a twitch are helpful in unco-operative animals. In very uncooperative horses, short acting sedation with xylazine or romifidine can be used, but there is always the possibility that the drug will interfere with the subsequent interpretation of the block and they are best avoided if at all possible.

Needle placement

As small a volume of local anaesthetic as will reliably block the nerve is deposited adjacent to it with as much accuracy as possible. The more proximal nerve trunks are thicker and more deeply situated within the limb tissues, making accurate placement more difficult. In general, the volume of local anaesthetic used is therefore greater for the more proximal nerve blocks. For proximal blocks requiring long needles (which are therefore of relatively wide gauge), it is helpful to place a small bleb of local anaesthetic subcutaneously using a fine gauge needle before positioning the larger needle.

A sterile needle held by the hub is placed through the skin rapidly. The tip is then repositioned to the required site and depth. Once any movement of the horse has ceased, the syringe is attached and injection made. *The syringe is attached to the needle firmly enough to prevent loss of fluid during injection, but loosely enough to enable it to be removed rapidly should the horse move, thus leaving the needle in position.* Excessive resistance to injection usually means that the tip of the needle is buried in dense connective tissue and that repositioning is required.

The limb to be injected may be weight bearing or held in a flexed position by the clinician or an assistant at the time of injection. The exact routine employed is largely a matter of personal preference. Holding the limb flexed for injection gives good control of the limb and this approach is used by the author for those distal limb blocks where the nerves themselves can usually be palpated, e.g. the palmar digital block and the abaxial sesamoid block in the forelimb. Injecting with the limb in a weight bearing position has the advantage of tensing the regional soft tissues which makes identification of landmarks easier and this approach is used by the author for all regional blocks proximal to the fetlock. If the limb to be injected is weight bearing, the opposite limb can be held up as a form of restraint. The disadvantage to this approach is that some horses will suddenly withdraw and flex the limb being blocked when the needle is placed through the skin. If the opposite forelimb is raised, the horse may collapse on its carpi. This problem can be avoided by placing the needle through the skin with both limbs on the ground and then lifting the contralateral limb for restraint during injection once the needle is in the correct position.

The peripheral nerves generally run in association with an artery and a vein as a neurovascular bundle. If a needle inadvertently enters a blood vessel on initial placement it should be withdrawn slightly and repositioned (usually a little more caudally). It is also prudent to withdraw on the syringe plunger prior to injection to double check that the needle is not in a blood vessel.

Distal limb blocks will usually take effect within 5–10 minutes. Because of the increased thickness of proximal nerve trunks, the more proximal blocks take longer to become effective and should generally be given at least 20 minutes. The efficacy of distal perineural analgesia can be tested to some extent by evaluating skin sensation distal to the block. This is best done using a blunt point such as a ball point pen. The response should be compared with that in the equivalent region of

the contralateral limb assuming that this has not been previously blocked. Some horses are very stoical to such stimulation and require quite considerable pressure even on unanaesthetized skin to elicit a response. In contrast, some horses, particularly after multiple nerve blocks, become extremely sensitive to any approach to the distal limb and withdraw the limb before it has even been touched. In these cases it is helpful to shield the horse's eye so that it cannot see the approach of the examiner and also to approach from the opposite side of the animal.

Perineural analgesia should be carried out in a sequential manner starting distally and working proximally if the lameness is still present. If a specific joint is suspected to be the source of the lameness from the initial physical examination, it is better to proceed to an intra-articular block of this joint first rather than a regional block proximal to the joint. The intra-articular block will not interfere with subsequent, more distal, regional blocks if the response is negative.

Sites of nerve block in the forelimb

Palmar digital nerve block (Fig. 13.2)

The palmar digital neurovascular bundle is palpable in many horses on the palmarolateral and palmaromedial aspects of the pastern. The nerve is the most palmar structure within the bundle.

The site for injection is subcutaneously on the palmarolateral/medial border of the digital flexor tendons just proximal to the margin of the lateral cartilage. A volume of 1–2 ml local anaesthetic is delivered through a 1 inch x 23G (25 x 0.65 mm) needle. It is usual to block both medial and lateral nerves but they can be done independently if uniaxial foot lesions are suspected as the cause of lameness.

The palmar digital block is traditionally regarded as anaesthetizing the palmar part of the foot. However, while skin desensitization is

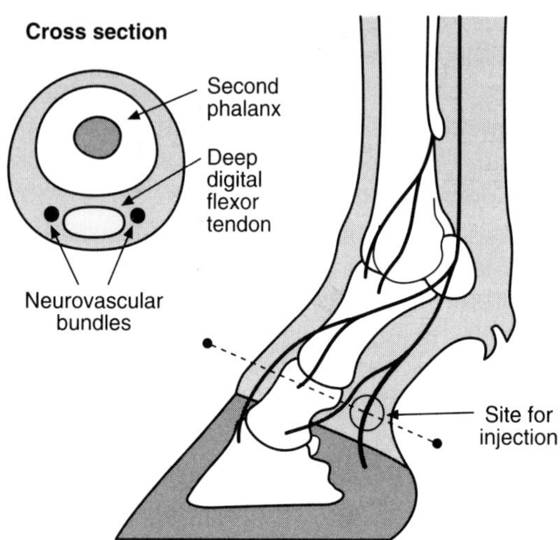

Figure 13.2   Site of palmar digital nerve block.

usually confined to the heels, deep sensation at more dorsal sites within the foot may also be lost since the nerves run forward within the hoof capsule. As a consequence, some cases of distal interphalangeal joint pain and even laminitis will show improvement in response to a palmar digital block.

Abaxial sesamoid nerve block
(Fig. 13.3)

The neurovascular bundle is usually palpable with ease where it runs over the abaxial surface of the proximal sesamoid bones, making this technique the easiest regional block to perform.

The site for injection is subcutaneously on the palmar aspect of the neurovascular bundle over the abaxial surface of the proximal sesamoid bones. A volume of 2 ml local anaesthetic is infiltrated on each side using a 1 inch x 23G (25 x 0.65 mm) needle.

Skin sensation is lost over the palmar pastern and the distal dorsal pastern. Deep sensation is lost from the foot and proximal interphalangeal joint. Partial desensitization of the palmar fetlock may occur.

Palmar and palmar metacarpal nerve block (four point block)

To desensitize the fetlock joint and all structures distal to it, the medial and lateral palmar nerves are usually blocked together with the medial and lateral palmar metacarpal nerves

Palmar nerves (Fig. 13.4)

The palmar neurovascular bundles run dorsolateral and dorsomedial to the deep digital flexor tendon in the metacarpus.

The site for injection is therefore subcutaneously just dorsal to the deep flexor

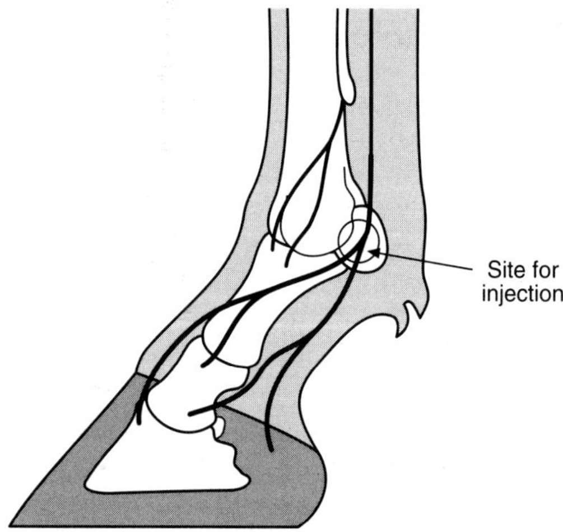

Figure 13.3   Site of abaxial sesamoid nerve block.

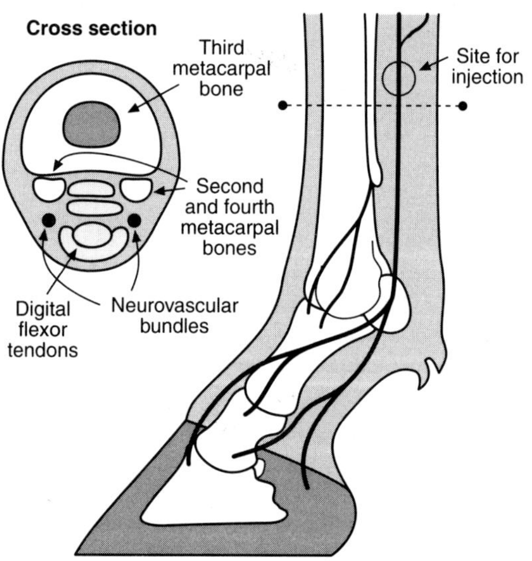

Figure 13.4   Site for blocking the palmar nerves.

tendon about 8 cm proximal to the fetlock. A volume of 3 ml local anaesthetic is infiltrated on each side using a 1 inch x 23G (25 x 0.65 mm) needle. In determining the optimal proximal-to-distal level for injection, consideration must be given to the presence of two anatomical structures:

(1) The digital sheath which surrounds the digital flexor tendons in the distal quarter of the metacarpus.
(2) A communicating nerve branch which runs from the medial palmar nerve distally and superficially around the palmar aspect of the flexor tendons to join the lateral palmar nerve. This is usually palpable on the palmar aspect of the superficial digital flexor tendon in the mid metacarpal region.

The injection sites for the palmar nerves should be above the level of the digital sheath, but below the communicating branch.

NB In the hindlimb the communicating branch is usually situated more distally and is generally more difficult to palpate. This leaves less room between the branch and the digital sheath and in this instance the injection is better made above the communicating branch.

The required number of needle penetrations of the skin can be reduced by injecting around both lateral and medial palmar nerves from the lateral side. This is done by performing the lateral injection as described above and then pushing the needle deeper right across the limb just in front of the deep digital flexor tendon to inject around the medial palmar nerve.

Palmar metacarpal nerves (Fig. 13.5)

The medial and lateral palmar metacarpal nerves are derived from the lateral palmar nerve at the level of the distal carpus and run distally, axial to the 2nd and 4th metacarpal (splint) bones. They emerge from under the distal button of the splint bone to supply the dorsal aspect of the fetlock joint.

The site for injection is subcutaneously just distal to the button of the splint bone on each side. A volume of 2 ml local anaesthetic is infiltrated on each side using a 1 inch x 23G (25 x 0.65 mm) needle.

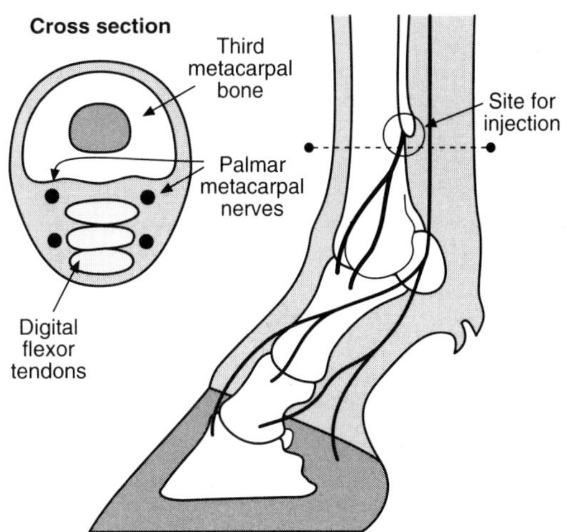

Figure 13.5   Site for blocking the palmar metacarpal nerves.

NB In the hindlimb the situation is complicated by the presence of medial and lateral dorsal metatarsal nerves (derived from the deep peroneal nerve), which contribute to the innervation of the dorsal aspect of the fetlock. Opinions vary on the necessity for specifically blocking these nerves to achieve adequate fetlock desensitization. The dorsal metatarsal nerves can be blocked via the same needle placement employed for the plantar metatarsal nerves by redirecting the needle one to two centimetres dorsally just under the skin and injecting a further 2 ml of local anaesthetic.

Subcarpal block

The subcarpal block involves anaesthetizing the medial and lateral palmar nerves and the medial and lateral palmar metacarpal nerves just below the carpus. This will desensitize the structures on the palmar aspect of the metacarpus in addition to the fetlock and digit.

Medial palmar nerve (Fig. 13.6)

The site for injection is on the dorsomedial margin of the deep flexor tendon beneath the carpal fascia just distal to the carpus. A volume of 6–8 ml local anaesthetic is infiltrated at a depth of approximately 1 cm using a 1 inch x 20G (25 x 0.90 mm) needle.

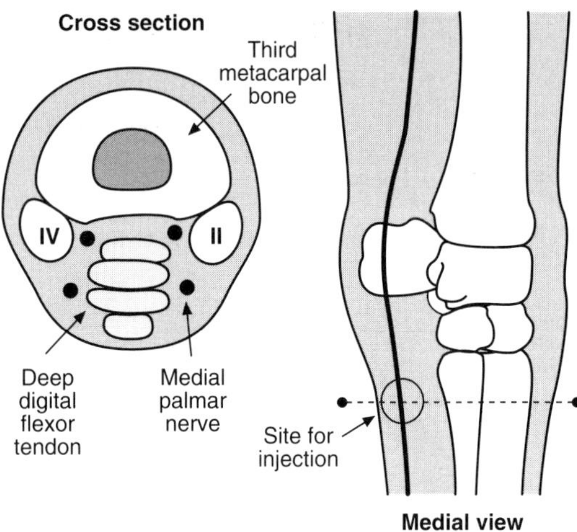

Figure 13.6   Site of medial palmar nerve block.

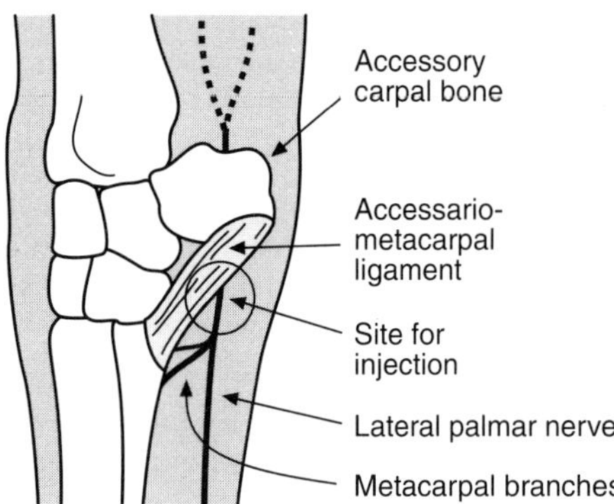

Figure 13.7   Site for blocking the lateral palmar nerve and the palmar metacarpal nerves.

Lateral palmar nerve and palmar metacarpal nerves (Fig. 13.7)

The lateral palmar nerve gives off a deep branch in the proximal metacarpus which in turn gives rise to the medial and lateral palmar metacarpal nerves. By blocking proximal to this branch the palmar metacarpal nerves are also blocked without the necessity for separate injections.

The site for injection is midway along and just distal to the ligament linking the palmar border of the accessory carpal bone to the head of the 4th metacarpal bone (the accessario-metacarpal ligament) and deep to the carpal

flexor retinaculum. A volume of 10 ml local anaesthetic is injected at a depth of 1–2 cm using a 1 inch x 20G (25 x 0.90 mm) needle.

Median and ulnar nerve block

Median and ulnar nerve blocks will desensitize the carpus and structures distal to it. As with tibial and peroneal blocks in the hindlimb, skin desensitization is not complete distal to the block but only affects certain areas (see below). It is therefore advisable to perform these proximal limb blocks on a different occasion to the more distal regional blocks in order to be able to demonstrate that the appropriate skin desensitization has occurred.

Median nerve (Fig. 13.8)

The site of injection is the caudomedial border of the radius just distal to the superficial pectoral muscle. The nerve lies cranial to the median artery and vein. A volume of 15 ml local anaesthetic is injected at a depth of 3–4 cm using a 2 inch x 19G (51 x 1.0 mm) needle. NB Skin desensitization involves only the medial aspect of the pastern.

Ulnar nerve (Fig. 13.9)

The site for injection lies in the groove on the palmar aspect of the antebrachium between the ulnaris lateralis and the flexor carpi ulnaris muscles, 10 cm proximal to the accessory

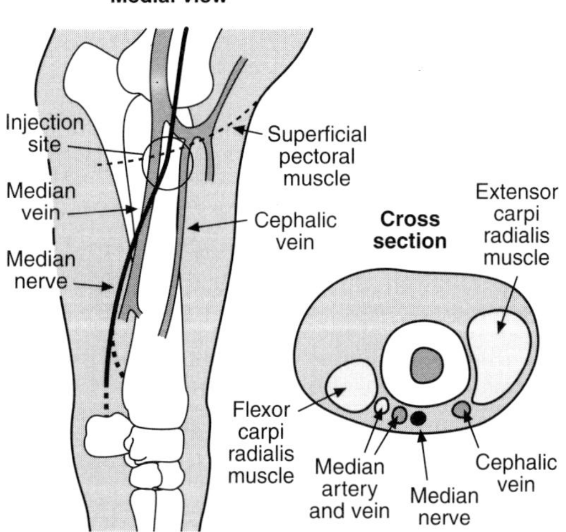

Figure 13.8   Site of median nerve block.

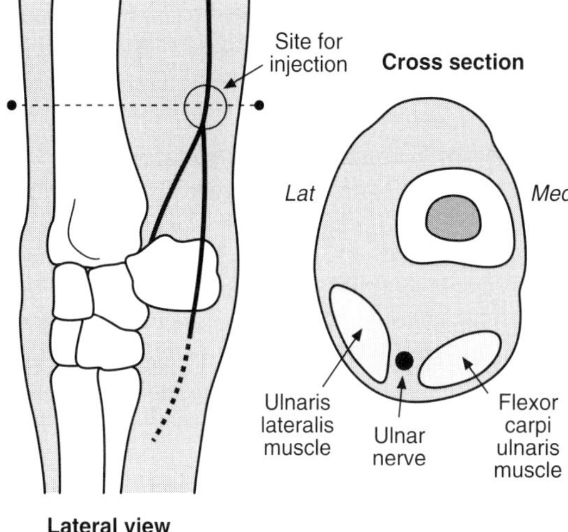

Figure 13.9   Site of ulnar nerve block.

carpal bone, at a depth of 1–2 cm. A volume of 10 ml local anaesthetic is injected using a 1 inch x 20G (25 x 0.90 mm) needle. NB Skin desensitization occurs on the dorsolateral aspect of the proximal metacarpus.

Sites of nerve block in the hindlimb

The distal hindlimb can be desensitized in very much the same way as the forelimb, as outlined above. When dealing with chronic hindlimb lamenesses, many clinicians will start with an abaxial sesamoid block, or even a four point block above the fetlock, as specific chronic foot lameness is generally less common in the hindlimb than in the forelimb. If a positive response is obtained to such a block, more specific regional or intra-synovial blocks distal to this level may be performed on a later occasion. Extra care should always be taken when performing hindlimb blocks owing to the greater potential for injury to the clinician.

Plantar and plantar metatarsal nerve block (four point block)

Details relevant to this hindlimb block are included under the distal forelimb four point block (above).

Tibial and peroneal nerve block

Tibial and peroneal blocks will eliminate deep sensation from the hock and structures distal to it. As with median and ulnar blocks in the forelimb, loss of skin sensation is limited to certain areas and may be inconsistent.

Tibial nerve (Fig. 13.10)

The site for injection is just caudal to the deep digital flexor tendon and cranial to the Achilles tendon about 10 cm proximal to the top of the tuber calcis on the medial aspect of the limb beneath the fascia. A volume of 15–20 ml local anaesthetic is deposited at a depth of 1 cm through a 1 inch x 20G (25 x 0.90 mm) needle. Skin sensation is usually lost between the bulbs of the heel.

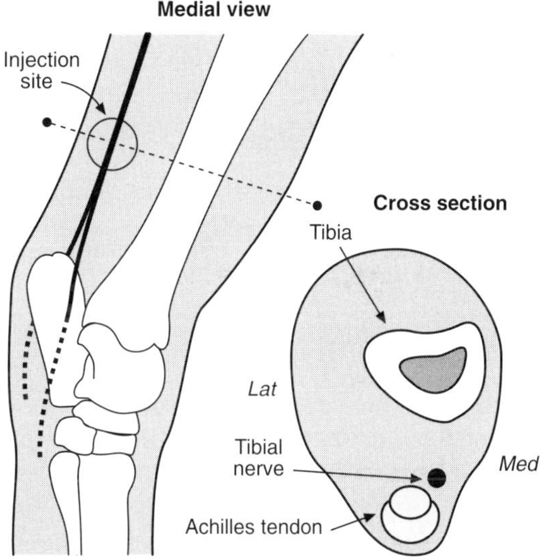

Figure 13.10   Site of tibial nerve block.

Peroneal nerve (Fig. 13.11)

The site for injection is between the long and lateral digital extensor tendons on the lateral aspect of the crus, 10 cm proximal to the lateral malleolus. The peroneal nerve has deep and superficial branches. A volume of 15 ml local anaesthetic is loaded into a syringe for delivery through a 2 inch x 19G (51 x 1.0 mm) needle. Ten ml is injected around the deep branch at a depth of about 2–3 cm, and 5 ml is delivered around the superficial branch during

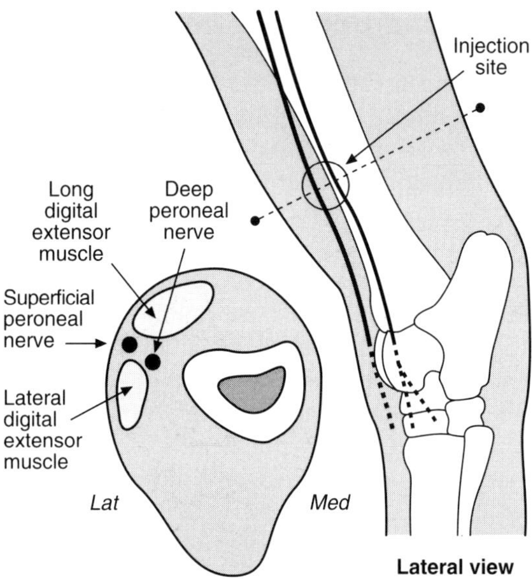

Figure 13.11   Site of peroneal nerve block.

withdrawal of the needle. Skin sensation is usually lost over the lateral aspect of the distal hock.

Intrasynovial analgesia — general considerations.

The general remarks made above in relation to perineural analgesia also apply for the most part to intrasynovial analgesia. However, a few additional points should be borne in mind. The consequences of inadvertent introduction of infection into a synovial cavity can be disastrous and it is therefore extremely important that all practical steps are taken to minimize this risk. The hair at the site of needle placement should, therefore, always be clipped and the skin thoroughly scrubbed with antiseptic solution prior to needle placement. The clinician should wear sterile gloves and fresh bottles of local anaesthetic solution should always be used for each injection.

The most reliable sign that the needle has been accurately placed within the synovial cavity is the appearance of synovial fluid at the hub of the needle. However, this will not always happen immediately for a number of reasons:

- Some of the smaller joints and bursae contain only a very small amount of synovial fluid (e.g. the navicular bursa or the distal intertarsal joint).
- Synovial villi may be sucked into the end of the needle and effectively prevent any synovial fluid escaping through it.

Twisting or slightly repositioning the needle may help to obtain synovial fluid and thus confirm accurate needle placement. It may also be possible to aspirate yellow synovial fluid into the syringe once a small amount of local anaesthetic has been injected. In some small synovial cavities local anaesthetic (sometimes tinged yellow by the synovial fluid) will reflux spontaneously into the syringe when pressure is taken off the needle, indicating that injection has been made into a closed cavity. In some situations the depth and direction that the needle has penetrated indicate that it must have entered the joint space (e.g. penetration of the tarsometatarsal joint). Other, less satisfactory, indicators of correct placement include the palpable contact of the needle with the cartilage of the articular surface and the lack of resistance to injection of the anaesthetic solution.

There is no reliable way of testing whether an intrasynovial block has taken effectively and thus it is important to be sure that needle placement is accurate in the first instance. In those cases where a positive response is seen, the time taken to achieve soundness varies from as little as five minutes for small distal joints (such as the distal interphalangeal joint), to up to an hour for large complex joints such as the stifle.

Intrasynovial analgesia in the forelimb

Distal interphalangeal (coffin) joint (Fig. 13.12)

The site for injection is in the dorsal midline approximately one centimetre proximal to the coronary band with the needle angled slightly more steeply than at right angles to the skin.

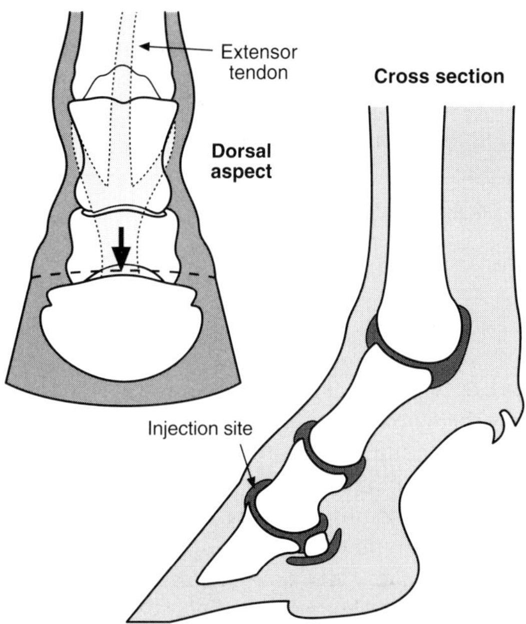

Figure 13.12   Position and direction of needle insertion to anaesthetize the coffin joint.

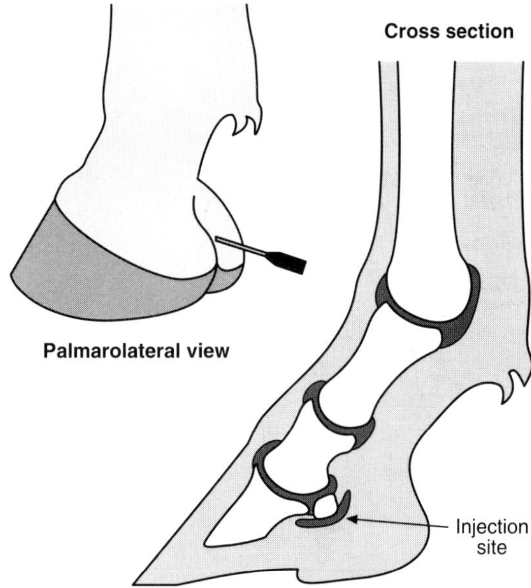

Figure 13.13   Position and direction of needle insertion to anaesthetize the navicular bursa.

The needle is advanced through the extensor tendon and correct placement is usually associated with an immediate flow of synovial fluid. A volume of 5–8 ml local anaesthetic is delivered through a 1 inch x 20G (25 x 0.90 mm) needle.

Navicular bursa (Fig. 13.13)

The site for injection is at the midline of the palmar aspect of the pastern between the bulbs of the heel. It is helpful to place a bleb of local anaesthetic subcutaneously using a fine needle before positioning a larger needle. A 3.5 inch x 19G (90 x 1.0 mm) disposable spinal needle is aimed to run through the digital cushion to the flexor cortex of the navicular bone.

The exact angle at which the needle needs to be inserted varies depending on the foot conformation of the horse. Radiographic guidance may be helpful in determining this — at specialist centres insertion can be monitored periodically by fluoroscopy. In practice, a plain film can be taken prior to needle placement with a small metallic marker taped to the site of intended skin puncture. This allows estimation of the necessary angle of insertion relative to the weight bearing surface of the foot.

Synovial fluid does not often appear at the hub of the needle initially, although passive reflux of local anaesthetic plus fluid usually occurs if pressure is released from the plunger after the injection of 2 ml of local anaesthetic. It is possible to inject a mixture of local anaesthetic and a small amount of a water soluble, non-ionic, organic iodine contrast material, e.g. iopamidol ('Niopam': Merck), or iohexol ('Omnipaque': Nycomed) and sub-sequently take a further lateromedial radio-graph of the foot. This should demonstrate the contrast material within the confines of the navicular bursa if the injection has been made correctly.

Proximal interphalangeal (pastern) joint (Fig. 13.14)

The site for injection lies in the dorsal midline approximately 3 cm proximal to the coronary band with the needle angled slightly more steeply than at right angles to the skin. Firm palpation may reveal the level of the dorsal

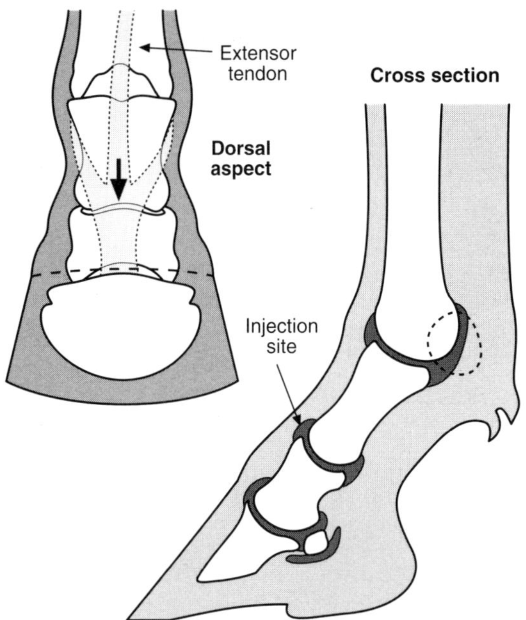

Figure 13.14   Position and direction of needle insertion to anaesthetize the pastern joint.

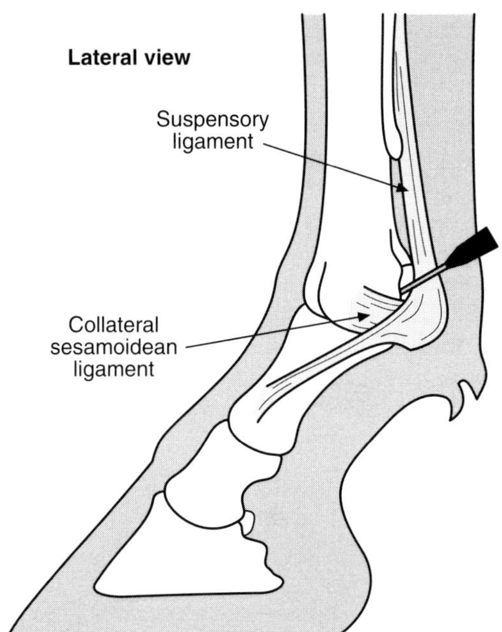

Figure 13.15   Site for anaesthetizing the fetlock joint.

joint margin and provide a further guide to the level for insertion of the needle. The needle is advanced through the extensor tendon until bone is reached. Synovial fluid usually emerges following successful placement. A volume of 5 ml local anaesthetic is introduced using a 1 inch x 20G (25 x 0.90 mm) needle.

Metacarpophalangeal (fetlock) joint (Fig. 13.15)

The site for injection of the proximal palmar pouch lies laterally between the palmar aspect of the third metacarpal bone and the suspensory ligament, just proximal to the collateral sesamoidean ligament that links the proximal sesamoid bone to the third metacarpal bone. The pouch is often distended in the presence of fetlock joint disease. A volume of 10 ml local anaesthetic is introduced through a 1 inch x 20G (25 x 0.90 mm) needle with the limb bearing weight, or with the joint flexed.

An alternative technique for arthrocentesis and/or intra-articular injection of the metacarpophalangeal joint has recently been

suggested. This involves placing the needle through the collateral sesamoidean ligament between the lateral sesamoid bone and the third metacarpal bone with the joint flexed.

Digital tendon sheath

Analgesia is usually performed only in the presence of synovial distension of the sheath. *The site for injection* is the most prominently distended part. A volume of 10 ml local anaesthetic is introduced through a 1 inch x 20G (25 x 0.90 mm) needle.

Midcarpal joint (Fig. 13.16)

The site for injection with the carpus flexed lies on the dorsal surface of the joint just lateral to the extensor carpi radialis tendon between the proximal and distal rows of carpal bones. The midcarpal joint usually communicates with the carpometacarpal joint, which will also be anaesthetized by this procedure. A volume of 10 ml local anaesthetic is introduced using a 1 inch x 20G (25 x 0.90 mm) needle.

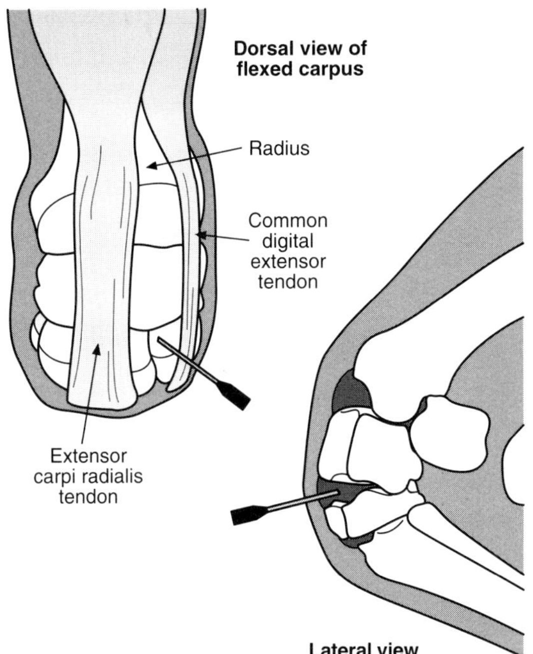

Figure 13.16 Site for anaesthetizing the midcarpal joint.

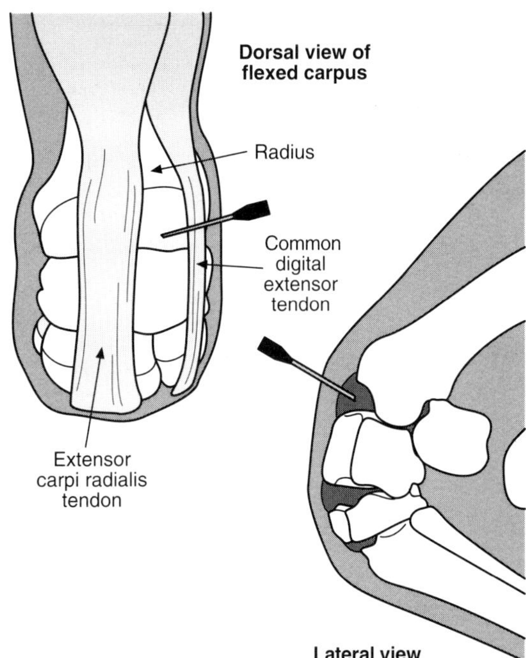

Figure 13.17 Site for anaesthetizing the antebrachiocarpal joint.

Antebrachiocarpal joint (Fig. 13.17)

The site for injection with the carpus flexed lies on the dorsal surface of the joint just lateral to the extensor carpi radialis tendon between the distal radius and the proximal row of carpal bones. A volume of 10 ml local anaesthetic is injected using a 1 inch x 20G (25 x 0.90 mm) needle.

Elbow (Fig. 13.18)

The site for injection lies just cranial or caudal to the lateral collateral ligament. The level of the joint space can usually be appreciated with careful palpation. A volume of 15 ml local anaesthetic is injected through a 2 inch x 19G (51 x 1.0 mm) needle.

Shoulder (Fig. 13.19)

The site of needle insertion lies horizontally between the cranial and caudal prominences of the lateral tuberosity of the humerus at 45 degrees to the long axis of the horse. A volume of 20 ml local anaesthetic is introduced through a 3.5 inch x 19G (90 x 1.0 mm) disposable spinal needle.

Intrasynovial analgesia in the hindlimb

Tarsometatarsal joint (Fig. 13.20)

The site for injection lies over the head of the fourth metatarsal bone, between this point and the fourth tarsal bone. A 1 inch x 20G (25 x 0.90 mm) needle is directed at 45 degrees distally and slightly axially. A volume of 5 ml local anaesthetic is introduced.

Distal intertarsal joint (Fig. 13.21)

The site for injection lies one centimetre proximal and slightly dorsal to the junction between the head of the second metatarsal bone, the third metatarsal bone and the distal row of tarsal bones. A volume of 5 ml local anaesthetic is introduced through a 1 inch x 20G (25 x 0.90 mm) needle.

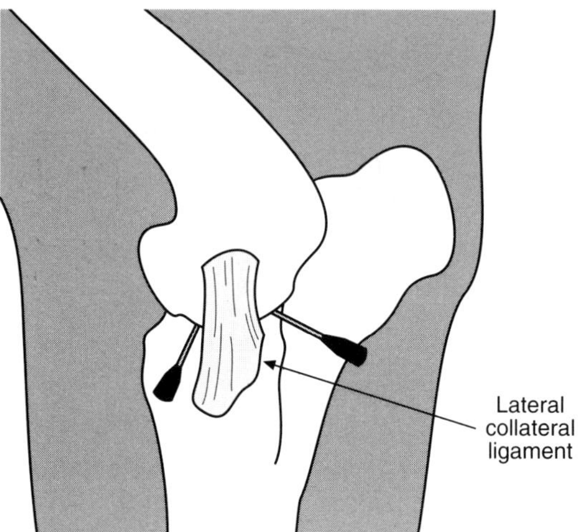

Figure 13.18   Site for anaesthetizing the elbow joint.

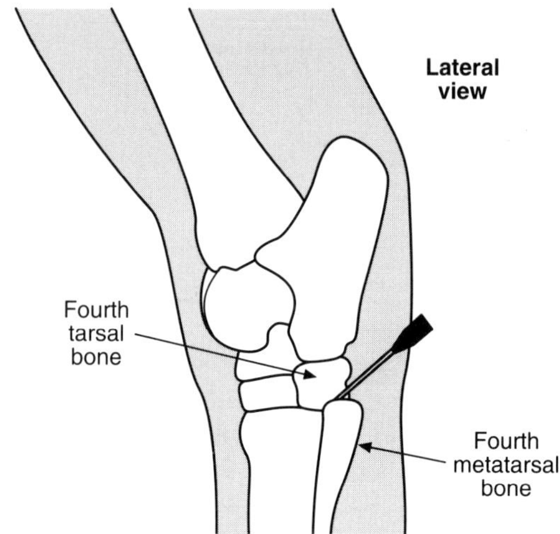

Figure 13.20   Site for anaesthetizing the tarsometatarsal joint.

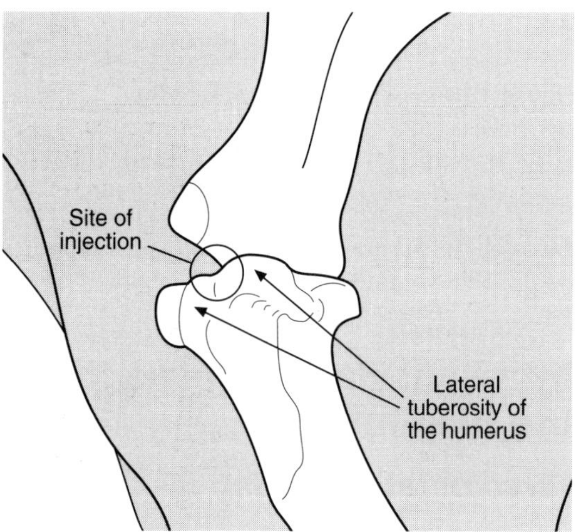

Figure 13.19   Position and direction of needle insertion to anaesthetize the shoulder joint.

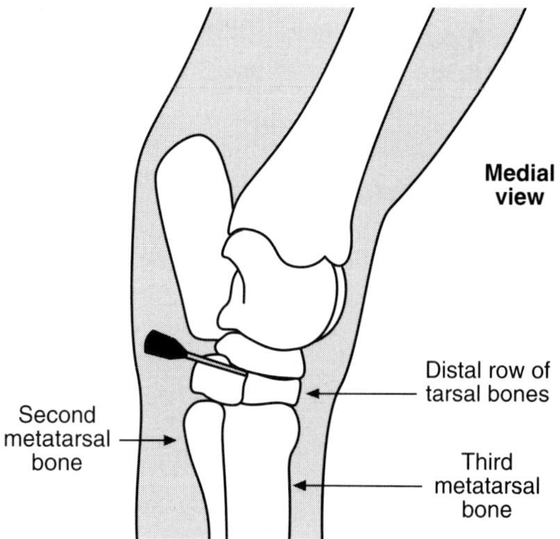

Figure 13.21   Site for anaesthetizing the distal intertarsal joint.

Tarsocrural joint (Fig. 13.22)

The site for injection is into the dorsomedial pouch of the joint just medial or lateral to the saphenous vein. A volume of 15 ml local anaesthetic is delivered through a 1 inch x 20G (25 x 0.90 mm) needle.

Femoropatellar joint (Fig. 13.23)

The site for injection is either medial or lateral to the middle patellar ligament. The needle is directed inwards and proximally. The femoropatellar joint communicates with the medial femorotibial joint in at least 65% of horses. A volume of 20 ml local anaesthetic is injected through a 2 inch x 18G (51 x 1.2 mm) needle.

An alternative approach involves injection into the lateral cul-de-sac of the femoropatellar joint, just caudal to the lateral patellar ligament and 5 cm proximal to the lateral condyle of the tibia.

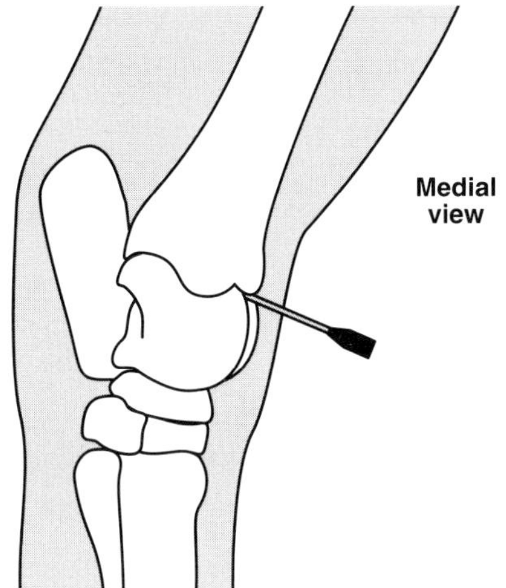

Figure 13.22   Site for anaesthetizing the tarsocrural joint.

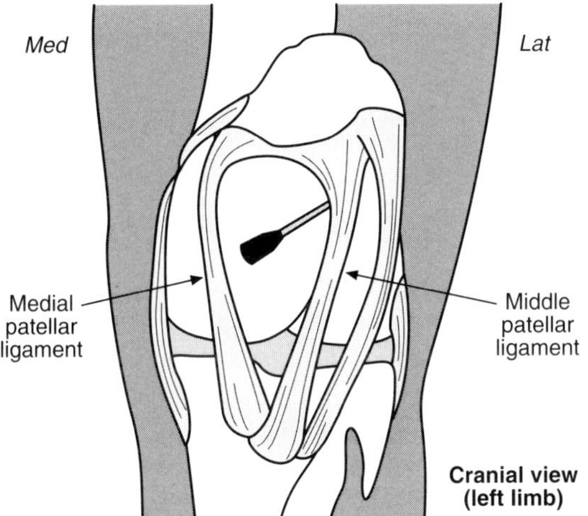

Figure 13.23   Position and direction of needle insertion to anaesthetize the femoropatellar joint.

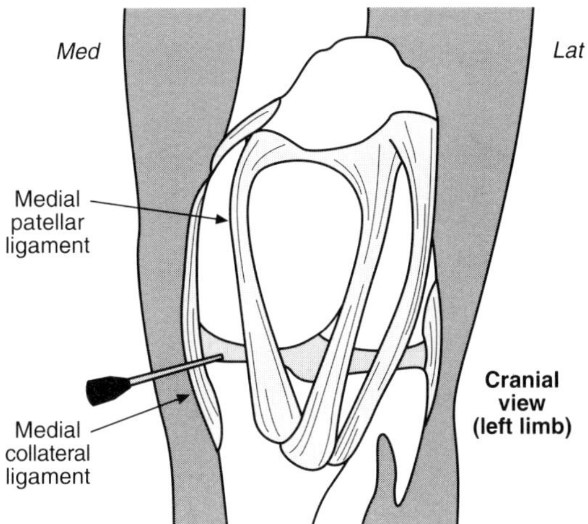

Figure 13.24   Site for anaesthetizing the medial femorotibial joint.

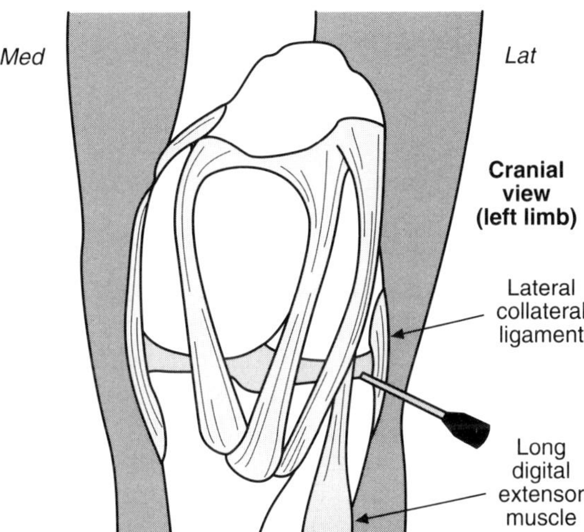

Figure 13.25   Site for anaesthetizing the laterial femorotibial joint.

Medial femorotibial joint (Fig. 13.24)

The site for injection lies between the medial patellar ligament and the medial collateral ligament just proximal to the tibial plateau. A volume of 20 ml local anaesthetic is delivered through a 2 inch x 18G (51 x 1.2 mm) needle.

Lateral femorotibial joint (Fig. 13.25)

The site for injection lies between the tendon of origin of the long digital extensor and the lateral collateral ligament of the femorotibial joint just proximal to the tibia. A volume of 20 ml local anaesthetic is delivered through a 2 inch x 18G (51 x 1.2 mm) needle.

III. Imaging techniques

Imaging techniques are most usefully employed once the site or sites of abnormality have been definitively established by physical examination and, if necessary, local analgesia. The last twenty years have seen the development of a variety of imaging procedures in human medicine but to date only radiography, ultrasonography and to a lesser extent nuclear scintigraphy have found routine clinical application in the horse.

Radiography

X-ray machines

Modern portable X-ray machines are capable of producing diagnostic images of most of the equine limb, particularly if used in conjunction with rare earth cassette screens for the more proximal regions.

The capacity to produce a reasonably high tube current (e.g. 60 mA) will enable short exposure times to be employed which will reduce the chance of movement blur. The machine should be easily and quietly manoeuvrable around the patient and the tube head should be capable of going down to the floor, to radiograph feet, and up to the height of upper cervical spine and head. A light beam diaphragm is essential for accurate collimation of the X-ray beam.

Intensifying screens and film

Rare earth intensifying screens are more sensitive than older calcium tungstate screens, enabling shorter exposure times and extending the capabilities of lower powered equipment. High definition rare earth screens should be used for distal limb radiography to produce highly detailed images. Single screen cassettes with single emulsion films are available which will give even better detail, but at the expense of slightly longer exposure times.

Supplementary equipment

Grids are employed to reduce the effects of scattered radiation on the film. They are most helpful when radiographing the thicker proximal parts of the horse which produce more scattered radiation, e.g. shoulders, spine and pelvis.

Cassette holders should be employed wherever possible to support the cassette while a film is being exposed. *There is no reason why a cassette need ever be hand-held for radiography of the carpus, hock or more distal limb structures.* For radiography of the feet, cassettes may be supported in wooden boxes which, for certain views, need to be strong enough to support the weight of the horse. Blocks to raise the foot off the ground are also essential, e.g. for lateromedial views of the feet (see later under: 'Laminitis'). Cassettes may be placed in a bag supported by a drip stand for radiography of the shoulder, spine or head.

Films should always be permanently labelled with the date, owner and animal identification, limb under examination, projection, and identification of lateral/medial aspects.

Positioning, centring and collimation

The part to be radiographed should be as close as possible to the cassette and parallel to it — thereby avoiding magnification and distortion of the resultant image. The beam should be centred on the area of primary interest — usually at the level of the joint space in the case of joint examination. The beam should be collimated to include only the area of interest and in such a way that it does not extend beyond the margins of the cassette at any point. This not only improves radiation safety but also image quality by reducing the amount of unnecessary scatter.

Exposure factors

Production of an exposure chart or log, based on experience with a particular machine and film/screen combinations, is an invaluable aid to the consistent production of high quality radiographs. As many factors as possible should be standardized, including films, screens, tube-film distance and development procedures and materials. The only variable to take into account should then be patient size.

Preparation for radiography

The degree of restraint which is required will depend upon the temperament of the patient and the projections required. Manual restraint with a headcollar or bridle and bit will be sufficient for most horses. Sedation with detomidine or a combination of detomidine and butorphanol will help in more difficult animals. Restraint should be sufficient to enable high quality films to be produced safely and quickly. In particular, it should be sufficient to eliminate patient movement which will otherwise degrade film quality and increase the physical and radiation hazards to personnel and subject.

Dirt on the coat and, in particular, the foot will cast confusing shadows on the film. The hair coat over the area of interest should be washed or brushed clean prior to radiography. Prior to radiographing the feet the shoes should be removed, the feet cleaned, superficial horn pared away and the frog sulci packed with a material of soft tissue density (e.g. soft soap) to even out the density of the soft tissues.

Personnel

All personnel involved in the radiographic examination should wear leaded rubber aprons — other people should be excluded from the area. Staff regularly involved in radiographic examination should wear a monitor badge. Everyone involved should be aware of the procedure to be undertaken and how to achieve the optimal result quickly and safely.

Radiographic projections

Equine bones are relatively thick and dense. This results in difficulty in appreciating subtle abnormalities when they are superimposed on the normal bone mass. Many abnormalities are easiest to see when 'skylined' on the edge of the bone.

A radiograph is a two dimensional representation of a three dimensional object. In order that any abnormality may be fully appreciated, it must be imaged from at least two directions. This explains the necessity for using multiple projections in equine limb radiography. In very general terms it is preferable to obtain views from in front, at the side, and at least two additonal oblique views taken at 45 degrees when radiographing distal joints.

There is no limit to the number of projections that may be obtained of any particular area of the equine limb. The decision as to which are regarded as routine and used in every examination of a particular area and which are used only in specific circumstances remains a matter of clinical judgement and to some extent personal preference. A balance must be struck between the risk of missing or incompletely understanding a lesion by obtaining too few views and the additional time, expense and radiation exposure if every conceivable projection is employed in every case under examination. The following list is therefore not intended to be comprehensive, but to act as a guide as to which views might be regarded as routine and what specific additional options are commonly used.

Not infrequently, additional views are obtained once the routine views have been examined. Slight variations in exposure factors or the angle of obliquity are attempted in order to demonstrate more clearly a lesion seen, or suspected, on the initial films. To some extent each radiographic examination is therefore unique and tailor-made for the circumstances surrounding the individual horse and should not be constrained by formal lists of possible views.

Terminology of projections

To avoid imprecision and consequent confusion, a specific nomenclature has been

the opposite limb may be helpful for comparison.

Ultrasonography

Diagnostic ultrasound provides a useful means of imaging soft tissue structures which is employed in the examination of the equine musculoskeletal system; particularly in the evaluation of flexor tendon and ligamentous injuries. However, the technique is equally applicable to other structures including muscle and to some extent joints.

The tendons and ligaments most commonly imaged are those on the palmar/plantar aspect of the metacarpus/tarsus. These are fairly superficial structures and are therefore best imaged using a high frequency transducer to give good image detail — 7.5 MHz transducers have been most commonly employed. Small linear array transducers are probably the best option as they give better longitudinal images than sector probes. A 'stand-off' to separate the transducer from the skin is essential when imaging the superficial digital flexor tendon in order to bring it within the focal zone of the transducer.

Restraint of the patient is as described for radiography. Preparation involves clipping the hair over the site to be 'scanned' and thoroughly cleaning the underlying skin.

Acoustic coupling gel is then applied to the skin and the transducer to enable sound to travel easily between the two.

When scanning the palmar metacarpus/metatarsus, both transverse and longitudinal images may be produced throughout the region. The individual structures to be identified include the superficial and deep digital flexor tendons, the accessory head of the deep digital flexor tendon (inferior check ligament) and the suspensory ligament (Fig. 13.29).

Each structure should be evaluated for its size, shape, position, echogenicity and margination. Slight alterations in the angle or pressure with which the transducer is held against the skin can markedly alter the image. In consequence, attempts should be made at each level to optimally image each structure in turn as it is difficult to produce an optimal image of all of them at once. If possible, hard copy images should be made and kept as permanent records of the images produced and these should be suitably labelled with the animal and owner identification, date, limb and level of the scan.

Any suspect abnormalities should be re-imaged several times to check that the appearance is consistently abnormal. 'Lesions' that can be made to disappear by altering the angle of the transducer are usually artefactual. As usual, comparison with the contralateral

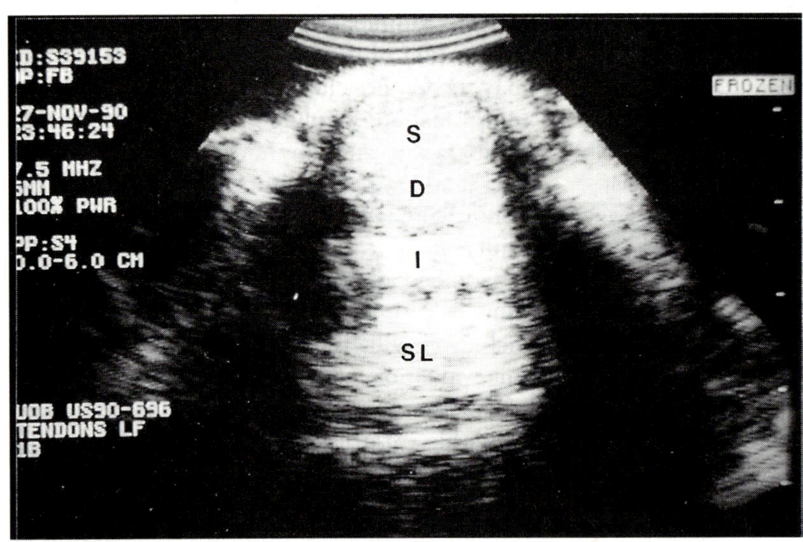

Figure 13.29
Ultrasonogram showing the superficial (S) and deep digital (D) flexor tendons in a healthy horse. This image was obtained at the proximal third of the cannon bone. Also seen are the inferior check ligament (I) and the suspensory ligament (SL).

limb is helpful in interpreting images in many cases.

Nuclear scintigraphy

Nuclear scintigraphy is limited to specialist centres but the principles are described here for general interest. The technique involves the administration of a radioactive nuclide which is conjugated to a compound which becomes preferentially located in a particular body system or lesion. The level of uptake at a particular site can then be determined using a detecting or imaging system which records the radiation emitted from that site at a particular time after administration.

In evaluation of the skeletal system the isotope most commonly employed is Technetium 99m. This emits gamma radiation at 140 KeV with a half life of 6 hours. This is usually linked to methylene diphosphonate which is taken up into the mineral lattice of bone at a concentration dependent upon the rate of bone turnover at a particular site. Sites that have a high rate of bone turnover for physiological or pathological reasons will therefore accumulate more of the nuclide than normal and this will be reflected in an increase in the amount of gamma radiation being emitted from that particular site.

The radiopharmaceutical is normally administered as an intravenous injection and the scan is performed several hours later. Tc99m–MDP is excreted via the urinary tract which has consequences for both imaging and radiation safety. Urine within the bladder and when voided contains a high concentration of nuclide.

Scintigraphy is probably most useful in the detection of relatively acute bone injuries which may be difficult to define in other ways in their early stages, e.g. stress fractures. More chronic entities such as degenerative joint disease may also result in variations in uptake, but these can be more subtle and therefore less easy to interpret.

Diagnostic arthroscopy

Arthroscopy allows direct inspection of synovial cavities, including joints and tendon sheaths. It therefore allows assessment of cartilage surfaces, synovial membranes and intra-articular ligaments; all of which may be difficult to assess fully by other means.

The drawbacks and limitations are firstly that the procedure necessitates general anaesthesia and therefore the usual attendant risks and expense. Secondly, while the range of areas that can be inspected using the arthroscope is constantly expanding, there are still limitations as to the joints that can be meaningfully evaluated and it is rarely possible to examine any joint in its entirety.

Within these limitations the technique can still be useful as a purely diagnostic aid. It is particularly useful in the examination of joints known to be a site of pain through the use of intra-articular analgesia, but where no explanation has been forthcoming using radiography or other imaging techniques, e.g. ligamentous injuries in the carpus or femorotibial joints.

IV. Laminitis

Laminitis has been mentioned earlier in this chapter but merits a separate section. The acute form represents an emergency that requires immediate diagnosis to enable appropriate treatment; otherwise the pedal bone is at risk of displacement within the foot.

Laminitis is essentially an interruption of the blood supply within the vascular dermis or *corium* which surrounds the pedal bone. The result is a painful disruption of the attachment between the corium (the sensitive laminae) and the hoof wall (the insensitive laminae). It affects all types of equidae, especially ponies and donkeys. One or more feet may be affected.

Associated history

There are various situations which predispose to laminitis and the associated history can be of diagnostic use:

- Overweight and inactive ponies and donkeys are metabolically predisposed to laminitis. The greatest risk in these individuals is associated with feeding highly nutritious grass, cereals, coarse mixes, compound nuts, etc.
- Prolonged or repeated concussion such as road work or jumping on hard ground will predispose.
- Toxaemia associated with sepsis, of whatever origin, will predispose.
- A high percentage of horses with pituitary adenoma (Cushing's disease) develop laminitis (see Chapter 5: 'Endocrine diseases').
- Corticosteroids can induce iatrogenic laminitis, particularly in protracted use.

Acute signs of laminitis

The early stages of laminitis involve vasoconstriction of the vascular bed in the corium. The result is a painful ischaemia and an increased resistance to blood flow within the foot. This obstruction to arterial flow opens arterio-venous shunts at the level of the coronet and increases the digital arterial pulse volume.

As well as being painful, the ischaemia denies adequate oxygen and nutrition to the sensitive laminae. This predisposes poor keratinization, resulting in a loss of attachment between the stratum germinativum of the sensitive laminae and the interdigitations of the insensitive laminae. In addition, capillaries within the sensitive laminae become leaky, allowing exudation between the laminar attachment, thus increasing pain and the tendency to separate. The animal's weight bearing on the compromised laminae gives impetus to their forced separation and adds to the pain. Separation of the laminae will cause the pedal bone to be displaced downwards within the foot.

These various changes are responsible for a number of acute clinical signs. The extent of the injury, and therefore the clinical signs, varies from mild and reversible to severe and progressive. In severe forms there is separation of the pedal bone from the hoof wall. The following signs are collectively diagnostic:

- The animal is unwilling to move and may lie down for protracted periods.
- The stance may reflect the horse's attempt to throw its weight back onto its heels in order to reduce the pain, i.e. to oppose the separation of the greatest area of laminae at the front of the pedal bone. If only the front feet are affected, the body's weight is thrown back over the hindlegs, producing a characteristic 'backward lean' stance. If all four feet are affected, the weight is transferred to the mid-back region and the stance appears more normal, but the back may be roached.
- In progression, the stride and arc of foot movement are reduced. There is a characteristic action in which the heel of an affected foot is always brought to the ground before the toe.
- There is a bounding digital pulse palpable over the proximal sesamoids behind the fetlock of each affected foot (Fig. 13.30).
- In early stages there may be heat in the coronet and upper hoof, but this is a variable and unreliable sign.

Within 24–48 hours of acute onset the pedal bone may start to displace within the hoof, giving rise to further dramatic signs:

- If the shape of the coronet at the dorsal wall has changed from a normal rounded bulge

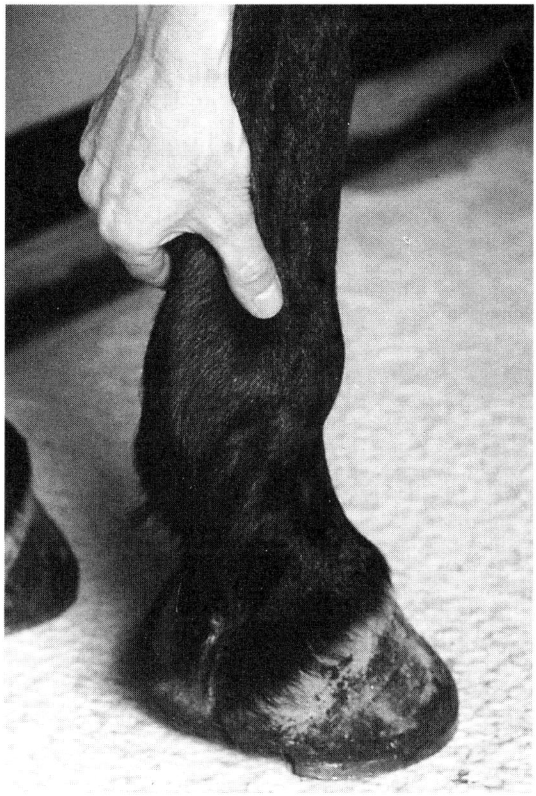

Figure 13.30   Location of the finger and thumb over the proximal sesamoids of the fetlock to appreciate digital pulsation.

to a sunken channel, then it is likely that the pedal bone has displaced, dragging the coronary corium with it. This distal movement of the front of the pedal bone is termed *'founder'*. If the coronet is palpably sunken beyond the dorsal wall, around the quarters and heels, then it is likely that there has been a total separation of interlaminar bonds with displacement of the entire pedal bone. This extreme condition is termed a *'sinker'*.

- Extensive laminar exudate may track upwards and break out at the front of the coronet.
- A pliability of the sole in front of the point of the frog indicates that the animal's weight on its displaced pedal bone has induced a pressure necrosis of the soft tissues at its toe, and that it has impinged on the solar horn. In extreme cases the sole is penetrated and the toe of the pedal bone may be visible.

The speed and severity of these changes varies enormously between cases. *In acute cases pedal movement can begin within 24 hours of onset and for this reason the condition constitutes an emergency.* More chronic cases may deteriorate gradually over weeks or months. If the pain of the acute case exceeds 48 hours then lateral radiographs should be taken to assess pedal movement.

Radiography in laminitis

To be of diagnostic use, radiographs must show the relationship of the pedal bone to the hoof wall and sole in order to judge whether it has moved from its normal position. A lateral view of the whole hoof is required with markers indicating the outside of the wall, the relative position of the frog to the base of the pedal bone, and the ground surface.

To achieve this a wooden block is required to raise the foot approximately 8 cm from the ground. A wire is embedded into the bearing surface of the block to provide a radiopaque ground reference.

The sole and frog are trimmed lightly to remove excess or flaking horn. A stiff wire of known length is then used to delineate the front and top of the hoof wall on the radiograph. This is fastened in position using adhesive tape with the top of the wire placed at the point where the wall starts to change from hard to soft horn (Fig. 13.31). Because the wire is of known length, it can be used as a reference for measurements on the radiograph, thus overcoming any artefacts of magnification. In this way the 'displacement distance' (see below) can be measured and compared with subsequent radiographs.

The position of the point of the frog in relation to the base of the pedal bone can be judged by inserting a shortened drawing pin into the frog approximately 2 cm behind its apex. Its position in the foot is marked by a line drawn across the trimmed sole with a felt pen, thus enabling cross reference between the pin image on X-ray and its position in the patient's foot. This is of particular relevance if it is intended that a 'heart bar' shoe will be fitted as

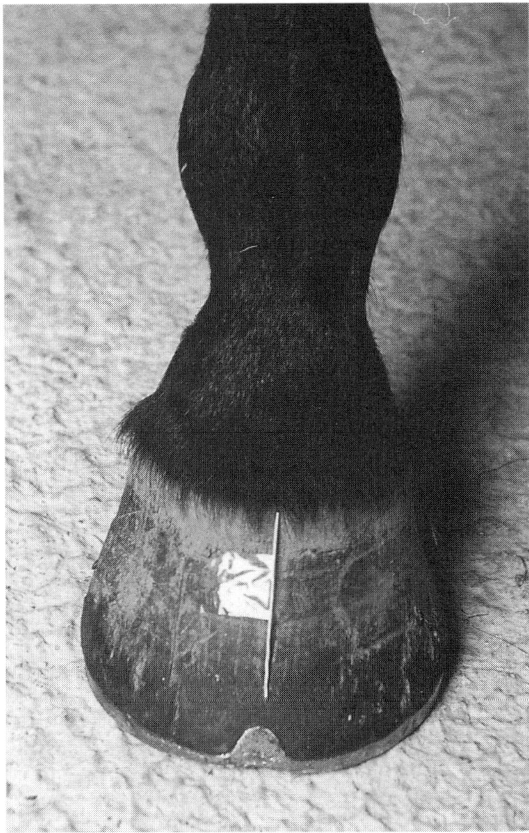

Figure 13.31   Placement of a wire marker at the front of the hoof prior to radiographic assessment of laminitis.

part of the management of the condition.

The radiograph is taken with the leg in a vertical standing position. This usually requires the opposite leg to be raised so that the horse stands straight on the foot under investigation. The beam should be parallel to the top of the block and perpendicular to the axis of the limb.

Interpretation

In the healthy foot the phalanges are in a straight line and the wire marker at the front of the hoof is parallel to the front of the pedal bone. The top of this wire is usually just above the top of the pedal bone at the extensor process (Fig. 13.32).

In pedal displacement there is an increased vertical distance between the top of the wire and the extensor process (displacement distance), and the front of the pedal bone is no longer parallel with the marker wire (Fig. 13.33). If the pedal bone is tipped out of straight alignment with the first and second phalanges, it is probably due to the pull of the deep digital flexor tendon — a condition frequently referred to as 'rotation' of the pedal bone. In the extreme case of total pedal displacement (a 'sinker'), the vertical distance between the top of the wire and the extensor

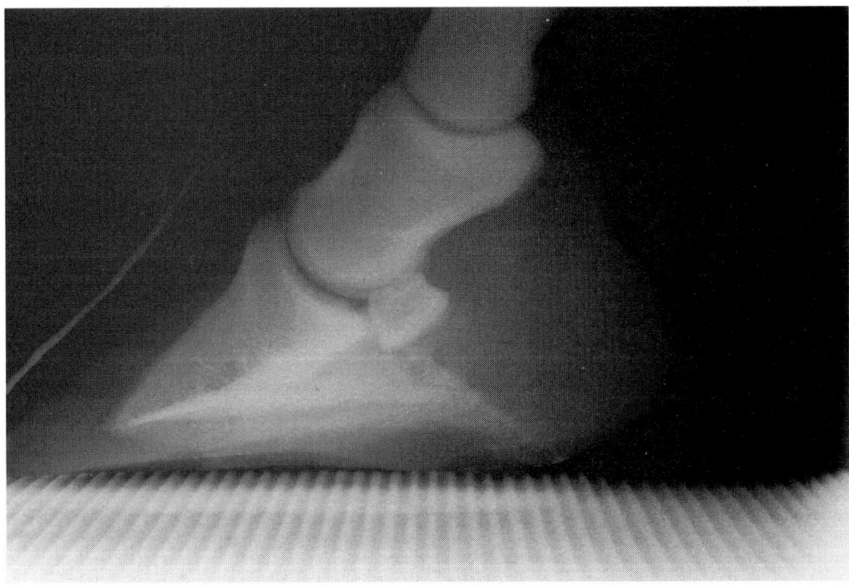

Figure 13.32
Radiograph showing the relationship of the wire marker to the pedal bone in a healthy foot.

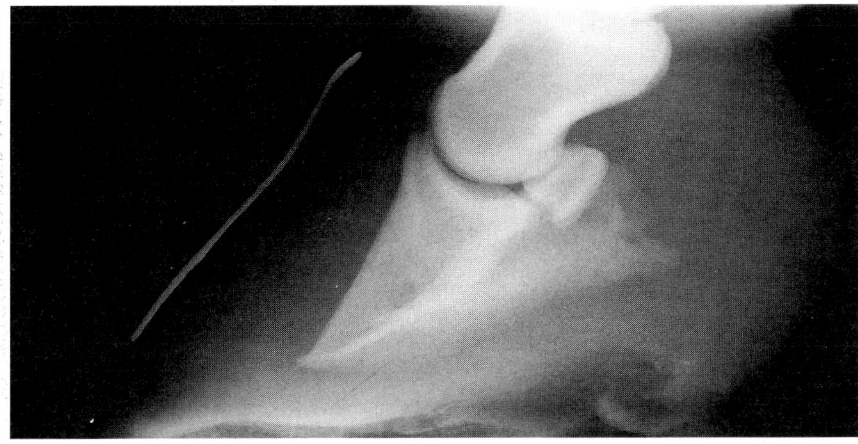

Figure 13.33 Radiograph showing pedal displacement. Note that the marker wire is not parallel with the front of the pedal bone and that the extensor process is well below the top of the wire.

process increases greatly and the toe of the pedal bone is brought close to the inside of the solar horn and may be seen pressing onto it.

Chronic signs of laminitis

A number of characteristic hoof changes are associated with chronic laminitis:

- There is a disproportionate growth between the heel, quarter and front regions of the coronet. Because the blood supply at the front of the coronet is usually under pressure from pedal displacement during the acute episode, the subsequent growth of hoof wall is slower than that of the heel, i.e. the growth rate at the front of the hoof is reduced.

- The disproportionate growth rates cause hoof rings to grow out divergent at the heel and close together at the toe ('laminitic rings'), unlike the parallel rings seen in the wall of the healthy foot.
- Looking at the sole, the white line becomes thickened at the toe as a result of the detachment of interlaminar bonds at the front of the foot. This thickening, combined with differential hoof wall growth from the coronet, provokes a 'curling' of the toe in the chronic laminitic patient.
- The normal concavity of the sole is lost and it assumes a flattened or even convex shape as a result of chronic pedal displacement.
- Radiographs will reveal the various disparities considered in 'Radiography in laminitis' (above).

V. **Myopathies**

The commonest myopathy encountered in equine practice is exertional rhabdomyolysis (synonyms: 'azoturia'; 'tying up'; 'set fast'). Less common are muscle infections, post-anaesthetic myopathy, an atypical form of myositis with myoglobinuria, and nutritional muscular dystrophy.

Exertional rhabdomyolysis ('azoturia')

This acute onset myopathy occurs during exercise and interferes with the normal gait. The hindlimbs become stiff, there is considerable pain and the horse may stagger or, in the extreme, collapse.

Clinical examination sometimes reveals a hardness of the gluteal and lumbar muscles and in severe cases the urine will show discolouration owing to release of the muscle respiratory pigment myoglobin.

Diagnosis

- The clinical signs associated with exercise are highly indicative. The immediate differentials are iliac thrombosis (see above under: 'Hindlimb — examination of the pelvis and hip'), vertebral or pelvic fracture associated with a fall, and colic.

- The serum muscle enzymes creatine phosphokinase (CPK) and aspartate aminotransferase (AST) are elevated as a result of muscle cell degeneration (see later).

- In severe cases the urine assumes a brown to black discolouration depending upon the amount of myoglobin released from damaged muscle cells.

Comments

- Serum muscle enzymes are an excellent monitor of recovery. The horse should be kept on a low plane of nutrition and not brought back into (gentle) work until both enzymes have returned to their normal ranges.

- Differential causes of urine discolouration include haematuria and haemoglobinuria. In the case of haematuria, red blood cells will settle out of a urine sample whereas haemoglobin and myoglobin will not. Because haemoglobinuria is invariably a result of intercurrent haemolysis, a blood sample will show red discolouration of the plasma (haemoglobinaemia) if allowed to settle for a few minutes. In contrast, horses suffering rhabdomyolysis do not show discolouration of the plasma despite evidence of myoglobinuria.

- Marked myoglobinuria indicates levels of myoglobin in the circulation that are toxic to the liver and kidneys. If myoglobinuria persists it is wise to check serum urea and creatinine as indicators of renal failure.

- There is compelling evidence that electrolyte imbalances render some individuals prone to exertional rhabdomyolysis. To a limited extent electrolyte balance in the patient can be investigated by assessing the *fractional excretion of electrolytes* (see later). On occasion this enables corrective supplementation of the feed.

Muscle infections

Muscle infection is a natural consequence of wounding. Puncture wounds, or iatrogenic infection associated with intramuscular injection, may result in abscessation.

In the worst instance, deep wounds with localized bruising may allow germination of clostridial spores producing a gangrenous myositis ('malignant oedema'). In these cases there is a localized oedema followed by necrosis, gas production (crepitus), a thin serosanguinous exudate and generalized toxaemia. All these signs can appear within 24–48 hours. The toxaemia causes severe depression, tachycardia, and a progressively weak pulse culminating in fatal shock. Diagnosis is essentially based on the clinical findings.

Post-anaesthetic myopathy

This is an uncommon complication of general anaesthesia in the horse. During anaesthesia the weight of the horse's body on its underlying musculature can provoke a myositis associated with reduced blood perfusion. The result seen post-operatively is a localized muscular swelling and pain.

Diagnosis

- The clinical findings, associated with recumbency under general anaesthesia, are highly indicative of myositis.

- The serum muscle enzymes are elevated.

Atypical myoglobinuria

This is a rare condition of ponies and horses at grass which is characterized by a generalized weakness, progressing to recumbency, and the production of myoglobinuria unassociated with exercise.

Isolated instances or small outbreaks have been reported since 1984 when the condition was heralded as a 'new' disease. However, identical clinical descriptions of isolated cases appear in older literature. The cause is unknown but an environmental mycotoxin is suspected.

Diagnosis

- The serum muscle enzymes are massively increased.

- The differential causes of discoloured urine (haematuria and haemoglobinuria) are easily investigated (see above under: 'Exertional rhabdomyolysis'). Myoglobinuria in a grazing animal coupled with massively increased serum muscle enzymes is diagnostic of atypical myoglobinuria.

- Post-mortem examination usually reveals evidence of rhabdomyolysis, but this is not always distinctive and submission of muscle for histopathology is essential to diagnosis.

Nutritional muscular dystrophy

This is a very rare problem encountered in the growing animal. *It is the only muscle disease of horses which has an unequivocal association with a primary deficiency of vitamin E and selenium.* The deficiency occurs in the dam during pregnancy but primarily affects the suckling foal during the first weeks or months of life.

Diagnosis

- The clinical signs in the young animal are suggestive: failure to suck, weakness, difficulty in standing, falling when exerted. In acute cases tachycardia and hyperpnoea are usual and foals may die of exhaustion associated with heart and circulatory failure.

- Serum muscle enzymes are elevated, reflecting myopathy in skeletal and cardiac muscles.

- At post-mortem examination the muscles show generalized pallor or white 'streaking'.

- Glutathione peroxidase activity of whole (heparinized) blood is low (see below under: 'Selenium and vitamin E').

VI. Clinical pathology

Haematology

Haematology has little application in the diagnosis of musculoskeletal disease except for the non-specific indicators of inflammation. The total white cell count may be raised in inflammatory conditions and an increase in the plasma fibrinogen concentration suggests sepsis. Whole blood in EDTA should be submitted to the laboratory.

Serum muscle enzymes

Skeletal and heart muscle cells release enzymes into the circulation following injury. The concentration of these serum muscle enzymes can be measured and in general terms there is good correlation between the severity of injury and the muscle enzyme profile.

The two enzymes most commonly monitored are aspartate aminotransferase

(AST) and creatine phosphokinase (CPK or CK). AST is present in the mitochondria and cytoplasmic fluid of all cells, but it is particularly concentrated in liver, heart and skeletal muscle cells. The serum concentration may therefore be raised by many forms of soft tissue injury, but it is markedly increased following liver, heart or skeletal muscle injury. In contrast, CPK is mainly found in heart and skeletal muscle and can be regarded as muscle-specific.

Following hard exercise in a healthy horse there is a physiological increase in the circulating concentrations of both enzymes. AST concentration peaks at about 24 hours and returns to normal range within 7–10 days. CPK increases to a peak at about 6 hours and returns to normal range within 2–3 days. These physiological changes amount to some four-fold increase in the concentration of their upper ranges, but in conditions of myopathy the concentrations increase by a factor of ten to many thousands. Persistent high concentrations indicate an ongoing myopathy; the enzymes will only return to their normal ranges once the lesion has resolved.

In cases where exertional rhabdomyolysis is suspected as a recurrent problem, serum muscle enzymes should be measured before and after exercise. The exercise regime should mimic a normal hard day's work for the horse at its current level of fitness. In a healthy horse the samples obtained before exercise and at 6 and 24 hours thereafter should compare with the physiological variations described above. Massive increases which are persistently raised for days afterwards are consistent with rhabdomyolysis.

Rhabdomyolysis and the fractional excretion of electrolytes

Muscle function is closely linked with intra- and extracellular electrolyte concentrations and electrolyte imbalance has therefore been implicated in the pathogenesis of rhabdomyolysis.

The estimation of electrolyte concentrations in the blood cannot be used to detect electrolyte deficiency or excess with any accuracy because of the homeostatic mechanisms which maintain normal blood concentrations. The most practical approach to evaluating electrolyte balance is the measurement of urinary electrolyte excretion.

Electrolyte balance is primarily regulated by the kidney and urinary electrolyte concentrations have been shown to reflect dietary intake. However, the direct determination of urinary electrolyte concentrations requires long-term collection of urine which is impractical in horses. A more realistic approach is to compare the renal excretion of an electrolyte with that of creatinine.

Endogenous creatinine is excreted by glomerular filtration alone and its rate of excretion thus approximates to the glomerular filtration rate. Creatinine excretion is therefore a convenient standard against which the excretion of an electrolyte may be compared. The ratio of these excretion values is known as the urinary fractional excretion (FE) of an electrolyte which is given as:

$$FE = \frac{[E]_u}{[E]_p} \times \frac{[Cr]_p}{[Cr]_u} \times 100\%$$

where $[E]$ = concentration of electrolyte and $[Cr]$ = concentration of creatinine in plasma (p) or urine (u).

The FE of an electrolyte is therefore calculated once the urinary and plasma (or serum) concentrations of both the electrolyte and creatinine are known. This approach eliminates the need for protracted collection of urine, but the urine and plasma samples must be obtained at the same examination time (within 30 minutes of each other). In horses fed a balanced diet the FE results tend to fall within consistent limits. The following FE ranges, determined for healthy horses on a balanced electrolyte intake, serve as a guide:

Sodium	0.04–0.52%
Potassium	35–80%
Inorganic phosphorus	0.0–0.2%
Chloride	0.7–2.1%

Technique

The optimal time for collection of blood and urine for FE estimation is at rest and before feeding. Free flow urine is best obtained after a brisk trot to stir the bladder contents. Urine cannot, of course, be obtained by request, but if a horse is rested for 2 hours in a box without bedding, then trotted briefly and introduced into a box with clean bedding, urination is likely to follow.

Urine should be submitted in capped, sterile containers to avoid artefactual changes in the phosphate and creatinine concentrations as a result of bacterial contamination. The plasma should be separated fairly soon, and both urine and plasma should be analysed as quickly as possible (certainly within 4 days). In cases of delay, high temperatures must be avoided.

Samples should not be collected during (or soon after) a rhabdomyolysis episode because circulatory disturbances and increased plasma myoglobin may affect renal function and produce spurious FE values. The animal should be investigated once it has recovered from the acute episode.

Interpretation

Low dietary intake of an electrolyte results in its conservation by the kidney and an abnormally low FE value. Thus a low FE for potassium could reflect the need for replacement therapy. An alternative interpretation of a low FE value is that the electrolyte intake is adequate, but that absorption/utilization is a problem. In either instance, dietary supplementation may restore the FE value. In the case of diets with a low calcium to phosphorus ratio, there is an increase in the FE of phosphate. Supplementing the diet to bring the ratio closer to 2:1 (Ca:P) should restore normal phosphate excretion.

Horses known to have suffered rhabdomyolysis, or thought to be susceptible to it, should be maintained on a proprietary feed (which is recommended as an adequate and balanced diet), for at least 2 weeks before collection of samples. A subsequent FE profile which is abnormal suggests an absorption/ utilization problem rather than a dietary imbalance. Appropriate supplementation can then be given and fine-tuned in accordance with FE monitoring. If, however, the balanced diet is associated with normal ranges of FE values, then any further rhabdomyolysis attacks in that individual are unlikely to be related to electrolyte imbalance.

Comments

- The urinary concentrations of electrolytes and their rates of excretion are also influenced by hydration, endocrine and renal factors. In consequence, FE values vary between horses and within the same individual throughout the day. *Tests producing abnormal results should therefore be repeated to confirm a trend.*

- Although raised FE values usually result from the increased dietary intake of electrolytes, significant increases can be associated with renal tubular damage (see Chapter 6: 'Urinary diseases').

- Delayed urine samples which have very low creatinine concentrations ($< 10\,000$ μmol/L) are probably contaminated and not worth analysing since the FE results will be spurious.

- Despite the fact that calcium is precipitated in urinary crystals which may be lost to analysis, its FE value can be of use. However, the colorimetric methods used in most commercial laboratories are unsuitable for urinary calcium estimation and its FE value is not considered here.

Selenium and vitamin E

Selenium is an essential mineral nutrient whose metabolism is closely linked with that of vitamin E. It has been suggested that the function of vitamin E is to prevent the oxidation of selenium. Although a deficiency of selenium has been associated with myopathy in many species, this has not been demonstrated unequivocally in the horse, except in the singular case of nutritional muscular dystrophy — which is a rare condition.

Tocopherol concentrations in the blood and liver provide good information on the vitamin E status of an animal, but they are difficult to assay and are not commonly undertaken. A deficiency of vitamin E is assumed if the animal is of low selenium status.

Selenium is incorporated into the glutathione peroxidase (GSH-Px) of red blood cells during erythropoiesis. In horses it has been shown that a direct relationship exists between erythrocyte GSH-Px activity and selenium levels in the blood and tissues. Consequently, GSH-Px is a sensitive indicator of dietary selenium intake and/or the response to selenium administration. However, increases in GSH-Px activity as a result of selenium administration will not be detectable until 5–6 weeks later. Whole blood should be submitted in heparin for GSH-Px estimation.

GSH-Px activity in foals reflects the amount of selenium taken up by the mare during pregnancy.

Serology

Brucellosis

Brucellosis in horses is now a rare disease, probably because of the success in eradicating the causal agent *Brucella abortus* from cattle.

As eradication in cattle proceeded in the UK, there were marked shifts in the clinical manifestations of equine brucellosis. Purulent bursitis of the supraspinous bursa ('fistulous withers') and/or occipital bursa ('poll evil'), gave way to inflammation of the joints and/or tendon sheaths. A systemic form of the disease, similar to that in humans, was also recognized and was characterized by a fluctuating body temperature ('undulant fever'), with a generalized stiffness and lethargy.

Nowadays equine brucellosis is hardly recognized, but it is worth investigating in cases of shifting lameness associated with synovial inflammation and cases of generalized stiffness where other (more likely) causes have been eliminated. In tick areas, patients with these clinical signs should also undergo serological investigation for 'Lyme disease' (see below).

Diagnosis

● Serological confirmation of circulating antibody is still undertaken by some commercial veterinary laboratories and, by arrangement, via government laboratories. A positive serum agglutination test (SAT) is indicative, but requires confirmation using more sensitive antibody detection systems: the complement fixation test (CFT) and the Coombs' test.

NB It is possible to obtain positive SAT titres without associated clinical signs. A definitive diagnosis is indicated by a high SAT titre with a confirmatory CFT and Coombs' test, or a rising SAT titre over 3–4 weeks of disease.

Comment

● In the author's experience, rare cases of suspected brucellosis (e.g. fluctuating synovitis) do occur in the absence of diagnostic titres, yet seem to respond to long-term treatment with potentiated sulphonamide. Synovial fluid aspirates from such cases contain high numbers of leucocytes, but are bacteriologically sterile.

Lyme disease (borreliosis)

Lyme disease is caused by the spirochaete *Borrelia burgdorferi*, which is transmitted by a tick vector. The disease is well characterized in man and the dog, but its importance in the horse is still unclear. In the UK a serological survey has indicated that asymptomatic infection in horses is probably quite common, particularly in tick areas, but there is little evidence of associated clinical disease.

In the USA borreliosis has been reported in association with diverse clinical signs such as arthritis, myositis, weight loss and fever. A number of unexplained lamenesses associated with fever and/or tick infestation have also shown positive titres in the UK, but it is difficult to prove disease when so many clinically healthy horses are also sero-positive.

In clinical practice it is almost impossible to demonstrate the presence of the organism in cases of suspected disease. Culture is notoriously difficult and although the presence of *B. burgdorferi* DNA can be detected by the polymerase chain reaction, this test is not routinely available. Diagnosis therefore relies upon the ambiguity of the serological test. Commercial laboratories offer an ELISA test, for which a serum sample is required.

Comments

- A raised titre to *B. burgdorferi* does not necessarily indicate active infection.

- Cross-reacting antibodies produced by other infections may interfere with the specificity of the test.

Synovial fluid samples

The approaches used for arthrocentesis of individual joints for the collection of synovial fluid samples have been described earlier under: 'Intrasynovial analgesia'. The remarks on adequate restraint and careful site preparation apply as equally to fluid collection as to injection of local anaesthetic. Fluid is aspirated using a sterile needle and syringe.

Gross appearance

Synovial fluid is normally yellow, clear, translucent and viscous. Gross evidence of discolouration (e.g. with blood), opacity or turbidity, low viscosity or clotting would be suggestive of abnormality. Recent trauma or infection will produce marked changes in gross appearance. Other joint diseases, e.g. osteoarthritis, do not generally have a marked effect on the gross appearance of the fluid.

Useful laboratory measurements

Cytology

Total and differential white cell counts are particularly useful; especially in the diagnosis of septic arthritis or tenosynovitis.

Normal: 0.2×10^9/l; < 10% neutrophils, some lymphocytes and mononuclear cells.
Trauma: $0.5–10 \times 10^9$/l; neutrophil ratio increased.
Degenerative joint disease: $0.5–1 \times 10^9$/l.
Infection: > 50×10^9/l; > 90% neutrophils.

Total protein

Normal: 10–20 g/l
Inflammation: 20–40 g/l.
Infection: > 40 g/l.

Gram stain and culture

Samples for culture should be submitted in sterile containers with a minimal air gap to support anaerobes. A better alternative is to inoculate a commercial culture medium that will sustain both aerobic and anaerobic growth. Sample collection and inoculation must be done under strict aseptic conditions to avoid contamination.

In approximately 50% of septic synovitis cases, no organisms are found in synovial fluid because bacteria are sequestrated in the synovial membrane, and/or antibiotics have been administered previously. A higher culture rate can be obtained by using enrichment broths, submitting anaerobic as well as aerobic culture samples, and culturing synovial membrane biopsies in addition to synovial fluid samples.

Markers of cartilage degeneration

The main disadvantage of synovial fluid analysis is that it does not allow for the recognition of cartilage damage. The search for a marker of osteoarthritis has lead to the attempt to analyse joint fluid for the presence of cartilage particles after filtration of the synovial fluid sample. Although this has proven to be an inconsistent technique, new and more promising biochemical markers of proteoglycan and collagen breakdown are presently under investigation.

Further reading

Butler JA, Colles CM, Dyson SJ, Kold SE and Poulos PW (Eds) (1993) *Clinical Radiology of The Horse*. London: Blackwell Scientific Publications.

Eustace RA (1990) Equine laminitis. *In Practice* (supplement to the Veterinary Record) **12**: 156–161.

Harris P and Gray J (1992) The use of the urinary fractional electrolyte excretion test to assess electrolyte status in the horse. *Equine Veterinary Education* **4**: 162–166.

McIlwraith CW (Ed.) (1990) *Diagnostic & Surgical Arthroscopy in the Horse*, 2nd edn. Philadelphia: Lea & Febiger.

Stashak T S (Ed.) (1987) *Adams' Lameness in Horses*, 4th edn, pp. 1–270 (chapters 1–4). Philadelphia: Lea & Febiger

Wyn-Jones G (1988) *Equine Lameness*, pp. 1–27 (chapters 1–2). London: Blackwell Scientific Publications.

14 Neurological diseases

I. Neurological examination

The aims of a neurological examination are to determine the presence or absence of neurological disease and, if present, to try to determine the site and cause of disease. A neurological examination always follows, and is often integral to, a thorough clinical examination. It is important to distinguish cases of primary neurological disease from cases showing neurological signs which are secondary to some other generalized or systemic disease, e.g. signs of hepatic encephalopathy in a case of liver failure.

General examination

A general neurological examination is usually incorporated into the clinical examination of any patient. Information concerning the animal's clinical history and the nature of the complaint should be obtained from the owner prior to the examination. This examination should include observation of the animal's behaviour, mental status, vision, and its head and body posture. Comment is often required from the owner/groom as to what is considered normal for an individual animal.

In the head region, the facial symmetry should be assessed together with inspection of the oral cavity and ocular structures, including pupillary light responses. The animal's stance is assessed as is the symmetry of muscle masses and bony landmarks over the body. The posture and gait are further evaluated by observing the animal when walking, trotting, circling and backing. Findings from these observations are related to findings from the general clinical examination to determine whether there are indications of neurological disease and whether other, more detailed, investigations are required. It is important that the more detailed examination is performed in a thorough and logical manner. For most cases, an examination starting at the head and moving caudally is preferable.

The head and cranial nerves

The animal's behaviour should be observed both at rest and when being handled. Any inappropriate behaviour, especially if repeated, should be noted. Mental status is a feature of both the animal's temperament and state of arousal. It may also be altered in the presence of systemic factors, e.g. exhaustion or weakness. Abnormalities of behaviour or mental state usually relate to cerebral dysfunction.

Head posture is assessed with particular reference to the presence of a head tilt or head turn. It is important to distinguish between a head tilt, where one eye and ear are usually higher than the others, from a head turn, where the eyes and ears are level but the head/neck is turned away from the long axis of the horse. Head tilts are typically a result of vestibular disease, whilst head/neck turns may result from cerebral or severe vestibular disease.

Evaluation of cranial nerve (CN) function should be performed in a logical manner and in cases of unilateral disease, any abnormal responses should be compared with the contralateral side.

CN I – Olfactory nerve

This is responsible for the animal's ability to smell. In general terms this can be assessed by its ability to respond to an odour. A positive response to a familiar smell such as the owner's hand or a hand containing feed, or a negative response to an unfamiliar smell such as a spirit-soaked swab, can be assessed with the horse blindfolded.

CN II – Optic nerve

This is responsible for vision and may be assessed by the response to a menace test. Here a threatening movement towards the eye results in rapid eyelid closure and withdrawal of the head. A normal response indicates an intact afferent pathway and a functional optic nerve. An abnormal response may result from a lesion anywhere along the afferent or efferent pathways, for example opacity of the anterior chamber of the eye. An ophthalmic examination forms part of the assessment of vision and is described in Chapter 15: 'Ocular diseases'. A further indication of visual impairment may be provided by observing the animal in its normal environment or when negotiating an obstacle course, such as straw bales placed in an indoor arena through which the horse is encouraged to walk.

CN III – Oculomotor nerve

This is responsible for innervation of the pupillary constrictor muscles and extraocular muscles. A lesion affecting this nerve will not affect vision but usually produces a dilated pupil (mydriasis). In addition, the pupillary light response will be absent when light is directed at the eye on the affected side and the consensual pupillary light response will be absent when light is directed at the contralateral eye. Signs of dysfunction of the extraocular muscles are described in CN IV below.

CN IV – Trochlear nerve

This innervates the extraocular muscles, which are responsible for normal positioning of the eye within the orbit and for normal eye movements. These can be assessed by observing the animal's eye movements and position at rest and during deliberate manual movement of the head. An abnormal eye position at rest (strabismus) may be a result of damage to CN III, IV or VI, damage to the extraocular muscles, or some other extraocular lesion.

CN V – Trigeminal nerve

This provides the sensory innervation for most of the head via its three branches: mandibular; maxillary and ophthalmic. In addition, the mandibular branch provides the motor pathway for the muscles of mastication.

Unilateral abnormalities of motor function may be seen as unilateral muscle wastage and occasionally a slight degree of dysphagia. If a bilateral lesion is present, a dropped jaw and marked dysphagia may be evident. Sensory function may be assessed by pricking the skin over the head in the regions supplied by each of the three branches of the trigeminal nerve. Gentle stimulation will usually produce local twitching of the ears, eyelids or lips, mediated via the facial nerve (CN VII). More sustained stimulation will usually induce a behavioural response. In addition, the ophthalmic branch can be tested by assessing the corneal reflex. Light digital pressure on the cornea through the closed eyelid should normally result in a reflex retraction of the globe.

CN VI – Abducens nerve

This is responsible for innervation of the extraocular and retractor bulbi muscles. Signs of dysfunction of the extraocular muscles are described above under CN IV (trochlear nerve). The ability to retract the eyeball may be assessed by applying light digital pressure to the globe, through the eyelid, and feeling the reflex retraction.

CN VII – Facial nerve

This nerve supplies motor function to the muscles of facial expression. It therefore controls movements of the eyelids, ears, lips and nostrils and is assessed during the menace test and the palpebral and corneal reflexes. Facial paralysis is usually recognized by drooping of the ear and lips on the affected side with ptosis of the upper eyelid. These changes are best assessed by a head-on visual inspection of the horse in which the facial features on each side of the head are compared. The normal muscle tone on the unaffected side of the face leads to deviation of the muzzle away from the affected side.

CN VIII – Vestibulocochlear nerve

This nerve has two sensory components, the auditory branch involved with hearing and the vestibular branch involved with balance. Hearing loss, unless bilateral and complete, is difficult to assess in the horse. Vestibular disease may present as abnormalities of balance, a head tilt, or nystagmus. Nystagmus may occur at rest or when the animal's head is manipulated. In general, disorders of the vestibular branch result in the head tilt and the fast phase of nystagmus being directed away from the side of the lesion. Signs of vestibular disease may be exacerbated by blindfolding the animal to remove any compensatory visual input.

CN IX (Glossopharyngeal)/CN X (Vagus)/CN XI (Spinal accessory)

These nerves collectively provide the sensory and motor input for normal pharyngeal and laryngeal function. Disorders of these nerves therefore result in pharyngeal and laryngeal paralysis. Normal pharyngeal and laryngeal function can be assessed by observing and listening during normal breathing and swallowing, and/or during an endoscopic examination of the pharynx and larynx. Pharyngeal paralysis usually results in signs of dysphagia, and laryngeal paralysis in signs of dyspnoea. In both cases bilateral involvement is associated with more severe clinical signs.

The laryngeal adduction test (slap test) may be used to assess the vagal nerve. In this test the normal response to a manual slap on the withers is a reflex adduction of the contralateral arytenoid cartilage. This can be assessed by digital palpation over the larynx or by direct observation with an endoscope.

CN XII – Hypoglossal nerve

This nerve provides motor function to the tongue. The tongue should therefore be evaluated for normal movement and tone, muscle mass and signs of atrophy. Often dysphagia will only be apparent with bilateral nerve damage.

Motor function/spinal cord function

A general evaluation of motor function/spinal cord function can be made by examining the animal's gait and posture. It is important to distinguish abnormalities of gait and posture caused by neurological disease from those caused by musculoskeletal pain/lameness. In cases of neurological disease, weakness and ataxia are the most common signs. These must be assessed for each limb in turn. General observations may be made with the animal at rest, when walking and trotting in hand, turning tight circles, and backing up. Mild neurological deficits may only become apparent with more specific investigations. These include: walking up, down and across a slope; walking with the head and neck raised; walking blindfolded, and performing specific manoeuvres when being ridden. In addition, signs of weakness may be determined by attempting to pull (via the tail) or push the animal off balance while it is stood still or walking forwards.

The tail and perineum should be assessed for tail tone and the presence of a normal perineal reflex. This involves pricking the skin of the perineum and watching for normal reflex anal sphincter contraction and clamping down of the tail. A rectal examination may be used to assess any abnormal faecal retention or bladder distension as a result of urinary retention.

II. Specific conditions

The brain and cranial nerves

Head trauma

If head trauma is witnessed then a direct report of the nature and extent of trauma may be available. In many cases, however, head trauma is only suspected. Evidence of local abrasions and contusions may support this conjecture. The signs shown are likely to vary depending on the site(s) of injury and its severity. Depression and dementia are the most common general signs. Visual deficits may occur due to indirect optic nerve and retinal damage. The vestibular system also appears more susceptible to the effects of cranial trauma than other areas.

Radiography of the head may be useful in cases of severe trauma and those with evidence of haemorrhage from the nose or ears. Epistaxis has been recognized in cases of cranial trauma where the animal has fallen over backwards fracturing the basisphenoid bone. However, epistaxis is a common sequel to major or minor cranial trauma in the absence of any fracture. Cerebrospinal fluid analysis may be necessary to confirm suspected head trauma (see later). However, care should be taken that a sudden drop in pressure (as fluid is released from the cisterna magna) does not lead to prolapse of the brain into the foramen magnum as a result of brain swelling or haematoma formation within the cranium.

Space occupying lesions

Space occupying lesions produce clinical signs related to damage of the adjacent structures. These are most apparent where skeletal structures restrict local expansion of a lesion as occurs within the cranial vault. The most common causes in horses are haematoma formation following trauma, abscess formation (usually involving *Streptococcus equi*) and neoplasia. In all these cases the onset of clinical signs is often acute, despite the insidious nature of the underlying lesion in many instances. A thorough neurological examination will often allow accurate localization of the lesion and cerebrospinal fluid analysis may be informative, but for many cases a definitive diagnosis is reached only at post-mortem examination.

Meningitis

Bacterial meningitis is rare in adult horses, except when infection has been introduced by direct trauma. It is more common in young animals, particularly neonatal foals, as a sequel to bacteraemia. Other causes of meningitis (viral, fungal, protozoal) are uncommon in the horse.

The main clinical signs include depression and ataxia/weakness. Stiffness, particularly of the head and neck, hyperaesthesia and seizures are also commonly seen, but pyrexia is an inconsistent finding. In an adult, trauma to the head may be apparent and in the neonatal foal there are signs related to systemic infection.

Haematology may show a neutrophil response and increased neutrophil numbers are usually present in the cerebrospinal fluid. In addition, the cerebrospinal fluid will usually have a raised protein concentration and decreased glucose concentration.

Narcolepsy

Narcolepsy is a rare neurological condition characterized by the inappropriate onset of episodic loss of muscle tone, associated with sleep. The severity of signs varies, but in horses the usual history is of cataplexy, the complete loss of skeletal muscle tone, leading to sudden collapse. Less severe signs include sudden lowering of the head, buckling of the knees, stumbling and ataxia. In many cases there is an apparent precipitating circumstance leading to onset of the condition. Typically, this involves a routine stable procedure being performed on the animal such as grooming, tacking up or leading out of the stable. The aetiology of the condition is unknown, although a familial occurrence has been reported in Miniature Shetland ponies.

Diagnosis of the condition is usually based on the description or observation of an attack. Clinical and neurological examinations should eliminate any other neurological disorder. Pharmacological testing using physostigmine salicylate as a provocative agent has been advocated but its reliability has recently been called into question. The test involves the slow intravenous infusion of 0.06–0.08 mg/kg physostigmine salicylate which supposedly induces an attack within 10 minutes in an affected horse. In the authors' experience this is not always the case, despite a convincing history which is consistent with narcolepsy. Care is needed with the test as the cholinergic effects of physostigmine may induce colic, diarrhoea, bronchospasm and bradycardia.

Hepatic encephalopathy

Hepatic encephalopathy is usually recognized as occurring in cases of severe liver disease which are progressing to liver failure. This may be of sudden onset in a case of acute hepatic necrosis, or a terminal event in more chronic liver disease such as that caused by the long-term ingestion of a hepatotoxic plant, e.g. ragwort. Much more rarely, signs of hepatic encephalopathy may result from abnormalities of hepatic vascularization. These are usually seen as portosystemic shunts in young animals.

Signs of hepatic encephalopathy include dullness, yawning, blindness, ataxia, aimless wandering, head-pressing, and terminally manic behaviour and seizures. The exact pathways involved in hepatic encephalopathy are unclear, but it is thought that hyperammonaemia, hypoglycaemia, altered ratios of branched chain to aromatic amino acids, increases in short chain amino acids and the induction of false neurotransmitters may be involved. Diagnosis is usually based on the clinical signs and laboratory confirmation of liver failure (see Chapter 4: 'Liver diseases'). In particular,

the measurement of plasma ammonia concentrations provides the most useful correlation with the severity of clinical signs.

Bracken poisoning

Bracken poisoning is rare in horses. It follows long-term ingestion and, although the plant is toxic at all stages of growth, the clinical signs in grazing animals are most common in the late summer when other forage is scarce. The toxic principle is a thermolabile thiaminase, which is destroyed by heat, but not by drying, and it therefore remains toxic in bedding or hay. The clinical signs are caused by a build up of pyruvate metabolites as a result of decreased carboxylase production. These signs include ataxia, depression, weight loss and severe muscle tremors leading to recumbency and death in many cases. Diagnosis is based on the clinical signs and history of access to the plant.

Horner's syndrome

Horner's syndrome results from damage to the sympathetic supply to the head and eyeball. This sympathetic supply may be damaged at any level but most usually the lesion is found in the guttural pouch, or along the neck (affecting the vagosympathetic trunk), or at the thoracic inlet. The clinical signs of Horner's syndrome may include miosis, enophthalmus and protrusion of the third eyelid. If the sympathetic supply to the head is also involved then hyperaemia of the mucous membranes of the head may be seen, together with hyperthermia of the face and localized sweating of the face and neck.

Head shaking

Head shaking is the term used to describe a condition involving excessive movements of the head and neck. These movements when performed sporadically are probably a feature of normal horse behaviour. However, in this condition the frequency and severity of these movements is dramatically increased. The signs may be apparent at rest and/or at exercise. In most instances the owner's complaint involves the condition occurring at exercise and in severe cases it renders the horse unrideable. The signs are characteristic for the condition and include: vertical head nodding and flicking; horizontal head flicking; rotary head movements; rubbing the nostrils on the ground, the forelegs or the rider's leg. Increased snorting and a mucoid nasal discharge may also be seen. In an individual horse the signs may be variable, but in most cases the signs increase with time during the period of exercise.

There appears to be a seasonality to the condition in that many cases show clinical signs during the summer months only and have an apparent respite during the winter. Signs may also vary in severity with the location and prevailing weather conditions. Diagnosis of the condition is based on clinical signs and the absence of any other discernible cause(s) of abnormal head movements. The aetiology is unknown but an infraorbital/trigeminal neuropathy, vasomotor rhinitis or allergic rhinitis have been suggested. Accordingly, further diagnostic investigations have included infraorbital/trigeminal nerve blocks, intradermal skin testing with putative allergens, and administration of various pharmacological agents; but at present the results are inconsistent.

Differentials of dysphagia

Dysphagia is a common condition in the horse. There are numerous potential causes of dysphagia, many of which are not primarily neurological disorders. These include cleft palate, oesophageal impaction ('choke'), oesophageal stricture and dental disorders. Neurological diseases which may cause dysphagia include guttural pouch mycosis, meningitis, botulism, tetanus, lead poisoning and grass sickness. The clinical signs associated with dysphagia include inability/unwillingness to eat, pain on eating, dropping food whilst chewing, 'quidding', drooling of saliva/food, nasal return of saliva/food and coughing.

Investigation of the dysphagic horse should include a clinical and neurological examination, oral examination, radiography and endoscopy (see Chapter 2: 'Alimentary diseases').

The spinal cord

Cervical vertebral malformation

Cervical vertebral malformation is a well recognized cause of the 'Wobbler syndrome' in horses. It can occur at any age and in any breed but most cases are seen in young Thoroughbreds, particularly fast growing individuals up to 5 years of age. The main signs are of progressive ataxia. This usually starts with the hindlegs and may also involve the forelegs; however, the hindlegs are invariably the more severely affected. The ataxia is usually apparent at the walk and trot and will be exacerbated by turning, backing, walking with the head raised, and walking on a slope. The laryngeal adduction reflex, as assessed by digital palpation or endoscopy, may be abnormal. Neck pain may also be present.

Diagnosis is based on clinical signs and confirmed by a radiographic examination of the cervical spine, including a myelogram. Details of the radiographic technique and changes seen in cases of cervical vertebral malformation are well reported and beyond the scope of this book (see 'Further reading'). Essentially, the lesion is a result of progressive spinal cord compression which is often only demonstrable with contrast studies.

EHV-1 myeloencephalopathy

Equine herpes virus 1 may occasionally cause signs of neurological disease. These signs involve an acute onset of ataxia which can quickly lead to recumbency. The progression is very rapid and will usually stabilize after 24–48 hours. The disease may occur in outbreaks, especially at breeding establishments, where concurrent signs of respiratory disease, pyrexia and abortion may be present.

Neurological examination will usually reveal hind limb ataxia. There is often associated faecal and urinary retention leading to constipation, bladder distension and urine dribbling. Diagnosis is based on the clinical signs. A rising EHV-1 antibody titre in the patient or contact animals provides strong supportive evidence of EHV-1 involvement, as does virus isolation from respiratory secretions or the buffy coat of a heparinized blood sample. Cerebrospinal fluid may show a yellowish discolouration (xanthochromia) and a raised protein concentration (see later).

Neuritis of the cauda equina (polyneuritis equi)

This condition is uncommon and is caused by a progressive demyelination of the sacrococcygeal and lumbar nerve roots of the cauda equina. Occasionally, there may also be involvement of cranial nerves. Clinical signs include faecal retention, urinary retention and overflow, tail rubbing and colic. Neurological examination usually reveals a flaccid paralysis of the tail, anal sphincter and penis. There is usually an area of analgesia around the perineum (Fig. 14.1), which is often surrounded by a ring of hyperaesthesia. Rectal examination will confirm the faecal retention and also the bladder distension. Individual cranial nerve involvement may also be present and usually affects the facial, vestibular and trigeminal nerves.

Diagnosis is based on the clinical signs, particularly if cranial nerves are involved. Many affected horses have been shown to have raised levels of circulating antibodies against P_2-myelin protein. These antibodies can be detected by an ELISA which provides supporting evidence for a diagnosis of cauda equina neuritis. Unfortunately, the test is not available commercially.

Equine motor neurone disease

This rare condition has now been recognized and described in the UK following earlier

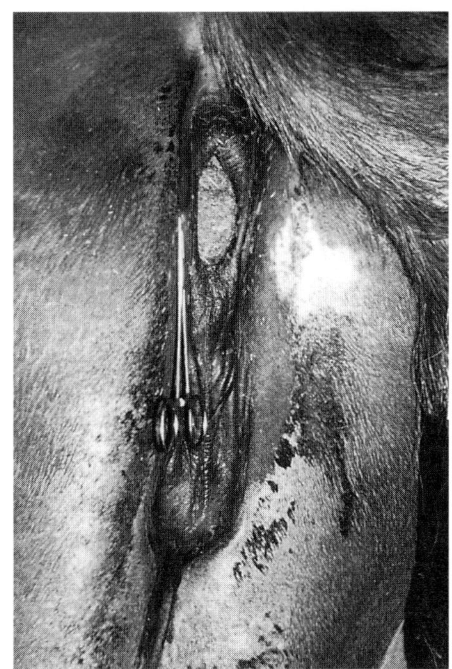

Figure 14.1   View of the perineum of a horse with neuritis of the cauda equina showing an area of perineal analgesia (forceps), loss of anal sphincter tone and faecal retention.

reports from the USA. Typically it is associated with weight loss and weakness despite a normal or increased appetite. Muscle tremors and fasciculations are also seen and may be accompanied by neurogenic muscle atrophy. Abnormal stance and head carriage, increased periods of recumbency and excessive sweating have also been recorded. Ataxia is not a feature of the disease. There may be moderate increases in serum muscle enzyme concentrations and cerebrospinal fluid analysis often shows an elevated protein concentration with occasional elevation of the creatine phosphokinase (CPK) concentration. Electromyographic studies are reported to show denervation responses in the affected muscles. There is no definitive ante-mortem diagnosis for the condition, but post-mortem examination at a specialist centre may confirm wide-spread degenerative changes in the motor nerve cell bodies in the ventral horn of the spinal cord. Certain brain stem nuclei are also affected.

Peripheral neuropathies

Specific peripheral neuropathies are uncommon in the horse. They usually occur as a sequel to trauma somewhere along the path of a nerve. Any peripheral nerve may be affected, but certain neuropathies occur more commonly than others.

Suprascapular nerve

Damage to this nerve is usually a result of the animal colliding with an object, most often the side of a doorway or passageway, and the resulting condition is known as 'sweeney'. The nerve innervates the supraspinatus and infraspinatus muscles of the shoulder and damage results in atrophy of these muscles producing apparent prominence of the spine of the scapula. The lack of collateral support to the shoulder, from the supraspinatus muscle, may result in lateral subluxation of the shoulder when weight bearing.

Radial nerve

Damage to this nerve is also a result of trauma. It may accompany a humeral fracture, a brachial plexus injury, or follow prolonged lateral recumbency in which the weight of the animal has been pressing on the affected side — typically during general anaesthesia. The animal tends to adopt a 'dropped elbow' stance and is unable to bear weight on the limb. The limb is often held forward, in a stance similar to grazing, or maintained with the carpus and fetlock semi-flexed (Fig. 14.2). In the absence of an accompanying orthopaedic injury, manual extension of the carpus will usually allow the animal to bear weight and take a stride on the affected leg.

Peroneal nerve

Damage to this nerve may occur in conjunction with a sciatic nerve injury or follow an injury to the lateral stifle. Peroneal neuropathy may also be seen after prolonged recumbency, as in general anaesthesia. There is an inability to flex

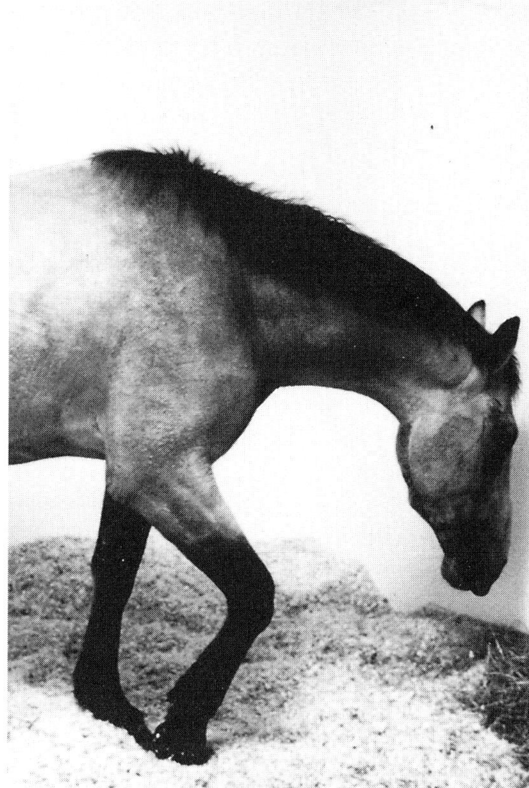

Figure 14.2   'Dropped elbow' stance in a horse with radial nerve dysfunction following prolonged general anaesthesia in lateral recumbency.

the hock and extend the digits, so that the animal will often bear weight on the dorsal surface of the hoof and fetlock. The fetlock is usually dragged along the ground when the animal attempts to walk.

'Stringhalt'

This uncommon condition occurs sporadically in individual horses in the UK. It has also been reported in Australia as outbreaks affecting several animals that show progressive signs. Typically, there is an acute onset of hyperflexion of one or both hindlegs during movement, the animal being normal at rest. The severity of the signs varies from case to case, and may resolve with time. In extreme cases the hindleg may hit the ventral body wall when the horse moves. Diagnosis depends on observing the typical clinical signs and ruling out other musculoskeletal disorders. Mild cases need to be differentiated from upward fixation of the patella.

'Shivering'

This rare condition is similar to stringhalt. It is seen as a muscular tremor affecting the hindlegs and tail during movement, particularly as the affected leg is raised off the ground. It is usually worse when the horse is backing and may affect one or both hindlegs. Heavy horses appear most prone to the condition and it is often progressive. Although little has been recorded in the literature about this condition, it appears to be well known amongst horse handlers who refer to affected horses as 'shiverers'.

Generalized neuropathies

Botulism

Botulism is a progressive muscular paralysis caused by an exotoxin of *Clostridium botulinum*. Compared with other species, the horse appears especially sensitive to the effects of botulinum toxin. In most cases it is preformed in the feed and is absorbed into the circulation following ingestion. One of the most important sources of intoxication to horses is big bale silage, in which contamination with soil-borne spores is common. In conditions of spoilage, secondary fermentation produces an alkaline pH which encourages spore germination and toxin production. Once absorbed, the toxin has an affinity for and binds to neuromuscular junctions where it interferes with the release and binding of acetylcholine, thus causing a diffuse muscular weakness.

The severity of the condition is variable and dependent upon the amount of toxin ingested. Typically the animal presents with a progressive muscular weakness. This is seen as depression, weakness and a shuffling gait. Lingual and pharyngeal paralysis cause dysphagia and the tongue may loll from the mouth in a flaccid state. In mild cases poor tongue tone may only be apparent with handling; when pulled to the side of the mouth it is not readily retracted. In severe cases the muscle paralysis leads to recumbency, and death follows paralysis of the respiratory muscles.

Diagnosis is based on the history and clinical signs. A toxin test can be performed on serum, gut contents or a suspected foodstuff. However, the toxin is extremely labile and is usually present in low concentrations, so that its detection is rarely successful. Ideally, serum samples should be collected early in the course of the condition and forwarded to a specialist laboratory by courier. In the case of big bale silage, contamination should be suspected if the product is alkaline, mouldy, or exhibiting an ammoniacal smell.

Tetanus

Tetanus in horses is usually associated with deep puncture wounds contaminated by the spores of *Clostridium tetani* in relatively anaerobic conditions which favour their germination. Clostridial spores are abundant in herbivore faeces and in the soil, but most wounds are relatively aerobic and do not promote their germination. The required anaerobic environment is usually found only in deep wounds, particularly those favouring local tissue necrosis and pus formation. The vegetative state of the bacterium produces a potent exotoxin. This is transported both in the circulation and by retrograde axonal migration to the central nervous system where it binds irreversibly to gangliosides in the ventral horn. The clinical signs are mainly associated with this toxic effect which prevents release of the inhibitory transmitter glycine at the spinal motor neurone, causing generalized muscle spasm.

An early sign is dysphagia due to spasm of the masseter muscles ('lockjaw'). Prolapse of the third eyelid is characteristic and may be induced by raising the head to the horizontal or gently tapping just below the eye. A stilted gait with a rigidly extended head and neck is also seen (Fig. 14.3). An anxious expression to the face appears as a result of eyelid retraction,

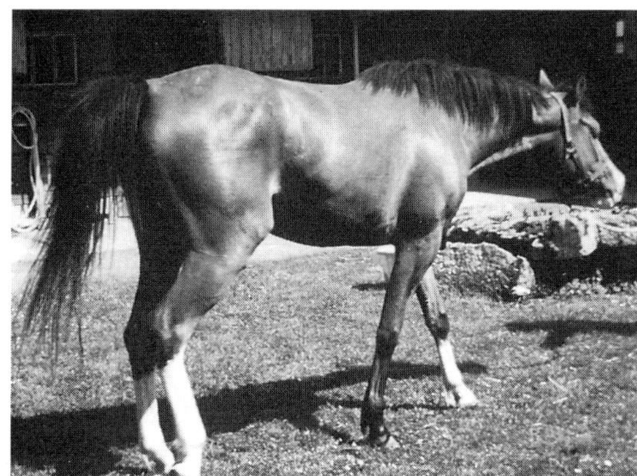

Figure 14.3 Typical appearance of a pony with tetanus, showing extensor rigidity of the limbs, raised tail head and extended head and neck.

nostril flaring and pricking of the ears. The tail head may be raised. In severe cases the extensor spasm of the limbs becomes more apparent and may lead to recumbency. Diagnosis is based on the clinical signs and may be supported by evidence of an appropriate wound, but the primary source is often not identified. Laboratory detection of either the organism or the toxin is difficult and rarely warranted.

Hypocalcaemia

Hypocalcaemia is relatively rare in the horse. Typically it can occur in one of three situations, although the clinical signs are similar in each case. 'Lactation tetany' occurs in breeding mares, usually 2–4 weeks after parturition or occasionally just after weaning. 'Transit tetany' occurs most commonly in ponies, but can occur in any animal following prolonged transit stress. Post-endurance tetany (synchronous diaphragmatic flutter or 'thumps') occurs in fatigued horses performing in endurance events.

The clinical signs relate to muscle tetany, and are seen as an anxious expression, muscle tremors, sweating and stiffness of the gait. Occasional cases will also show dysphagia, synchronous diaphragmatic flutter and intestinal ileus. Untreated cases may progress to recumbency and terminal convulsions. Diagnosis is confirmed by the response to treatment and the retrospective determination of serum calcium, magnesium and phosphorus concentrations (see 'Hypocalcaemia' in Chapter 5: 'Endocrine diseases').

III. **Practical techniques**

Cerebrospinal fluid collection

Cerebrospinal fluid may be obtained via the atlanto-occipital or lumbosacral spaces. However, it is important to realize the limitations of CSF analysis before attempting the procedure. Any lesion which is confined to the grey or white matter of the CNS, i.e. which does not impinge on the subarachnoid space, is unlikely to cause the leakage of pigments or protein, or the exfoliation of cells into the CSF. Space occupying lesions such as neoplasia, abscessation or haematoma may produce only scant haemorrhage and most toxic and metabolic neurological diseases are associated with normal CSF analysis. However, infectious diseases and trauma of the spinal cord are associated with increased protein concentrations and cellularity.

The atlanto-occipital space

Collection of fluid via the atlanto-occipital space requires the animal to be positioned in lateral recumbency. For all adults and most foals this necessitates general anaesthesia, although heavy sedation and manual restraint may be sufficient for some foals. Padding should be used to ensure that the long axis of the cervical spine and the head are horizontal and parallel with the ground. In addition, the long axis of the head should be positioned perpendicular to the long axis of the cervical spine.

The skin over the dorsal aspect of the atlanto-occipital joint should be clipped and surgically prepared and sterile gloves should be worn during the procedure. A 3 inch x19G (76 x 1.0 mm) spinal needle with stylet is ideal for adult horses, but a 1.5 inch x 20G (38 x 0.9 mm) disposable needle, without stylet and having a clear hub, is preferred for foals. The site of insertion of the needle is the same in both foals and adults. The needle should be inserted perpendicular to the long axis of the cervical spine and parallel to the ground through a point in the midline at the centre of a triangle formed between the external occipital protuberance and the cranial borders of the wing of the atlas (Fig. 14.4). The needle is inserted with little resistance to a depth of 5–7 cm, at this level a 'popping' sensation may be appreciated as the needle penetrates the atlanto-occipital membrane and dura mater. Beyond this point there is reduced resistance to further passage of the needle. When this 'popping' sensation is felt, or it is assumed that a suitable depth has been reached, the stylet should be removed and the hub watched for the appearance of clear, watery cerebrospinal

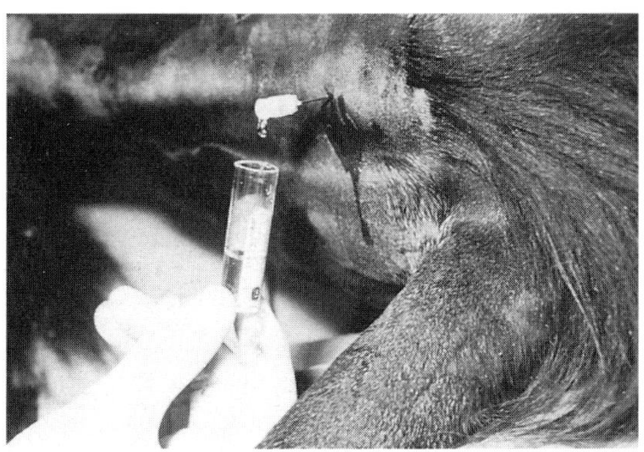

Figure 14.5 Collection of cerebrospinal fluid via the atlanto-occipital space. The stylet has been removed and cerebrospinal fluid is dripping from the hub of the needle.

fluid (Fig. 14.5). If none appears the needle may be rotated 90 degrees between finger and thumb and the hub observed again. If no cerebrospinal fluid appears the stylet should be replaced and the needle advanced again. If a depth of 10 cm is reached without encountering fluid, or the needle comes into contact with bone, it should be almost completely withdrawn before being redirected. At the subsequent attempt more attention should be paid to ensure the correct alignment of the needle with the bony landmarks and the long axis of the cervical spine. Once correctly positioned, cerebrospinal fluid will freely drip from the hub of the needle and can be collected into both EDTA and plain containers for cytology and biochemistry respectively.

The lumbrosacral space

Collection of fluid from the lumbosacral space is usually performed in the standing animal. The technique can be used in the recumbent patient but is more difficult to perform. Sedation is rarely required and should be used only in very uncooperative animals as the subsequent unsteadiness results in the animal not standing evenly and squarely on its hindquarters.

With the animal standing squarely, a 30 x 30 cm area over the lumbosacral space is clipped

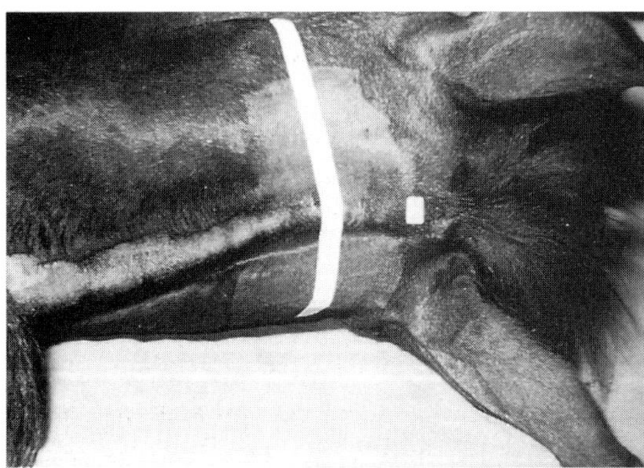

Figure 14.4 Landmarks for cerebrospinal fluid collection via the atlanto-occipital space. The tape joins the cranial borders of the wings of the atlas and the rectangular marker identifies the external occipital protuberance.

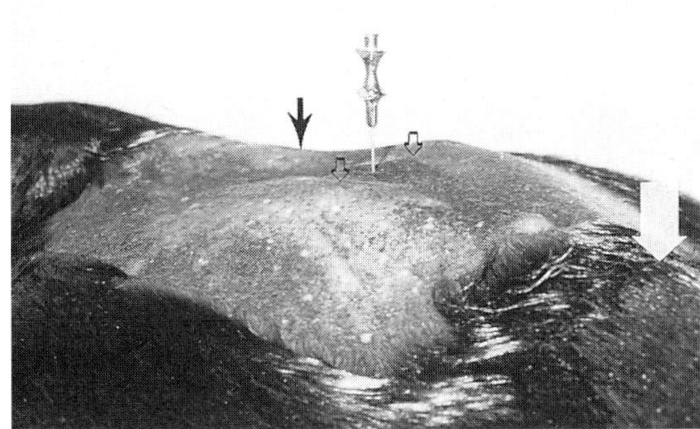

Figure 14.6   Site of needle insertion for collection of cerebrospinal fluid via the lumbosacral space in a standing horse. The tuber sacrale (short arrows), dorsal spinous process of the 5th lumbar vertebra (long arrow), and tail head (thick arrow) are identified.

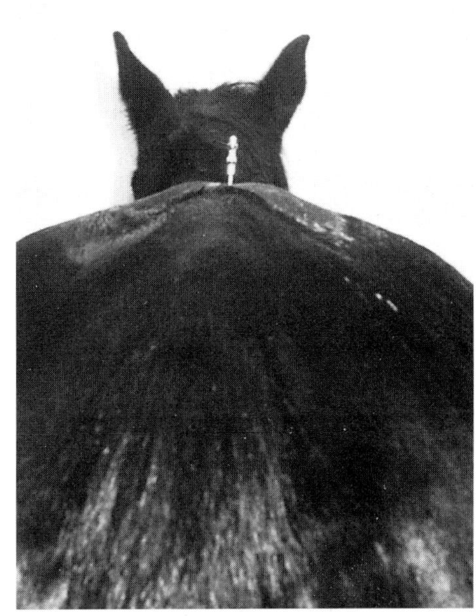

Figure 14.7   Collection of cerebrospinal fluid via the lumbosacral space. Caudal view during insertion of the needle to ensure that a vertical orientation is maintained.

and surgically prepared. Sterile gloves should be worn for the procedure. In most horses the dorsal spinous processes of the last lumbar (L6) and first sacral (S1) vertebrae are not palpable as they are shorter than L5 and S2 respectively. The site of needle insertion is in the midline immediately caudal to the dorsal spine of L6 (Fig. 14.6). If this is not palpable, and there is only a depression caudal to L5, then the position and length of L6 are estimated from the position and length of L5. The authors find that in most horses the site is level with a line between the cranial edges of the tuber sacrale and invariably cranial to a line between the caudal edges of the tuber coxae.

A bleb of local anaesthetic is inserted under the skin at this site and a number 10 scalpel used to make a small skin incision. A 6 inch x 18G (150 x 1.2 mm) spinal needle with stylet is ideal for most adult horses although a shorter needle (10 cm) with stylet may be sufficient in a pony. The clinician should stand to one side of the animal and insert the needle with the hand(s) firmly positioned against the animal's back to prevent any inadvertent movement of the needle if the patient moves unexpectedly. It is useful to have at least one assistant standing back from the horse and observing the direction and angle of the needle to ensure that it maintains a vertical position (Fig. 14.7). Beneath the skin incision there is usually little

resistance to passage of the needle to a depth of 12–13 cm. At this level, penetration of the lumbosacral interarcuate ligament is met with an apparent loss of resistance, and the simultaneous penetration of the dura mater and arachnoid usually produces a mild local response from the horse. Typically this is just a reflex tail movement and slight flexing of the hindlegs accompanied by a conscious pain response. If bone is encountered, rather than the interarcuate ligament, the needle should be almost fully withdrawn before being reinserted. Once the arachnoid has been penetrated, as indicated by the local response, the stylet can be withdrawn and cerebrospinal fluid should appear at the hub of the needle. This can be collected into an appropriate container or aspirated from the top of the hub. If no cerebrospinal fluid is forthcoming, the needle should be gently rotated through 90 degrees and, in addition, the intraspinal pressure can be

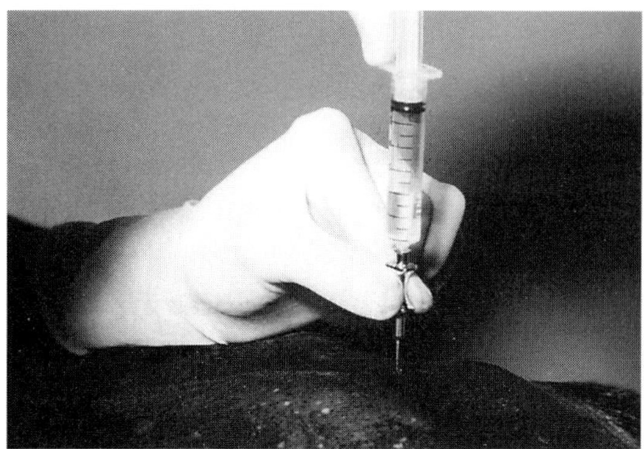

Figure 14.8 Collection of cerebrospinal fluid via the lumbosacral space. Gentle aspiration with a syringe attached to the needle.

raised by an assistant occluding both jugular veins. Alternatively, a small syringe may be connected to the hub of the needle and gentle suction applied directly to the needle (Fig. 14.8).

If cerebrospinal fluid is still not apparent, the stylet should be replaced and the needle inserted farther into the subarachnoid space at which point bone will be felt on the needle's tip. The stylet is again removed and the hub observed for the presence of cerebrospinal fluid. If none is forthcoming the needle is again rotated through 90 degrees, the intraspinal pressure is raised, or syringe aspiration is attempted. The needle can be gradually withdrawn a few millimetres and the process repeated until either a sample of cerebrospinal fluid is collected or the needle is withdrawn through the interarcuate ligament. At this stage the needle should be completely withdrawn and the procedure repeated with a new needle.

Cerebrospinal fluid analysis

Normal CSF appears clear and colourless. On analysis it contains no blood and few leucocytes (< 6/µl). The protein concentration is variable over a range of 0.4–1 g/l. Infectious diseases of the central nervous system are associated with an increase in protein concentration and cellularity. Bacterial diseases produce a neutrophilia whereas viral diseases may be associated with a mononuclear response. In both instances there may be yellow discolouration (xanthochromia) caused by red cell extravasation. Haemorrhage and xanthochromia can also be associated with trauma.

Further reading

Fordyce PS, Edington N, Bridges GC, Wright JA and Edwards GB (1987) Use of an ELISA in the differential diagnosis of cauda equina neuritis and other equine neuropathies. *Equine Veterinary Journal* **19**: 55–59.

Mayhew IG (1989) *Large Animal Neurology.* Philadelphia: Lea & Febiger.

Papageorges M, Gavin PR, Saude RD, Barbee DD and Grant BD (1987) Radiographic and myelographic examination of the cervical vertebral column in 306 ataxic horses. *Veterinary Radiology* **28**: 53–59.

15 Ocular diseases

I. Examination techniques

Examination protocol

This chapter describes the techniques for clinical examination of the eye and the routine sequence in which they should be undertaken. In all cases it is essential to keep accurate and sequential records of ocular findings and this is most simply done using standard annotated diagrams. The eye and adnexa (i.e. the eyelids, lacrimal apparatus, orbit and paraorbital areas) are first examined by naked eye in the light, assisted by a focal light source such as a pen light and some form of magnification such as a magnifying loupe. To enable a more detailed examination, particularly of the deeper structures of the eye, a second examination is then performed in the dark. Again, the naked eye, a light source and magnification are necessary, but the deeper structures additionally require the use of indirect and direct ophthalmoscopy techniques. These techniques and the associated equipment are well within the range of the non-specialist.

Restraint and local anaesthesia

On occasion an adequate examination of the eye and adnexa may only be possible using twitch restraint or sedation. These can be augmented by the use of local anaesthesia; either topical and/or regional.

Sedation

Lively or intractable patients should be sedated with 10–30 µg/kg detomidine hydrochloride ('Domosedan': SmithKline Beecham) by slow intravenous injection. Xylazine ('Rompun': Bayer) at 0.5–1 mg/kg and romifidine ('Sedivet': Boehringer Ingelheim) at 40–100 µg/kg, are suitable intravenous alternatives. If pain is prominent the sedative should be combined with some form of systemic analgesic such as butorphanol ('Torbugesic': C-Vet) given by slow intravenous injection at a dose rate of 25–50 µg/kg. The two injections (sedative and analgesic) should be separated by an interval of 5 minutes, although some practitioners combine these drugs in the same syringe.

Topical anaesthesia

If the eye is painful, topical anaesthesia may be required to densensitize the ocular surface. As it is difficult to avoid the contamination of multidose bottles when used between horses, a local anaesthetic such as 0.5% proxymetacaine hydrochloride ('Opthaine': Squibb) should be administered via a 1 ml syringe (Fig. 15.1). Alternatively, single use preparations are available such as 1% amethocaine hydrochloride ('Minims'; Smith and Nephew).

Local nerve blocks

Auriculopalpebral nerve block

This motor nerve block is of value when there is a risk of expulsion of the intraocular contents because of a full thickness penetrating injury, or when blepharospasm, which may be associated with handling or ocular pain, makes examination of the eye difficult. It prevents eyelid movement, but trigeminal sensation is not affected and invasive procedures therefore require additional, topical anaesthesia.

The auriculopalpebral nerve is a branch of the facial nerve which may be blocked at a

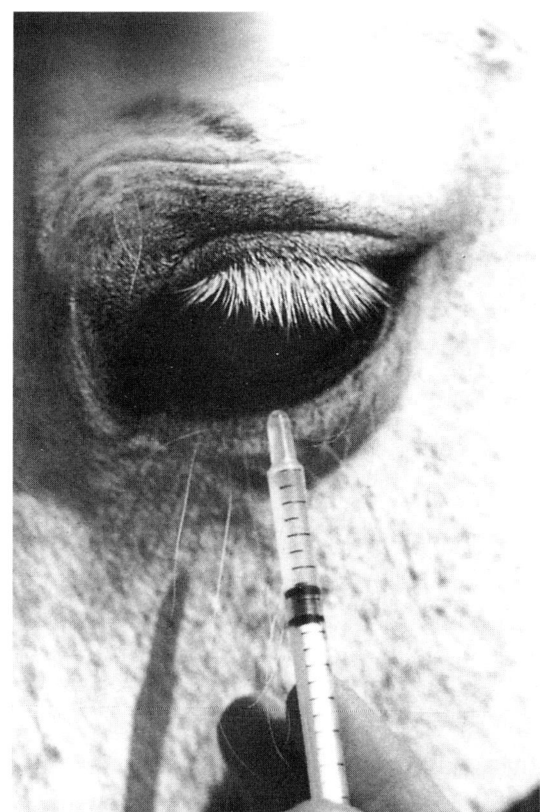

Figure 15.1   A 1 ml syringe being used to deliver local anaesthetic to the eye. The same technique can be used to deliver other types of liquid medication. Most horses tolerate this method of application, but a small proportion may react violently.

number of sites (Fig. 15.2). It originates deep to the parotid gland and passes dorsally to innervate the ear muscles. The palpebral branch passes anteriorly and obliquely over the zygomatic process of the squamous temporal bone and then courses forwards in subcutaneous tissues along the dorsomedial edge of the zygomatic arch towards the upper eyelid. In a proportion of animals, sedation will be required prior to administering the nerve block, and it is worth noting that in some cases sedation alone will be so effective that the nerve block is no longer necessary.

Using a 1 inch x 22G (25 x 0.7 mm) needle, 5–7 ml (up to 10 ml) of 1% prilocaine hydrochloride or 2% mepivacaine hydrochloride are injected deep to the skin in one of the following sites:

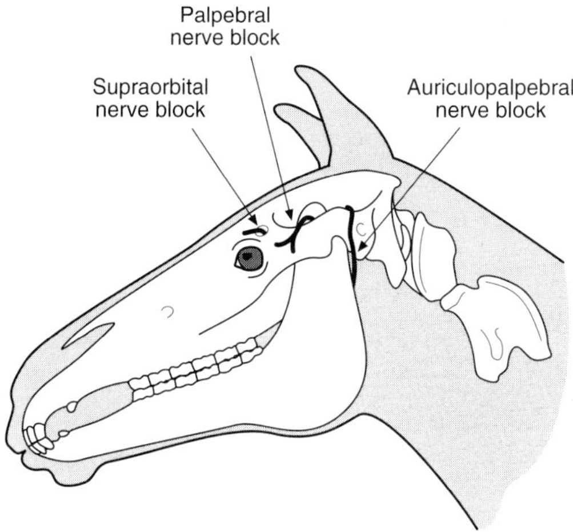

Figure 15.2 The sites for auriculopalpebral, palpebral and supraorbital nerve block.

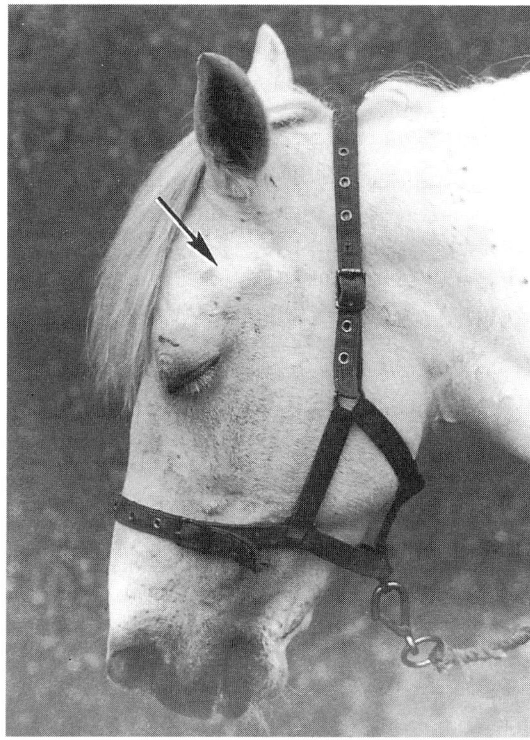

Figure 15.3 Mild ptosis of the upper eyelid and eversion of the lower eyelid denote a successful block of the palpebral nerve. The arrow denotes the site of injection.

- The auriculopalpebral nerve is blocked by infiltrating local analgesic into the depression caudal to the vertical ramus of the mandible approximately one inch (2.5 cm) below its highest point (Fig. 15.2). If the eye is particularly painful, this is a slightly easier and safer site for injecting local anaesthetic but it may, on occasion, produce mild facial paralysis. The needle is directed obliquely upwards and inwards towards the highest point of the zygomatic arch. A successful block is indicated by mild ptosis of the upper eyelid and eversion of the lower eyelid. The ipsilateral ear may also droop.
- The palpebral branch of the nerve is blocked by infiltrating a similar volume of anaesthetic immediately medial and slightly rostral to the highest point of the zygomatic arch, approximately halfway between the eye and the ear (Figs 15.2 and 15.3). The palpebral nerve is palpable at this point as it crosses the zygomatic arch in a ventromedial direction. The efficacy of the block is indicated within 10 minutes by ptosis and a much reduced or absent palpebral reflex.

Supraorbital nerve block

The supraorbital or frontal nerve is a branch of the trigeminal nerve and supplies sensory innervation to the medial and middle two-thirds of the upper eyelid. The supraorbital block is useful for minor eyelid surgery, including biopsies.

It is blocked by injecting 3–5 ml of 1% prilocaine hydrochloride or 2% mepivacaine hydrochloride using a 1 inch x 22G (25 x 0.7 mm) needle placed through the supraorbital foramen to a depth of approximately 1 cm (Fig. 15.2). The foramen can be palpated as a depression in the frontal bone on the dorsal aspect of the orbit. The efficacy of the block is indicated by desensitization of the upper lid within 10 minutes of injection. This block may also produce some motor paralysis of the palpebral branch of the facial nerve.

Examination in the light

Assessment of visual acuity

Complaints concerning the visual acuity of horses present a major diagnostic problem.

Except in cases of complete blindness, it is extremely difficult to define a level of visual capacity. Ophthalmic examination may define ocular lesions, but their significance in terms of the animal's ability to see is often uncertain.

Tests of visual acuity in horses are empirical. The pupillary light response is unreliable (see later under 'Examination in the dark'). A positive menace response, such as blinking or shying to a threatening visual stimulus, requires normal function of both peripheral and central visual pathways and therefore confirms some degree of visual capacity. However, the observer must take care not to create sounds or air currents that may stimulate other sensory pathways with the same result. The ability of a horse to negotiate unfamiliar surroundings may be tested in a simple obstacle course. These should be designed to avoid undue apprehension or injury. The same or a similar course may be repeated under varying light conditions, for example in an indoor school. In addition, each eye may be tested in turn using a cloth blindfold tucked under one side of the halter.

General examination

Apart from the naked eye, the most useful instruments for examination in the light are a magnifying lens and a pen light. All observations should be recorded on annotated diagrams.

Appearance of the eye and adnexa

The general appearance of the eye and the adnexa (eyelids, lacrimal apparatus, orbit and paraorbital areas) should be assessed and the symmetry of each side compared. Abnormal elevations, depressions or deviations of the skull or soft tissues of the head should be evaluated (Fig. 15.4). In particular, it is important to check that the supraorbital fossa is normal on both sides. Swelling in this region may indicate a retrobulbar or retro-orbital space occupying lesion. The presence of abnormal ocular or nasal discharges should be noted; excessive lacrimation suggests pain;

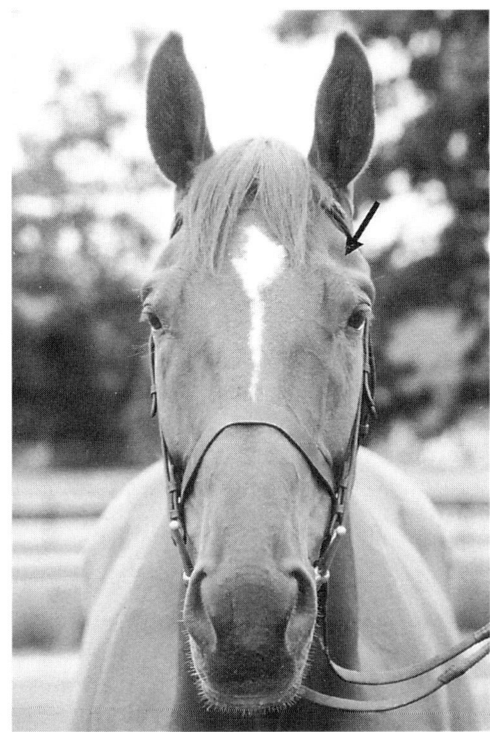

Figure 15.4   Initial naked eye assessment of the eye and adnexa should concentrate on the symmetry of the right and left sides of the face, including the obvious depression of the supraorbital fossa (arrowed) and whether or not any abnormal ocular or nasal discharges are present.

epiphora (tear overflow) suggests blockage.

The angle of the upper eyelashes should be examined. Normally they should be at almost 90 degrees to the cornea (Colour Plate 1). Downward deviation may well indicate *enophthalmos* (backward displacement of the eye into the orbit). Alternatively, an upward deviation may indicate *exophthalmos* (abnormal protrusion of the eye). Either of these situations may not otherwise be obvious.

The lacrimal apparatus

The presence of the upper and lower lacrimal puncta and the nasal ostium should be confirmed. The pre-ocular tear film should be assessed visually. A Schirmer tear test (see later) can be performed if there is any suggestion of abnormality.

The eyelids

The margins, outer and inner surfaces of the upper and lower eyelids should be examined. Non-pigmented eyelids should be examined carefully as they are more susceptible to solar blepharodermatitis and squamous cell carcinoma. The outer surface of the third eyelid should be also be inspected once it has been protruded by applying thumb pressure on the globe through the upper eyelid. The inner surface of the third eyelid is not examined routinely, but following the application of a local anaesthetic it may be everted using atraumatic tissue forceps. The inner surface of the third eyelid should be examined when neoplasia (e.g. squamous cell carcinoma) or a foreign body is suspected. In many horses there is also an obvious fleshy protruberance, the caruncle, located in the medial canthus proximal to the third eyelid which is a transition zone containing both subcutaneous and mucous membrane elements. It may be a potential site for squamous cell carcinoma when it is unpigmented.

The ocular surface

The ocular surface is the continuous epithelium which begins at the lid margins, extends onto the back of the lids, into the fornices and onto the globe. It includes the conjunctival, limbal and corneal epithelium. Naked eye examination will indicate if the appearance of the ocular surface is normal. The visible conjunctiva (bulbar and nictitating) should be examined with particular care, especially when it lacks pigment, because this is another site where squamous cell carcinoma can develop. The limbus should be examined next. In many horses this junction between the 'white' of the eye (bulbar conjunctiva with underlying episclera and sclera) and the clear cornea is well defined by a narrow rim of pigment. The cornea should be lustrous and transparent, allowing the fine structure of the iris to be visualized clearly (Colour Plate 1). A pen light can be used to assess the non-sensory corneal reflex, in which the light from the pen light should be reflected on the corneal surface without disruption. Irregularities of the preocular tear film or the ocular surface cause the reflection to 'break up'. The normal equine cornea is distinguished by its large size and prominence. In most horses there is an obvious grey line on the corneal side of the medial (nasal) and lateral (temporal) limbus which represents the insertion of the pectinate ligament into the posterior cornea at the termination of Descemet's membrane (Colour Plate 1). In shape the cornea is a horizontally elongated ellipse and the medial cornea is slightly wider than the lateral cornea.

The anterior chamber and iris

These can be examined briefly with a pen light at this stage, but it is easier and more rewarding to examine these regions in the dark. The pupil should be an almost symmetrical horizontal ellipse and black pigmented masses (the granula iridica or corpora nigra) are usually obvious on the dorsal pupillary border (Colour Plate 1). Variations in iris pigmentation are common (Colour Plate 2).

Examination in the dark

At this stage specific abnormalities detected in the first part of the examination can be looked at in more detail without the presence of distracting reflections. The eye, adnexa and the anterior and posterior segments are examined in sequence. A pen light, magnifying lens, condensing lens of +20 to +30 dioptre (D), and a direct ophthalmoscope are required.

Pen light examination

Eye and adnexa

The eye and adnexa are examined by pen light (Fig. 15.5), using magnification if necessary. Corneal opacities and lesions such as foreign bodies, abrasions, lacerations, ulcers or puncture wounds should be apparent using this technique. A useful light source with low power magnification can also be obtained by using an otoscope with the speculum removed (Fig. 15.6).

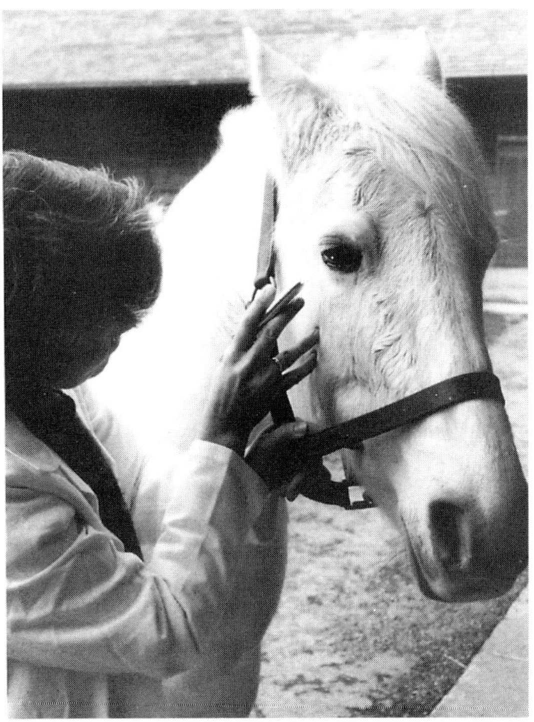

Figure 15.5 Pen light examination of the eye and adnexa (mainly performed in darkness).

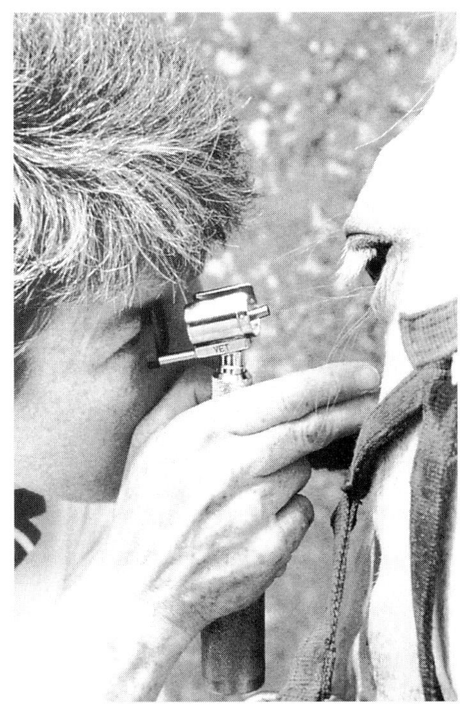

Figure 15.6 Illumination and magnification provided by using an otoscope with the speculum removed (mainly performed in darkness).

Anterior segment

The anterior segment (the internal structures of the globe up to and including the lens) is examined using the same equipment. The light should be shone from a number of different angles for evaluation of the anterior chamber, iris, lens and aqueous humour. The anterior chamber and iris should be examined for evidence of foreign bodies, cysts, neoplasia, uveitis or complications of uveitis such as synechiae. The latter may cause an irregular pupil shape and size.

Pupillary light response

The pupillary light response and the position, shape and size of the pupils are checked. The normal equine pupil responds somewhat sluggishly and incompletely, especially in comparison with that of the cat and dog, unless the light is particularly bright. NB The presence of a pupillary light response is not synonymous with vision, nor does the absence of a response necessarily indicate that the horse is blind. A reduced or absent pupillary light response is usually indicative of an ocular problem or a sub-cortical lesion. In more centrally located CNS disease, the pupillary light response may remain intact despite blindness.

For comprehensive examination of the lens and beyond, a mydriatic is necessary. Atropine should not be used as its effects are very long lasting in the normal equine eye. Topical application of 1% tropicamide ('Mydriacyl': Alcon) is perfectly satisfactory and will produce a dilated pupil within 20–30 minutes; its effects last for 8–12 hours.

The pen light may be used to demonstrate the anterior and posterior surfaces of the lens. An image of the light source may be readily identified on the anterior cornea (the corneal reflex) and with decreasing clarity on the anterior lens capsule and the posterior lens capsule. These are the *Purkinje–Sanson images* and their relative movement in relation to the light source (parallax) is a simple way of establishing the depth of anterior segment opacities. In cataract formation, there may be a loss of one or both lens images, depending on the site of the cataract.

Slit lamp biomicroscopy of the anterior segment

The slit lamp biomicroscope (Fig. 15.7) provides a refined means of examining the equine anterior segment in great detail. Its use may be essential to a definitive diagnosis, but for the most part it is usually employed at specialist centres and only the principles of its operation are given here. It consists of a light source which can produce diffuse illumination or a narrowed slit beam, and a binocular microscope which can move independently with respect to the light source.

Focal examination of the anterior segment can be performed using either diffuse or direct illumination (Fig. 15.8). Diffuse illumination is used initially to detect gross lesions involving the cornea, anterior chamber, iris, lens or anterior vitreous. The beam is then narrowed to a slit and directed obliquely so that an optical section of, for example, the cornea or lens may be observed. The slit beam illuminates any opaque structures and throws into relief minute optical differences in the transparent media. This is the easiest method of slit lamp examination to use in horses.

Indirect lateral illumination or scleral scatter utilizes a slit beam which is displaced laterally so that the light falls onto the limbus while the microscope is focused centrally onto the cornea (Fig. 15.8). With this method the light is transmitted within the cornea by total internal reflection and exits at the opposite limbus. If the cornea is normal no light is seen. If the light is obstructed by an opacity the lesion will become illuminated because it alters the path of the internally reflected light beam. This technique is particularly useful for the detection of subtle opacities and mild corneal oedema, but it is difficult to use effectively in horses.

Retro-illumination utilizes the reflection from the iris or the lens (especially if it is cataractous), so as to illuminate the cornea from behind (Fig. 15.8). This method of examination allows the detection of fine epithelial and endothelial changes, small blood vessels and opacities on the posterior corneal surface and, with practice, is rewarding to use in horses.

Indirect and direct ophthalmoscopy

The posterior segment (the internal structures of the globe beyond the lens) is examined using

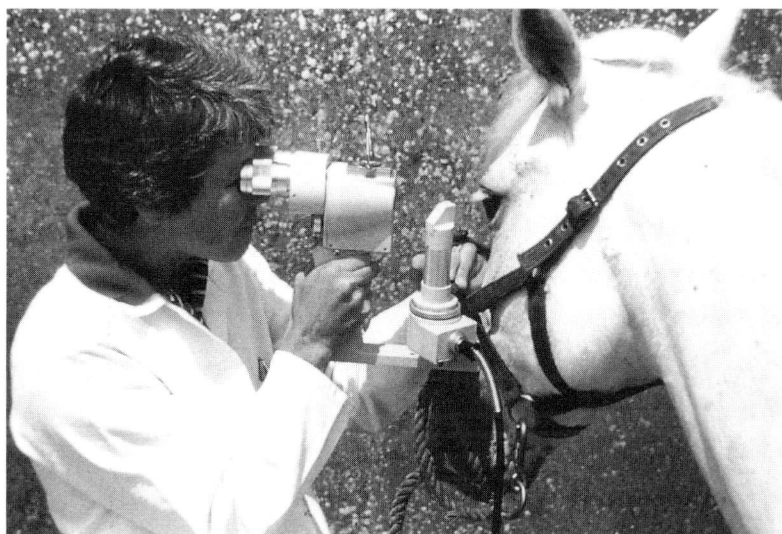

Figure 15.7 Slit lamp biomicroscopy (performed in darkness).

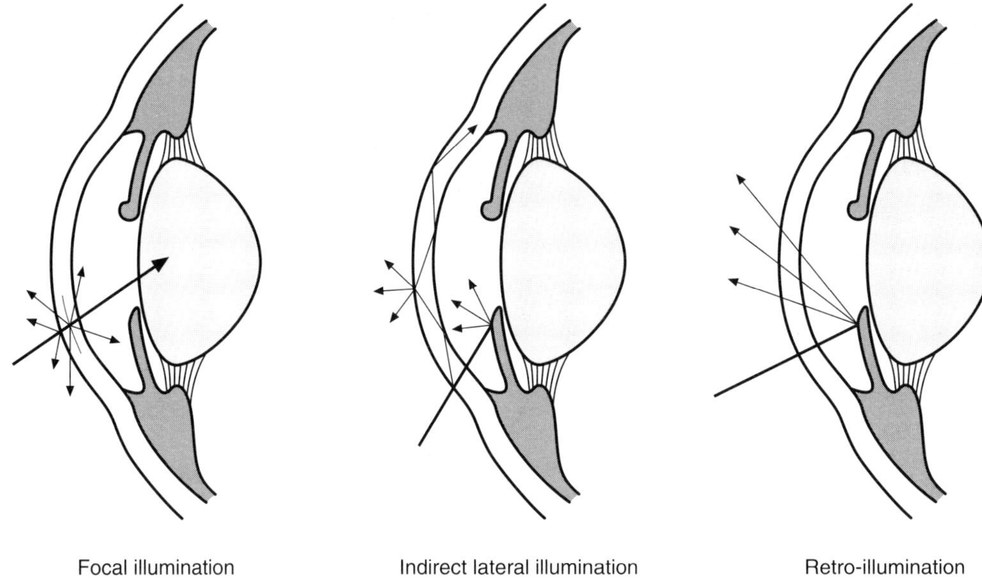

Figure 15.8 The technique of slit lamp biomicroscopy.

indirect ophthalmoscopy followed by direct ophthalmoscopy. The two methods are complementary rather than exclusive.

Indirect ophthalmoscopy

This is an efficient technique for screening the ocular fundus and can be performed most simply using a pen light and a condensing lens. The system produces a reversed, inverted, virtual image of low magnification, but the main advantage is that a large field of view is afforded which is not affected by major refractive errors in the patient's eye. It can therefore be very useful when the ocular media are opaque. Corneal, anterior chamber, vitreous and lens opacities are silhouetted against the tapetal reflection. Mydriasis and darkness are essential for detailed examination.

Monocular indirect ophthalmoscopy. In horses a +20 to +30 dioptre (D) condensing lens is the most versatile in use. A strong lens (high plus) produces a small, bright image whereas a weaker lens (lower plus) produces a larger, less bright image. The condensing lens is held some 2–8 cm from the patient's eye and the light source is held level with the bridge of the observer's nose. The aim is that the observer's eye, the light source, the lens and the patient's pupil should all lie in the same axis.

The plane of the lens must be parallel to that of the patient's iris and pupil (Fig. 15.9). The light is directed into the patient's eye so that the tapetal reflection is obtained and the lens is moved to and fro until a sharp image is produced. The observer–patient distance is approximately 50–75 cm.

A commercial monocular indirect ophthalmoscope is available (American Optical Company) which gives an erect image (Fig. 15.10).

Binocular indirect ophthalmoscopy. Binocular indirect ophthalmoscopes have an integral light source and a prism system for delivery of separate images to the observer's eyes. They are mounted on a headpiece or spectacle type frame. The working principle is the same as for monocular indirect ophthalmoscopy, but the instruments have the benefits of stereopsis and more powerful light sources. They also allow the observer one free hand. Spectacle models are probably most comfortable for extended use and many types are available.

Direct ophthalmoscopy

The use of a standard direct ophthalmoscope produces an upright image of greater magnification than is possible with the indirect

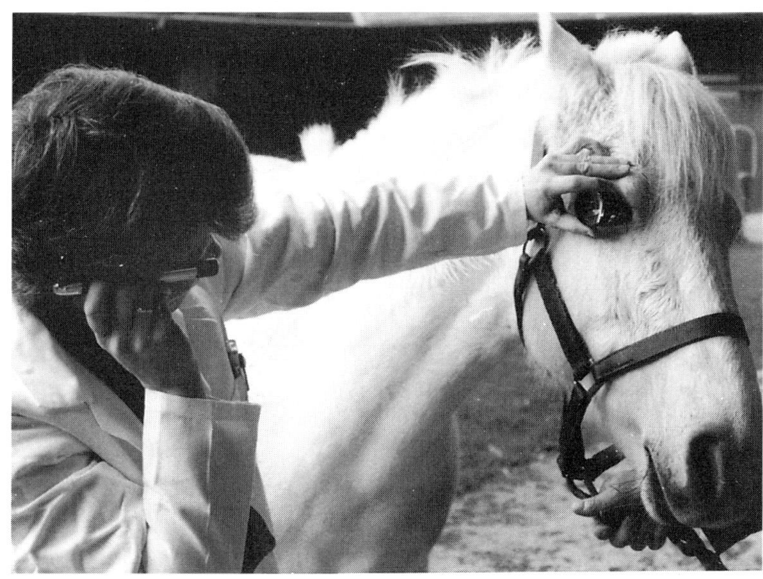

Figure 15.9 Monocular indirect ophthalmoscopy using a pen torch and condensing lens. The condensing lens is held 2–8 cm from the patient's eye. The observer to patient distance is approximately 50–75 cm (performed in darkness).

ophthalmoscope when used close to the patient's eye. However, viewing the fundus directly along a beam of light necessarily restricts the diameter of the field of view. Both distant direct ophthalmoscopy and close direct ophthalmoscopy should form part of direct ophthalmoscopic examination.

Distant direct ophthalmoscopy. This technique uses the tapetal fundus as a means of retro-illuminating the structures anterior to it. The ophthalmoscope is set to 0 dioptre (no magnification) and directed to find the tapetal reflex in the pupil at an observer–patient distance of 25–40 cm (Fig. 15.11). It is a useful way of assessing whether there are any opacities between the observer and the fundus and is usually used as a quick screening method prior to more detailed assessment. Any opacities present in the ocular media (cornea, aqueous, lens, vitreous) will appear as black forms against the fundus reflex. Assessment of comparative pupil sizes may also be made using this technique.

Close direct ophthalmoscopy. This can be used to examine all aspects of the eye and adnexa. The aperture of the instrument must be held as close as possible to the observer's eye and the subject's eye (Fig. 15.12). The lens range is approximately +30D (magnifying lenses) to –30D (reducing lenses). The image is real, erect and magnified up to 15-fold. As the

examiner reduces the strength of the plus lenses, the focus of observation gradually extends posteriorly, so that magnified details of the lids, cornea, aqueous, iris, lens and vitreous are successively visualized until features of the fundus are brought into focus. For detailed

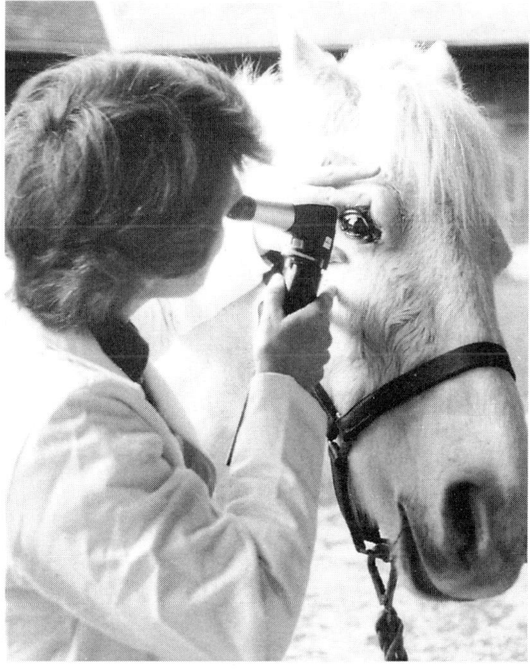

Figure 15.10 Monocular indirect ophthalmoscopy using a commercial instrument (performed in darkness).

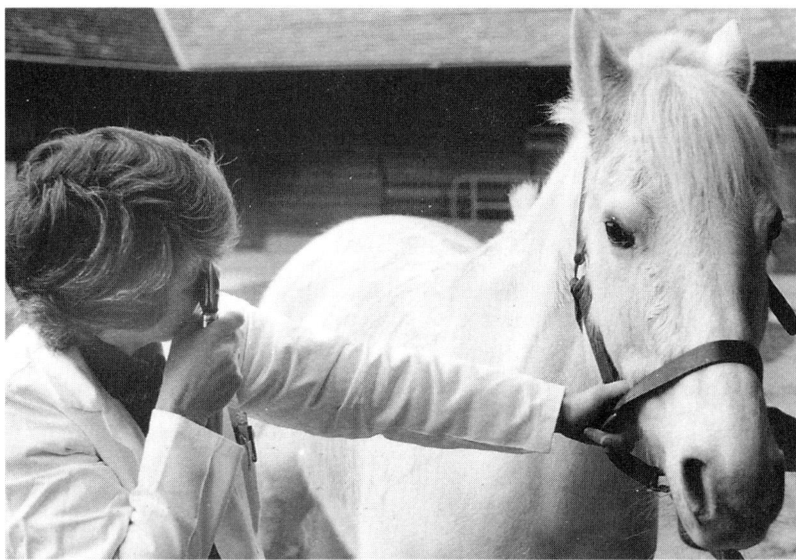

Figure 15.11 Distant direct ophthalmoscopy (performed in darkness).

examination darkness is essential and mydriasis is helpful.

The observer should remove spectacles when

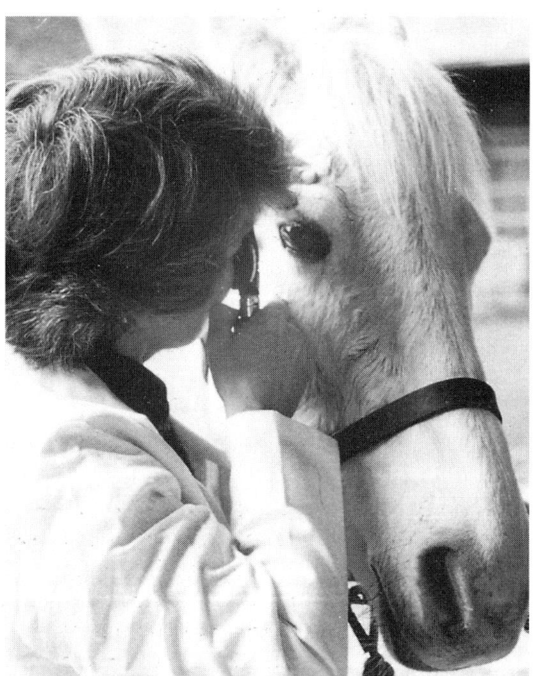

Figure 15.12 Close direct ophthalmoscopy (performed in darkness).

performing close direct ophthalmoscopy. A spectacle lens prescription can be set on the direct ophthalmoscope by trial and error and will compensate for any refractive error in the observer's vision during the examination.

For examination of the external eye and adnexa a setting of +20 to +15D is required. The iris may be examined with a setting of +15 to +12D. For the lens, the setting will be about +12 to +8D depending on whether the anterior or posterior parts are being examined. Intermediate settings will be required for the aqueous and vitreous. Close examination of the fundus is usually performed with the ophthalmoscope placed some 2 cm from the eye and a setting of between +2D or –2D (usually 0) is required. The examination is often made easier and safer if the hand holding the ophthalmoscope is rested lightly against the horse's head, so that sudden movements do not damage the eyes of the horse or the examiner.

The fundus should be examined in logical fashion, the tapetal fundus (when present), non-tapetal fundus, optic disc and visible vasculature should all be assessed and both eyes should be compared and contrasted (Colour Plates 3 and 4).

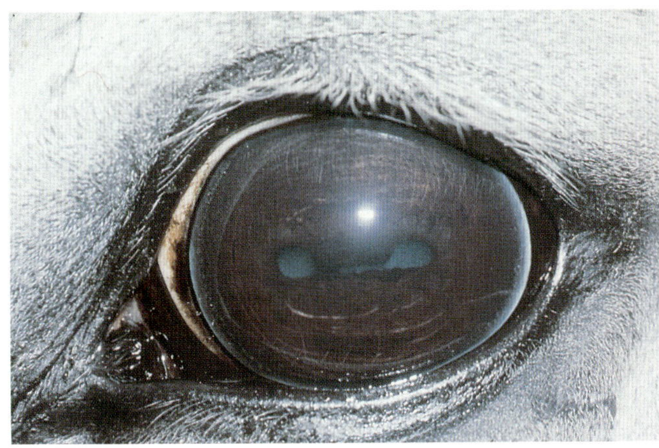

Plate 1. Closer naked eye examination of the eye and adnexa should note external details shown here such as the angle of the cilia on the upper eyelid, the dorsal and ventral orbital sulci (which divide the eyelids into tarsal and orbital portions), the position of the third eyelid and caruncle, and the amount of pigmentation present on the eyelids and conjunctiva. The limbus should be clearly defined; note the pigmented rim in this animal. The cornea should be transparent, allowing the fine structure of the iris to be clearly visualized. In this horse the grey line which marks the insertion of the pectinate ligament into Descemet's membrane and the cornea is very obvious laterally, less so medially.The pupil should be an almost symmetrical horizontal ellipse and granula iridica are usually obvious on the dorsal pupillary border, less so on the ventral pupillary border. In order to appreciate internal details beyond the pupil, examination must be continued in the dark.

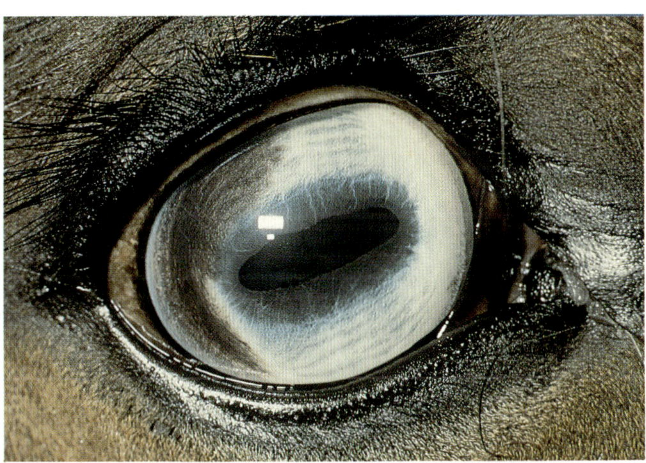

Plate 2. This horse shows a normal variant of iris colouration known as heterochromia iridis, whereby different sectors of the iris are of different colours, reflecting the degree of iris pigmentation. When the deficiency of pigment is marked and generalized the albinotic iris may be so hypoplastic that it is possible to view details of the underlying lens equator and zonule.

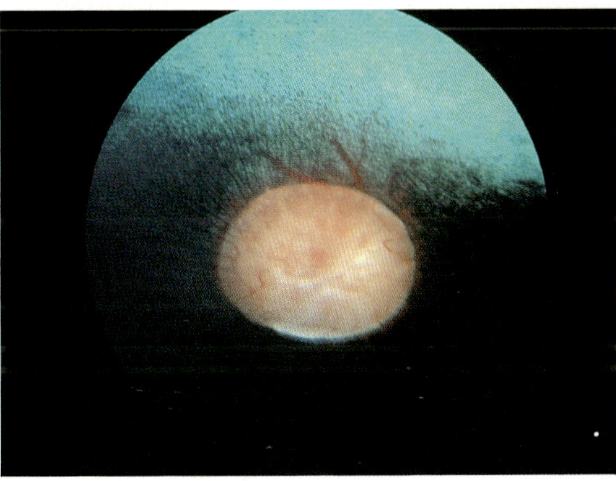

Plate 3. Normal fundus in a horse with a heavily pigmented iris. The optic disc (papilla) is located within the non-tapetal fundus. Note the fine peripapillary retinal vessels which radiate from the optic disc; they are deficient in the 6 o'clock position (a normal variation which marks the site of the original foetal fissure). Choroidal vessels are visible dorsal to the papilla because of suprapapillary hypopigmentation. The discrete black dots ('stars of Winslow') distributed throughout the green tapetal fundus represent choriocapillaris vessels viewed end on.

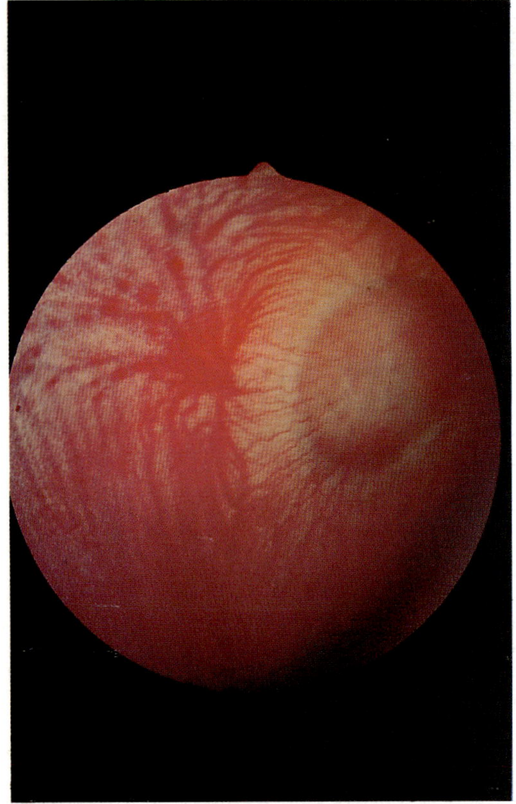

Plate 4. Normal fundus in a horse with a pale (subalbinotic) iris (china eye or wall eye). In this subalbinotic fundus there is no tapetum and very little pigment, hence both retinal and choroidal vessels are clearly visible against the creamy white of the sclera. The confluence of the choroidal vessels to form a vortex vein are very obvious in this animal.

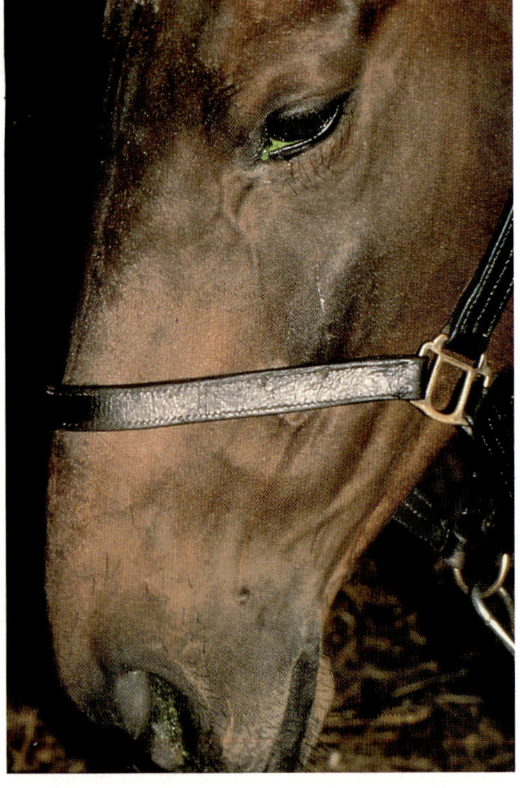

Plate 6. Fluorescein applied to the conjunctival sac should appear at the ipsilateral nostril within 1–5 minutes of application.

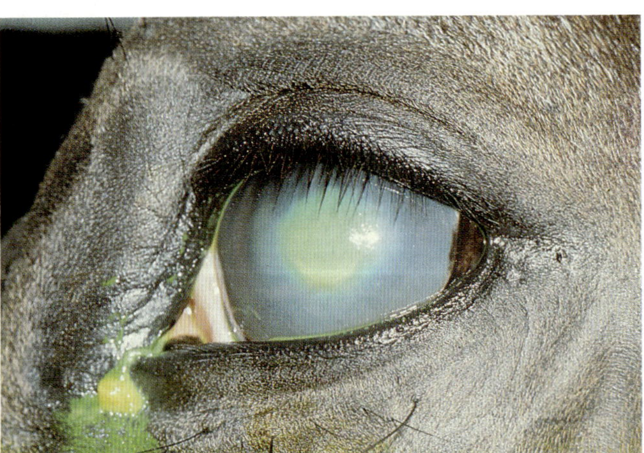

Plate 5. Fluorescein has been used to stain the large ulcer which is present in this horse's cornea.

II. Supplementary techniques

Swabs, scrapes, smears and biopsies

Swabs, scrapes and smears are most usefully taken from the eyelid margins, conjunctiva (Fig. 15.13) and cornea; the affected area being that which is sampled. For the conjunctiva and eyelid margins local anaesthesia is unnecessary, whereas precise sampling of corneal lesions requires topical anaesthesia. If corneal ulcers are sampled it is the edge of the ulcer which will yield replicating bacteria and a Kimura spatula is the best instrument to use for this technique.

Swabs and scrapes are useful for bacterial identification and sensitivity testing, but are of much less value in attempting to establish putative viral aetiologies.

Impression smears can be used to establish the nature of problems which involve the ocular or adnexal surface, such as squamous cell carcinoma. A clean dry glass slide is pressed gently, but firmly, against the abnormal area and the preparation is air-dried, fixed in methanol and submitted to a reliable histopathologist for staining and interpretation. At least two smears should be prepared.

Biopsies may be taken from the eyelids and conjunctiva following adequate topical anaes-thesia. Several applications of local anaesthetic will be required before the biopsy is performed. Fine needle aspiration or surgical excision (partial or complete) may be used. For surgical excision the normal tissue at the edge of the lesion is grasped with fine toothed forceps and an adequately sized sample is snipped off with fine pointed scissors or excised with a scalpel. It is important to avoid crushing and distorting the tissue when obtaining the sample and the correct orientation is often most easily maintained if the sample is placed on very thin card before immersion in fixative. Neutral buffered formaldehyde is acceptable for routine light microscopy and immunohistochemistry, whereas 2.5% glutaraldehyde in 0.1 M cacodylate buffer is the fixative of choice for electron microscopy. Always consult the laboratory before taking the samples if there is any doubt as to which fixative to use.

Topical ophthalmic stains

Fluorescein

This is an orange dye which changes to green in alkaline conditions. In horses it is primarily used to detect corneal ulceration as it is rapidly absorbed by the exposed hydrophilic stroma in such cases (Colour Plate 5). It does not stain the lipid-rich epithelium or the posterior lining membrane of the cornea (Descemet's membrane).

Fluorescein may also be used as a means of checking the patency of the naso-lacrimal drainage apparatus (see below) and, less frequently, for detecting the leakage of aqueous humour following penetrating injury or corneal repair (Seidel test).

Impregnated strips or single dose vials may be used and in horses it is often simplest to place the strip or solution in the lower conjunctival sac and allow the blink to distribute the fluorescein. To avoid false positives and

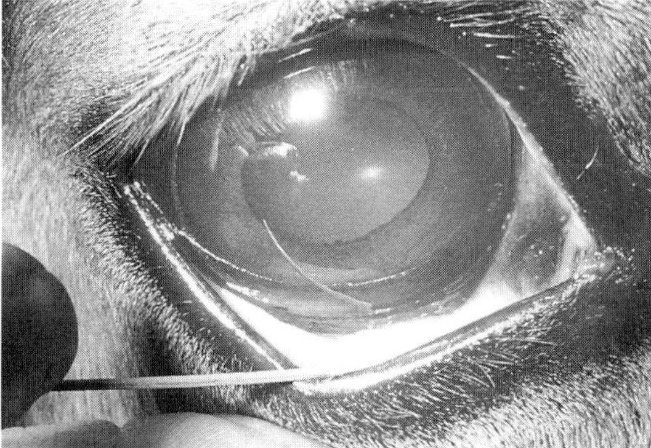

Figure 15.13 Conjunctival culture. The swab is placed in the lower conjunctival sac and rotated firmly against the palpebral conjunctiva.

provide sufficient moisture for adequate staining it is sometimes necessary to irrigate the eye with sterile saline or water. It is easier to detect subtle staining with a blue light source.

Rose bengal

This is a red dye which stains damaged or devitalized epithelium and mucin. It is irritant to the eye and its use is therefore reserved for the detection of subtle epithelial defects. It is seldom used in horses.

Schirmer tear production test

Few disorders of the pre-ocular tear film have been described in horses and testing tear production is not regarded as a routine part of equine ophthalmic examination. However, the Schirmer I tear test is the method most commonly employed for this purpose. A standardized strip of filter paper is inserted into the conjuctival sac and the length of paper which has become wet after a specific time is measured. Values of more than 15 mm in 30 seconds or 20–30 mm per minute are obtained in normal horses. Values of less than 10 mm per minute should be regarded with suspicion and repeated values of less than 5 mm are indicative of a lack of tear production, clinically manifest as *keratoconjunctivitis sicca*.

The test is easily performed using commercially available test strips which are up to 60 mm in length with a notch some 5 mm from the tip. Topical local anaesthetic solution is not used for the Schirmer I test. The strip is bent at the notched region and the tip is placed just within the conjunctival sac (Fig. 15.14). The strip is usually removed after 30 seconds and the value is read immediately, as measured from the notch in mm.

Investigation of naso-lacrimal drainage

The upper and lower lacrimal puncta and the nasal ostium are readily visible in horses and

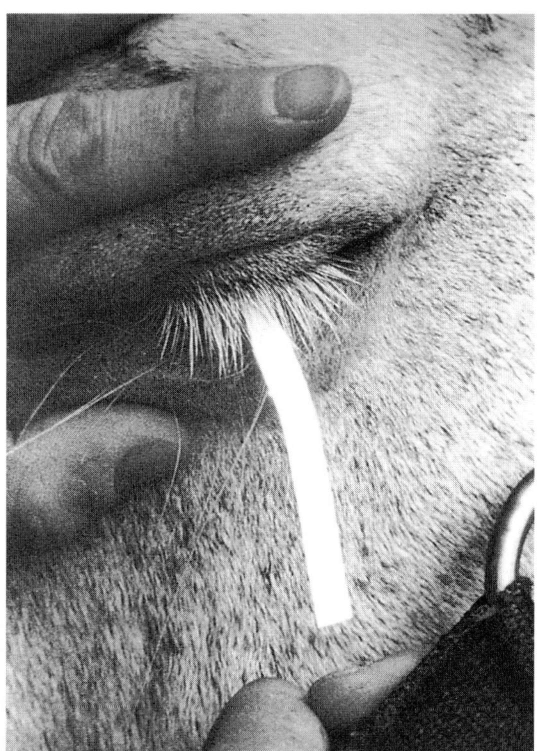

Figure 15.14   A Schirmer I tear test being performed on the conscious unsedated horse (sedation and anaesthesia will reduce tear production).

this means that investigations can be performed from the proximal (puncta) and/or distal (ostium) parts of the system.

Visual inspection

Initial examination consists of visual inspection of the nasal ostium (Fig. 15.15) and the lacrimal puncta. The upper and lower lacrimal puncta are identified as fine, slit-like openings about 2 mm long situated close behind the free edge of their respective eyelids, about 8 mm from the medial canthus. Their presence, size and position should be checked.

Cannulation/catheterization

If samples are required for culture and sensitivity they may be obtained by irrigation with sterile water following topical local anaesthesia and cannulation/catheterization of

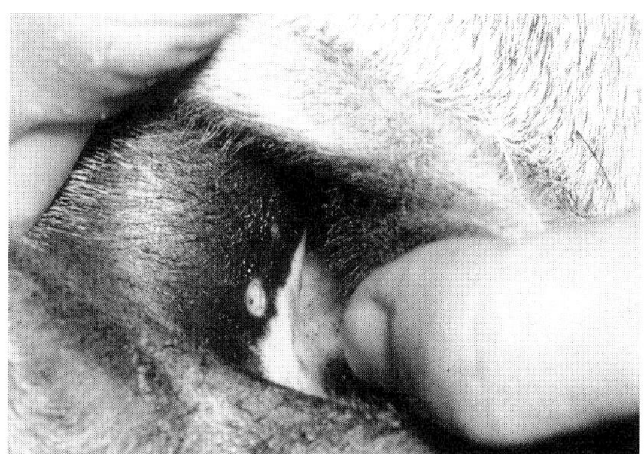

Figure 15.15 Visual inspection of the (left) nasal ostium which is located medially on the floor of the nostril close to the mucocutaneous junction.

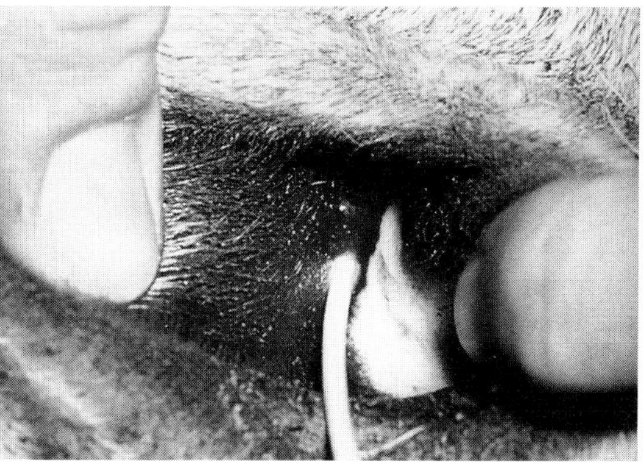

Figure 15.17 A catheter has been inserted into the nasal ostium and nasolacrimal duct after the application of local anaesthetic drops to the upper or lower lacrimal puncta and local anaesthetic (usually as gel or spray) to the nasal ostium.

the upper lacrimal punctum (Fig. 15.16). The upper lacrimal punctum is located and the upper eyelid is stabilized by tensing it upwards and everting it slightly, so as to move the canaliculus into a more vertical position. A silver cannula or plastic cannula/catheter can then be passed into the canaliculus via the the punctum. Sedation may be required in addition to local anaesthesia. Alternatively, samples may be obtained by retrograde flushing with sterile water after cannulation/catheterization of the nasal ostium (Fig. 15.17). Again, local

anaesthetic is applied to both the conjunctival sac and nasal ostium a few minutes before catheterization; sedation or application of a twitch may be necessary. These irrigation techniques will also indicate the patency of the duct.

Fluorescein drainage

If culture is not required, patency can be tested using fluorescein drops instilled into the lower conjunctival sac. These should appear at the ipsilateral nostril within 1–5 minutes of application (Colour Plate 6). Both sides should be tested.

Dacryocystorhinography

Dacryocystorhinography (contrast radiography of the nasolacrimal duct) is a useful technique for establishing the extent of congenital or acquired abnormalities of patency and, as the technique may confirm the necessity for surgical intervention, it is best performed under general anaesthesia. It is usual to cannulate/catheterize the upper lacrimal punctum and to inject approximately 5 ml of an iodine based contrast agent. Lateral and oblique radiographs are taken (Figs 15.18a and b).

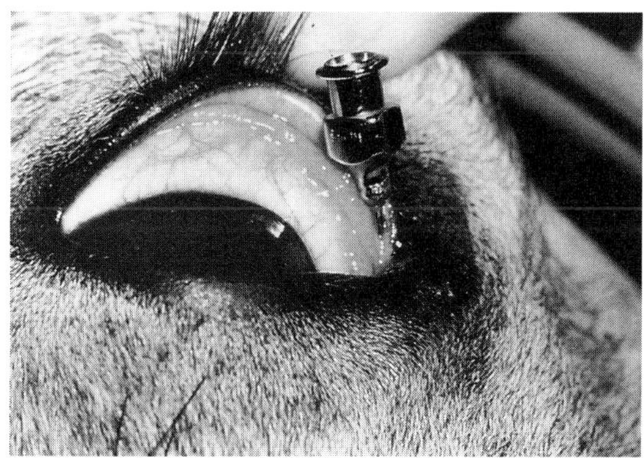

Figure 15.16 A nasolacrimal cannula has been inserted into the upper lacrimal punctum and canaliculus after applying several drops of local anaesthetic to the upper punctum. The cannula is made of silver, a relatively soft and malleable metal, which is unlikely to damage the canaliculus.

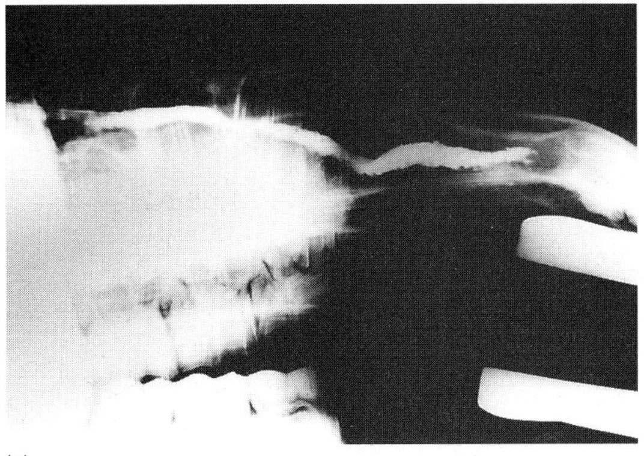

(a)

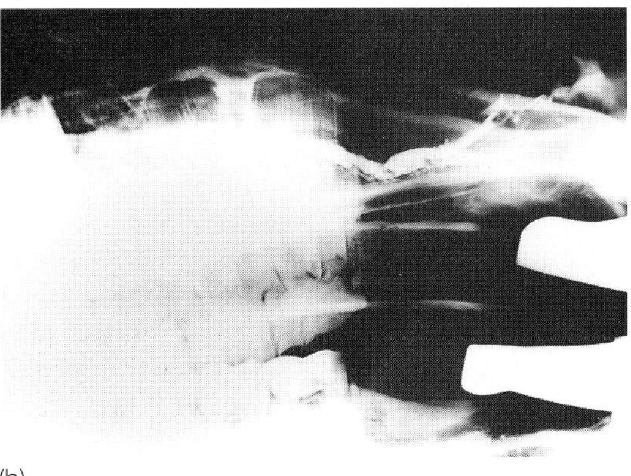

(b)

Figure 15.18(a) Dacryocystorhinography with an iodine based contrast agent has been used to confirm the results of clinical examination which showed that the nasal ostium was absent. The contrast agent delineates the extent of congenital atresia of the nasolacrimal drainage system prior to surgery. **(b)** The post-operative contrast radiograph demonstrating patency of the drainage system.

Tonometry

Tonometry in horses is most reliably performed with some form of electronic applanation tonometer (Fig. 15.19). The 'MacKay–Marg', 'Pro Ton' (Tomey Technology) and 'Tono-pen' (Carleton Medical) are all suitable for use in horses. The MacKay–Marg is no longer commercially available and requires a mains electricity supply, but it is accurate and second-hand models can occasionally be obtained. Pro Ton and Tono-Pen tonometers are portable but expensive.

The normal intraocular pressure of unsedated horses is between 16 and 32 mm Hg.

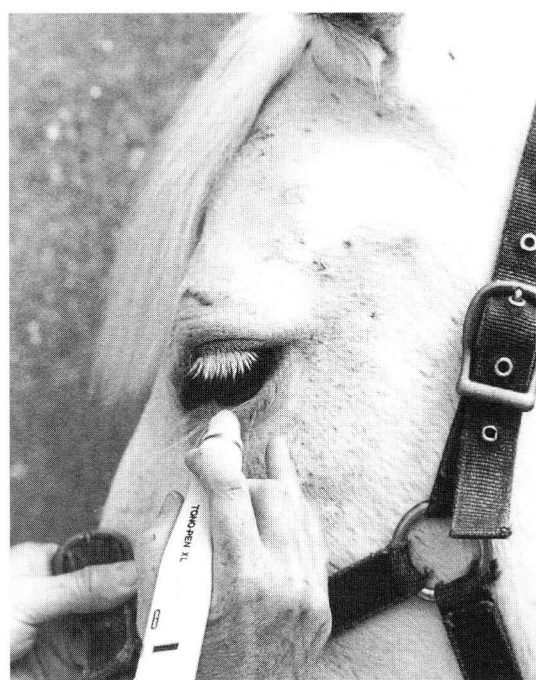

Figure 15.19 Tonometry being performed on the conscious unsedated horse (sedation and anaesthesia may affect intraocular pressure). Topical local anaesthetic drops are applied prior to the procedure.

In conscious animals, increased intraocular pressure is associated with glaucoma (which is rare in horses), whereas decreases in intraocular pressure are a feature of acute uveitis and the use of sedatives.

Diagnostic imaging

Radiography is of limited value in aiding diagnosis of soft tissue problems in and near the eye, but can be useful when there is a bony abnormality. However, B mode ocular ultrasonography is a valuable technique for soft tissue imaging and is best performed with a high frequency transducer of 7.5–10 MHz. Most horses tolerate the procedure well and general anaesthesia is rarely necessary.

Topical local anaesthesia and sedation may both be of value in providing good conditions for diagnostic imaging of the eye and retrobulbar tissues. The examination is carried out with the horse standing and the head held.

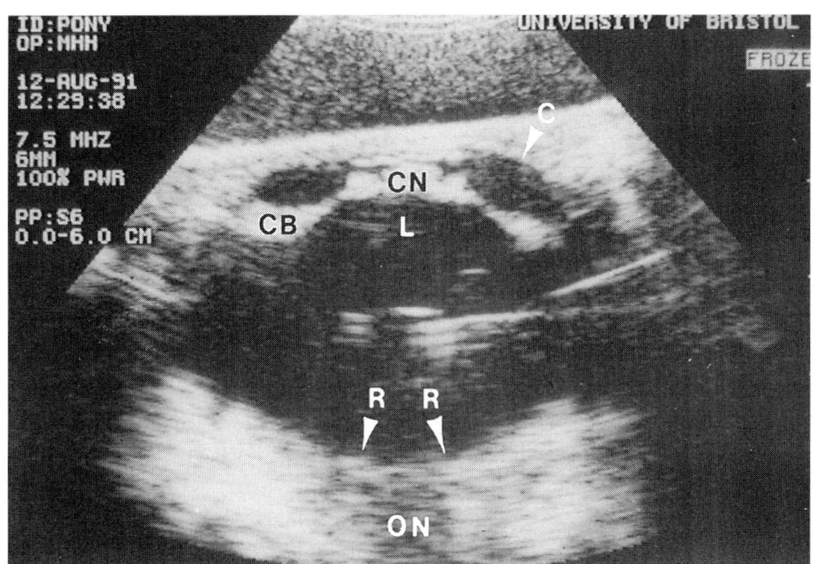

Figure 15.20
Ultrasonography of the normal equine eye. In addition to showing normal features of the globe in reasonable detail, the technique is of value in demonstrating whether the retrobulbar tissues are also normal. C: cornea; CB: ciliary body; CN: corpora nigra; L: lens; R: retina; ON: optic nerve.

Acoustic gel is applied to the transducer head before it is applied directly to the eye or to the closed eyelids; clipping is not necessary. However, image quality is reduced significantly when the transducer is applied to the closed eyelids and it should be applied directly to the cornea whenever possible.

The eye is examined in both horizontal and vertical section and it is sensible to examine both eyes so that an unaffected eye can be used as a normal control. Excess acoustic gel is wiped away gently at the end of the procedure.

The normal eye is clearly demarcated and the aqueous and vitreous compartments are anechoic so that they appear black on conventional scans (Fig. 15.20). The cornea, anterior chamber and lens are more clearly defined when a 'stand-off' is used to separate the transducer head from the cornea. In normal animals, the cornea is a smooth echogenic layer which appears white on conventional scans. The curved shape of the lens produces scattered reflections, so that only the central part of the lens is echogenic when the incident sound beam is perpendicular to the reflecting surface. The tissues at the back of the globe (retina, choroid and sclera) are identifiable as a curved white line.

The retrobulbar tissues are well defined in normal horses as the orbit contains much retrobulbar fat. The optic nerve may be recognized as a hypoechoic channel passing through the more echogenic retrobulbar tissues. The optic nerve will therefore appear dark grey and the retrobulbar tissues white.

Further reading

Barnett KC, Crispin SM, Lavach JD and Matthews AG (1995) *Colour Atlas and Text of Equine Ophthalmology*. London: Mosby-Wolfe.

Cooley PL (1992) Normal equine ocular anatomy and eye examination. In: *Veterinary Clinics of North America: Equine Practice* 8: 427–449.

Crispin SM, Matthews AG and Parker J (1990) The equine fundus I: Examination, embryology, structure and function. *Equine Veterinary Journal Supplement* 10: 42–49.

Hillyer MH (1993) Ocular ultrasonography in the horse. In: Raw ME and Parkinson TJ (eds) *Veterinary Annual*, 33rd Issue, pp. 131–137. London: Blackwell Scientific Publications.

16 Fat diseases

Fat diseases occur infrequently in equine practice. They include hyperlipaemia, fat tumours and steatitis/fat necrosis. Of these, the commonest is hyperlipaemia, a disturbance of fat metabolism to which ponies and donkeys are particularly susceptible. Tumours of the fat occur relatively commonly in the abdomen of older horses, but they do not invariably cause problems. Generalized steatitis and necrosis are recorded rarely and almost exclusively in foals. On very rare occasions a generalized or subcutaneous steatitis is seen in adults.

Hyperlipaemia

Hyperlipaemia is a disturbance of fat metabolism which is characterized by an abnormally high level of lipid in the circulation. This results in fatty infiltration of the tissues, circulatory failure and extensive vascular thrombosis. The disease is fatal unless the underlying cause is identified and treated successfully.

The cause is usually some form of stress or nutritional deprivation which is imposed upon susceptible animals. The most susceptible are ponies, especially Shetland ponies, during late pregnancy or early lactation. It is less commonly seen in non-pregnant animals, but in this category obese ponies and donkeys are at most risk. Many factors can constitute a stress and typical examples include climatic extremes, poor husbandry, and intercurrent disease — particularly gastrointestinal disease.

The pivotal event in the development of this metabolic disease seems to be inhibition of insulin activity. Insulin normally promotes the deposition of fat, but interference with its activity leads to fat mobilization from adipose depots. Ponies and donkeys, and more especially *obese* ponies and donkeys, have an inherent physiological insensitivity to insulin. In addition, hormonal changes (associated with pregnancy and lactation), and increases in circulating cortisol levels (associated with disease or other stresses), also act to antagonize insulin activity, thus compounding the inherent insensitivity in these animals. In summary, ponies and donkeys are metabolically predisposed to fat mobilization and conditions of pregnancy, obesity, disease, stress and/or reduced feed intake, act to promote this tendency.

Diagnosis

The clinical signs are non-specific. Progressive hyperlipaemia is associated with drowsiness, depression, reluctance to move, dysphagia and circulatory congestion. Ventral oedema is common, but not pathognomonic. Signs of hepatic encephalopathy may follow fatty infiltration and failure of the liver. *A pony in advanced pregnancy showing inappetance or depression should immediately be investigated for evidence of hyperlipaemia.*

In other cases, the clinical signs of hyperlipaemia may be masked by the more obvious signs of some primary disease which induces inappetance and/or a stress response. Any disease process which is associated with a reduced food intake has the potential to predispose to hyperlipaemia as a secondary complication. It should also be noted that healthy but overweight ponies or donkeys with a history of being put on an abrupt diet are prime candidates for hyperlipaemia.

In health, serum triglyceride concentrations are usually less than 1 mmol/l. In hyperlipaemic states they are greater than 5 mmol/l and can exceed 75 mmol/l in severe cases. Once the triglyceride concentration exceeds 5 mmol/l, the serum or plasma develops a visible opacity. Hyperlipaemia is easily demonstrated during clinical examination by taking a blood sample into anticoagulant. In a clear tube the light is reflected from the blood surface with a characteristic steel blue sheen. More obviously, when the tube has stood for a few minutes to allow the red cells to settle out, the plasma reveals a cloudy, milk-like appearance.

Post-mortem examination shows extensive fatty change in tissues. There may also be evidence of some primary disease process which has predisposed to the hyperlipaemic state.

Comments

- Hyperlipaemia in horses is not accompanied by dramatic increases in blood cholesterol concentration and its estimation is not diagnostically useful in this species.

- In advanced cases there is biochemical evidence of hepatic and renal failure. This takes the form of raised serum liver enzymes and developing azotaemia. However, lipaemic serum or plasma is often unsuitable for biochemical analyses and these developments can be missed.

- Animals at risk, such as pregnant Shetland pony mares, can have their serum triglyceride levels monitored during late pregnancy to ensure that the energy intake is adequate and that stressors such as parasitism are held in check.

NB Short-term fasting in ponies (e.g. in transit) may produce a physiological lipaemia which is reversible and without clinical sequel. This physiological state is sometimes referred to as *hyperlipidaemia*.

Fat tumours

Lipomas of the mesentery are relatively common in older horses/ponies. Those which develop on a lengthy pedicle have the potential to become entwined around the small intestine, thus causing an acute, often strangulating, obstruction. Much less commonly, the small colon may be obstructed. Lipomas are one of the commonest causes of strangulating obstruction in older horses, and ponies seem particularly predisposed.

Diagnosis

The clinical presentation is colic of acute onset, usually in the older horse or pony (> 9 years), and examination indicates a high obstruction. Definitive diagnosis requires laparotomy. Rectal examination will probably reveal turgid loops of small intestine within a few hours of onset, but it is most unlikely that a discrete lipoma will be palpable. Sometimes several loops of intestine are drawn together into a large palpable 'knot-like' mass.

Steatitis and fat necrosis

Steatitis and fat necrosis occur together as two extremes of an inflammatory condition, but they are extremely rare in the adult horse. The disease is characterized by widespread lesions within adipose tissues and is recognized externally by the appearance of firm plaque-like swellings beneath the skin. The generalized condition is invariably fatal because progressively indurated fat lesions impinge on vital functions such as heart activity.

Panniculitis, an unusual form of steatitis which is limited in distribution to the subcutaneous tissues, has also been described in the adult horse.

Diagnosis

Subcutaneous swellings of variable size, consistency and number are distributed over the body surface. The firmer, plaque-like masses are immobile and may have a soft, liquefied centre. Clinical examination and haematology indicate a wasting, inflammatory condition. Diagnosis is easily achieved by biopsy of a solid subcutaneous swelling. A small wedge removed from beneath a skin incision reveals foci of fat necrosis and possibly mineralization. However, biopsy alone cannot indicate the extent of fat lesions within the body. Post-mortem examination shows widespread discolouration of body fat with patchy induration and focal areas of liquefaction.

Comment

- In other species, generalized steatitis and fat necrosis are associated with a vitamin E deficiency which is part of the diagnostic criteria. In horses, vitamin E estimation is likely to be normal and the aetiology, pathogenesis and treatment of the disease remain a mystery.

Further reading

Watson T (1994) Hyperlipaemia in ponies. *In Practice* (supplement to the Veterinary Record) **16**: 267–272.

Edwards GB and Proudman CJ (1994) An analysis of 75 cases of intestinal obstruction caused by pedunculated lipomas. *Equine Veterinary Journal* **26**: 18–21.

Taylor FGR, Mair TS and Brown PJ (1988) Generalised steatitis in an adult pony mare. *Veterinary Record* **122**: 349–351.

17 Skin diseases

I. Assessing the problem

Skin lesions are very common in horses, but few can be diagnosed on appearance alone and many have a similar appearance despite a variety of causes. Careful evaluation of the history followed by a thorough clinical examination should help to limit the differential diagnoses and simplify the choice of practical investigative techniques. The first part of this chapter is concerned with assessing the problem in order to select a diagnostic route and the second part gives details of the investigative techniques.

History

There are a number of helpful questions which must be included in the history:

- Are other horses affected? If so, what is the common link: direct contact; tack; grooming equipment; feedstuffs? It is also worth checking whether any of the handlers/riders are suffering skin lesions.
- Is the lesion seasonal?
- Is it pruritic?
- Whereabouts on the body did it start; has it spread?
- What did it look like originally (i.e. the primary lesion); has it changed in appearance?
- Is there a recent history of using topical or systemic drugs?

Look at the horse's environment as a source of potential irritants or allergens and consider the distribution of lesion(s) on the animal. For example:

- Bedding material — contact areas are the lower limbs and belly.
- Dust from rafters/loft — falls over the head, neck and back.
- Feed positions — from above, food material falls over the face and neck; from below, it contacts the muzzle and lower limbs.
- Rugs and/or blankets — these will either

protect the skin underneath from lesions, or alternatively provoke lesions in that area.

Clinical examination

This should include a general examination, quite apart from the scrutiny of skin lesions, since systemic diseases are associated with some dermatoses. The principal features of the lesion(s) and their distribution are considered next. It is most useful to record details of the lesions and map their distribution on an annotated diagram.

Features of the lesion

The size, morphology and presenting characteristics are considered in an attempt to establish differential diagnoses. The principal features of lesions may be described as follows:

- Pruritis
- Crusting, scaling and hair loss
- Swellings: nodules, papules and urticaria
- Changes in hair growth: alopecia/hirsutism
- Pigmentation changes
- Congenital disorders

NB It must be emphasized that none of these features are mutually exclusive; for example, pruritis is frequently associated with hair loss and crusting. In consequence, it is often impossible to define a lesion from the principal features alone. Nevertheless, it is useful to consider the potential causes of each principal feature in attempting to narrow the differential diagnoses. Guidelines to differentials and selection of the appropriate diagnostic techniques are given below.

Pruritic lesions

Pruritis is usually associated with ectoparasites and contact irritants or hypersensitivities.

However, it may occasionally be a feature of infectious conditions (folliculitis/furunculosis), early photosensitization and urticarial lesions; all of which are described under other principal features. Pruritis associated with self-mutilation invariably leads to hair loss, exudation and crusting.

Ectoparasites

Lice

Lice are a late winter/early spring problem associated with crowded housing conditions. In a good light they may be seen with the naked eye, aided by a magnifying glass, at the base of the mane and tail. Biting lice (*Damalinia equi*) are fawn in colour and may be distributed in the dorsolateral trunk area. Sucking lice (*Haematopinus asini*) are a darker blue-black as a result of blood intake. The presence of copious scaling is likely, as are signs of rubbing. Shiny eggs ('*nits*') are seen attached to the hair.

Biting flies

Biting flies are probably the commonest ectoparasite causing pruritis. They are a summertime cause of annoyance, local skin eruption in the form of papules or wheals, and pruritis. Lesions are exacerbated by individual hypersensitivities (allergies) to the bite. *Horse flies (Tabanidae)* inflict painful bites which can result in large wheals. *Stable flies (Stomoxys calcitrans)* inflict severe bites to feed on blood/tissue fluids and can cause multiple wheals which develop into crusts along the neck, trunk and legs. *Black flies (Simulium)* attack the more sparsely haired areas such as the axillae, ventral midline and inguinal areas, producing a papular response. *Horn flies (Haematobia irritans)* are associated with a ventral midline dermatitis characterized by foci of hair loss, inflammation and scaling under the belly.

It is difficult to differentiate between these causes and a diagnosis of 'fly bite' may be achieved by the response to daytime stabling in a fly-proofed box. Biopsy of an early (primary) lesion will reveal a variety of tissue changes characteristic of an arthropod bite, but it will not distinguish between them. In theory, hypersensitivity tests should identify specific allergies (see later).

Bees and wasps

Bees and wasps may attack as swarms producing multiple papules and plaques which are painful rather than pruritic.

Culicoides species

Culicoides species are associated with the development of a common skin hypersensitivity known as 'sweet itch'. Predilection sites are the mane, croup and tail base. Affected areas show hair loss with exudation and the formation of hard, dry crusts of a few millimetres to several centimetres in diameter. As a result of rubbing, the mane and tail hairs are broken and there may be marked excoriation. Diagnosis is based on the appearance, seasonality and distribution of lesions, together with the marked pruritis. Biopsy is unrewarding since the histopathology will typify many arthropod reactions. Hypersensitivity tests can identify an allergy to *Culicoides* but should seldom be required to confirm diagnosis.

Mange mites

Mange mites uncommonly produce infestations in horses.

Chorioptic mange is caused by non-burrowing *Chorioptes* mites. The condition is uncommon and tends to be seen in the winter. Lesions are usually confined to the lower limbs and are predisposed by 'feathering' of the hair. Hair around the fetlock and pastern becomes matted with dried exudate. The mites are numerous and may be identified in a superficial skin scraping.

Demodectic mange (Demodex equi) is a follicular dermatitis which is very rare in horses and its diagnosis suggests a serious underlying systemic disease and/or immunosuppression. A few mites are commonly found as commensals and infestation is judged on the basis of large numbers being found in a deep skin scraping. Lesions present as hair loss and scaling over the face (eyes and muzzle), neck, shoulders and forelimbs. Pruritis may not be marked unless secondary infection is associated with pustule formation.

Psoroptic mange (Psoroptes communis) does not presently occur in the UK horse population. However, psoroptes mites are occasionally found in the aural canal, but the absence of associated lesions makes their significance doubtful.

Sarcoptic mange (Sarcoptes scabei) is extremely rare in the UK horse population. Lesions are associated with hair loss, skin thickening and dry scab formation. However, the possibility exists of spread from other species, notably cattle, and diagnosis is by deep skin scraping.

Harvest mites (Trombicula autumnalis; 'chiggers') cause pruritis and irritation about the horse's heels and muzzle following invasion from the herbage in autumn. The red/orange mite is visible to the naked eye, assisted by a magnifying lens. There are no marked skin lesions.

Forage mites are commonly found in hay and straw, but are a rare cause of pruritis. In this instance the mite is probably provoking a contact dermatitis (see below). The distribution of pruritic lesions is about the face and neck if fed from above, and about the muzzle and lower legs if fed from below. Diagnosis is by changing the feed and feeding position.

Warble flies (*Hypoderma* species)

Cattle are the usual hosts of warble fly larvae and since their eradication they are not currently seen in the UK horse population. The lesion is a hemispherical swelling of variable diameter, usually over the back. There may or not be a central 'breathing hole'. Diagnosis is based on the appearance of the lesion and careful removal of the grub following fomentation. Biopsy should not be attempted since this is likely to result in a severe local reaction.

Endoparasites

Onchocerciasis

Onchocerciasis (*Onchocerca cervicalis*) is a widespread filarial nematode endoparasite of horses. Adults live in the ligamentum nuchae, producing microfilariae which migrate out to connective tissues of the upper dermis. Many horses are infected, but few ever show evidence of clinical disease and it is rarely reported in the UK.

In clinical cases, hair loss, depigmentation, erythema and scaling are seen, particularly in the ventral midline region. Facial, cervical and proximal forelimb lesions are also described. Pruritis varies from mild to severe. Extraction of large numbers of microfilariae from finely chopped biopsy material provides a diagnosis, but it must be remembered that some microfilariae are to be expected in the skin of healthy horses. A more pragmatic diagnosis is the response to treatment with ivermectin, which resolves the inflammation within three weeks of treatment. However, the adult worm is unaffected and repeated anthelmintic treatment for microfilariae may be necessary.

Oxyuris equi

Oxyuris equi is a relatively common gut parasite. The adult female causes intense perianal irritation by depositing eggs on the perineum. Large numbers of eggs may be seen at the anal sphincter ('anal rust'). Smaller numbers may be detected microscopically using an adhesive acetate sampling technique (see later).

Contact dermatitis

Most contact dermatitis is caused by irritants damaging the skin as a result of persistent exposure. Examples are chemical sources such as tack treatments, drugs, certain plants, or body fluids such as urine. The distribution relates to the points of contact with the irritant, typically the head, limb extremities, ventral body surfaces and tack-associated areas. Lesions progress from erythema, serum ooze, crust formation and pruritis, to skin thickening and varying degrees of hair loss. In some cases the initial contact response is urticaria. Contact dermatitis of the lower limbs may progress to the 'greasy heel' reaction (see later).

Much less commonly contact dermatitis is allergic in nature. In this situation the sensitizing agents act as haptens, forming allergens with skin proteins. Allergy may arise to an agent which has been present in the horse's environment, without harm, for years. Once sensitivity is established, contact produces a pruritic dermatitis within 1–3 days. The lesions produced are similar to those seen in contact dermatitis due to irritants (above). Diagnosis is by maintaining the horse in an 'allergen-free' area (see below under 'Elimination tests for irritants and allergens'). Biopsy is usually unrewarding.

Crusting, scaling and hair loss

Hair loss is a common sequel to pruritis (above) and inflammatory reactions such as folliculitis and photosensitivity. It is frequently associated with exudation which may dry to form a solid, adherent crust. Scaling is the excessive production of thin flakes of cornified epithelial cells. It is the result of abnormal sebum production and keratinization (seborrhoea), which may be provoked by a number of inflammatory lesions. The appearance varies from that of 'dandruff' to the formation of greasy scales and crusts with accompanying inflammation.

Folliculitis/furunculosis

Folliculitis is an inflammation of the hair follicles, often suppurative in nature, which may be associated with *Staphylococcus aureus*, *Dermatophilus congolensis*, dermatophytes (*Trichophyton* and *Microsporum* species) and parasites (*Demodex equi*). If the lesion spreads into the surrounding dermis and subcutis, the more severe lesion is termed furunculosis. Pruritis is occasionally a feature of folliculitis, but not invariably.

Bacterial folliculitis

Bacterial folliculitis usually occurs in summer and may be associated with areas subject to sweat and friction from tack. The initial lesions are papules and pustules. Causative organisms, particularly *Staph. aureus* or streptococcal species, may be identified on culture. Impression smears demonstrate neutrophils surrounding cocci.

Dermatophilosis

Dermatophilosis is a common form of bacterial folliculitis associated with wet weather in the autumn and winter months. It is an extensive, exudative infection caused by *Dermatophilus congolensis*. There is usually a symmetrical distribution of lesions over the hindquarters, commonly termed 'rain scald'. In muddy conditions the same lesions may occur in the lower limbs ('mud fever') and may also affect the belly.

In appearance, the exudate mats the hairs giving a tufted, 'paintbrush' appearance to crusts. When removed the crusts are large in diameter and the underside is coated with purulent material. Diagnosis is by demonstrating the organism in a freshly lifted crust by impression smear or culture. NB Old lesions may be overgrown by staphylococci.

Dermatophytosis

Dermatophytosis or 'ringworm' is usually caused by *Trichophyton equinum*, or *T. mentagrophytes* and occasionally *Microsporum equinum*. Most cases occur in the autumn and winter in crowded housing conditions. The lesion appears as areas of erythema, scaling and crusting with broken hair shafts, giving a 'moth-eaten' appearance. It is not always pruritic and appears most commonly in areas rubbed by tack. Diagnosis is by fungal culture although direct microscopy is possible (see later). Wood's light examination is rarely positive in the horse.

Demodicosis

See 'Ectoparasites' above.

Photosensitivity

Photosensitivity is recognized as erythema, oedema, serum ooze, crusting and, in the extreme, skin necrosis in white, non-pigmented or flesh coloured areas such as the star, muzzle, coronets etc. Lesions are severe but localized. It is seen during the summer months and the initial erythema is associated with pruritis. Sunburn has a similar appearance but is not a photosensitization.

Primary and secondary photosensitization

Primary photosensitization occurs in conditions of high ultraviolet exposure and is associated with the grazing of plants which contain photodynamic agents (e.g. St. John's wort; perennial rye grass). Several horses in a group may be affected. Alternatively, secondary photosensitization is associated with liver failure where there is a decreased excretion of phylloerythrin, a product of bacterial activity on chlorophyll. This substance is photodynamic and provokes erythematous reactions in susceptible areas of skin. An extreme form of facial photosensitization is termed 'blue-nose disease' in which the affected areas show a faint blue tinge of cyanosis. In all cases of suspected photosensitization, serum liver enzymes should be checked for evidence of liver-associated disease (see under: 'Diagnostic techniques for the investigation of liver diseases'). Otherwise, diagnosis is by transferring the animal to shade and checking the pasture for implicated plants.

Photoaggravated vasculitis

Photoaggravated vasculitis ('pastern leucocytoclastic vasculitis') is a relatively common inflammatory lesion of unpigmented extremities, most usually the pasterns, which occurs during the summer months. This suggests that UV radiation has a role in the pathogenesis, but the condition is not a true photosensitization. It occurs in the absence of exposure to photosensitizing compounds and is not associated with liver disease. In the acute presentation the lesion is painful, with erythema, oozing and crusting. In more chronic cases it has a roughened 'warty' appearance. Diagnosis involves ruling out primary and secondary forms of photosensitization (see above) and determining the characteristic histopathological changes in a biopsy specimen.

Eosinophilic dermatitis

This is a rare multisystemic disease of horses involving the infiltration of various epithelial tissues with eosinophils. Also known as *eosinophilic granulomatosis* and *multisystemic eosinophilic epitheliotropic disease*, the aetiology is unknown, but it is presumed to be a hypersensitivity reaction. The skin and gastrointestinal tract are most usually involved. The presentation is of a chronic dermatitis with weight loss and depression.

The skin shows widespread symmetrical hair loss with exudation and crusting; secondary infection is usual. The coronets are also involved and marked pruritis is reported. Diagnosis is by skin biopsy which demonstrates eosinophil infiltration. Infiltration of the gastrointestinal tract produces a malabsorption syndrome resulting in weight loss and, if the hindgut is involved, diarrhoea. Investigative techniques include the oral glucose tolerance test (infiltration of the small intestine) and rectal biopsy (infiltration of the hindgut). See Chapter 2: 'Alimentary diseases'.

Pemphigus foliaceus

Pemphigus foliaceus is a rare autoimmune dermatosis of horses. The primary lesions are vesicles and pustules, but these quickly rupture and may be missed at presentation. Exudation follows with crusting and hair loss. The distribution is initially limited to the head and neck and/or limbs, but spreads over the entire body. Lesions are painful and sometimes pruritic. Systemic signs of depression, lethargy and inappetance are usual. Diagnosis is by biopsy of a recent lesion which shows loss of cohesion between epidermal cells (acantholysis), resulting in intradermal clefts and vesicles. An additional biopsy submitted for immunofluorescence may demonstrate widespread immunoglobulin deposits, but histopathological evidence is more reliable.

The 'greasy heel' reaction

The so-called 'greasy heel' describes an intractable, painful, exudative dermatitis affecting the back of the pasterns. There is exudation of a greasy seborrhoeic material which mats the hair and predisposes to secondary infection. It is a common sequel to a number of primary inflammatory causes already described above. Horses with feathering of the lower limbs are particularly prone. Among potential initiators are:

- Dermatophilosis
- Chorioptic mange
- Bacterial folliculitis
- Dermatophytosis
- Contact dermatitis (e.g. grasses; bedding)
- Photosensitivity
- Eosinophilic dermatitis
- Pemphigus foliaceus
- Photoaggravated vasculitis

Generalized seborrhoea

Generalized seborrhoea featuring dry scaling ('dandruff') or the production of large greasy flakes is occasionally seen in horses. In this instance the body has a rancid odour and erythema and thickening of the skin is possible. Proposed aetiologies are confusing, but in the absence of a defined skin insult, internal disorders of digestion or endocrine function should be suspected and investigated. Biopsy may show hyperkeratosis.

Cannon keratosis

Cannon keratosis is an uncommon dermatosis of obscure aetiology which affects the dorsal surface of the cannon region of both hindlimbs. The appearance is of a non-pruritic, non-painful scaling with matting of the hair in crusted plaques. Diagnosis is largely based on clinical appearance. Skin biopsy will show chronic inflammatory changes but is not definitive. Bacterial and fungal infections should be eliminated in the diagnostic procedure.

Nodules, papules and urticarial swellings

As the term suggests, nodular diseases present as hard circumscribed tissue masses of varying size. Their causative origins may be classified as idiopathic, neoplastic or infectious. Small masses, less than 1 cm in diameter, are frequently referred to as papules. They are the early (primary) lesions associated with bacterial folliculitis and, in many instances, fly bites. Urticarial swellings are common in horse skin and appear as multiple elevated patches of varying diameter.

Idiopathic nodules

Nodular necrobiosis

Nodular necrobiosis (synonyms: *collagen necrosis*; *eosinophilic granuloma*; *collagenolytic granuloma*) is probably the commonest nodular dermatosis of horses. Lesions occur as single or multiple nodules, 1–2 cm in diameter, over the withers and back and sometimes extend beyond these regions. The underlying cause is unknown. Diagnosis is by biopsy which demonstrates foci of degenerating collagen surrounded by an eosinophilic granulomatous reaction.

Aural plaques

Aural plaques (aural hyperkeratosis) are small areas of raised, depigmented, papillomatous skin composed of hypertrophied epidermis. They are commonly seen in the ears of horses in the absence of any discomfort or irritation. They are believed to be entirely benign and do not warrant invasive diagnostic procedures.

Nodular panniculitis

Nodular panniculitis is a rare multifocal inflammatory condition of the subcutaneous fat (steatitis). The nodules assume a large size, several centimetres across, and eventually become cystic in their centre. At this stage they may ulcerate, discharging an oily material. Needle aspiration of a cystic centre yields a sanguinous fluid containing inflammatory cells. Cultures of this fluid are negative. Diagnosis is by biopsy of a solid nodule (see Chapter 16: 'Fat diseases').

Amyloidosis

Amyloidosis is a rare condition in which multiple, hard, painless plaques of amyloid are deposited in the skin over the head, neck and shoulders of horses. Diagnosis is by biopsy.

Neoplastic nodules

Equine sarcoid

This is one of the commonest equine tumours. It is found around the eye, the paragenital region and the limbs. The clinical appearance is variable: verrucous (wart-like) tumours; fibroblastic tumours; mixed verrucous and fibroblastic tumours, and flat tumours characterized by hair loss, scaling and crust formation. Diagnosis is by biopsy, but it is preferable to submit a whole excised lesion. Flat tumours and verrucous tumours, if quiescent, are best left undisturbed by biopsy, otherwise further activity may be provoked.

Melanoma

Melanomas are common in aged grey horses. Pigmented lesions are seen under the tail, around the anus, on the ears and around the eyes. Diagnosis is usually based on appearance alone.

Squamous cell carcinoma

This is a relatively common tumour and is usually located in poorly pigmented, sparsely haired regions which are subjected to chronic ultraviolet light stimulation. In more temporate regions they may predominate in the penis and prepuce. Lesions appear as non-healing ulcerated plaques with indistinct borders, or as cauliflower-like masses. Diagnosis is by biopsy.

Cutaneous mast cell tumour

These tumours are uncommon and are probably a hyperplastic rather than a neoplastic process. They may be found on the head and limbs and are hairless, hyperpigmented and occasionally ulcerated. Diagnosis is by fine needle aspiration or excision biopsy.

Cutaneous lymphosarcoma

Although lymphosarcoma is probably the commonest internal tumour of horses, the cutaneous form is very rare. Multiple nodules are distributed over the body surface and may achieve large diameters. Diagnosis is by biopsy.

Infectious nodules

Equine viral papillomatosis

This is a common epithelial hyperplasia of yearlings and two-year-old horses. They are distributed about the muzzle and head and occasionally spread farther. They are pedunculated and verrucose and may achieve a size of 2 cm. The age incidence and appearance are diagnostic. Since they resolve spontaneously in 4–5 months, biopsy is unwarranted.

Warble fly nodules (*Hypoderma*)

See 'Ectoparasites' above.

Habronemiasis

Habronemiasis is a granulomatous nodular condition caused by tissue reaction to the intradermal migration of the larvae of stomach worms (*Habronema* species). Larvae are deposited in areas of moisture, or in wounds, by stable or house flies, which are intermediate hosts for the parasite. Lesions are reported in the medial canthus of the eyes, the prepuce and in wounds. The condition is extremely rare in the UK. Diagnosis is by biopsy which demonstrates the parasite in section, surrounded by eosinophils.

Papules

Bacterial folliculitis and fly bites

These often begin as papular lesions (see appropriate sections above).

Urticarial lesions

Urticarial reactions are very common in horses. They are often idiopathic and may not be worth investigating unless they persist for several weeks or recur regularly. Pruritis may or not be a feature. Biopsies are usually unhelpful, except to rule out other skin pathologies, and diagnosis leans heavily on the associated history. Secondary serum exudation and crusting may develop, leading to hair loss. In these cases urticaria may be mistaken for dermatophytosis.

Systemic drug reactions

The most common drug-induced urticarial responses are to antibiotics (especially penicillin) and non-steroidal anti-inflammatory drugs; but arguably any drug has the potential, as have proprietary products for topical use and vitamin/mineral feed supplements. The response may or may not be immune-mediated. Drugs may also be associated with non-urticarial skin reactions such as alopecia, pruritic dermatoses and erythema multiforme. Diagnosis is largely based on the associated history.

Food allergy or reaction

Urticaria, with or without pruritis, may be associated with a change in feeding practice. The culprit is usually grain rather than hay. Grazing allergies are also recognized. Diagnosis is by elimination diet testing (see later).

Contact urticaria

Wheals may develop at the site of topical administration of a drug or other substance shortly after application. The mechanism is usually toxic irritation rather than immune-mediated. Such reactions may occur in the absence of urticaria (see above under: 'Contact dermatitis').

Seasonal recurrent urticaria

Summertime wheal and papule formations are most commonly associated with ectoparasites and may be the result of irritant or hypersensitivity reactions. Much less often they are associated with individual hypersensitivities to inhaled allergens such as pollens or moulds. Such atopies may alternatively present as generalized pruritis without urticaria. In all cases a potential diagnostic approach is hypersensitivity testing (see later).

Systemic disease

Occasionally urticarial type lesions are a feature of *purpura haemorrhagica*, an immune-mediated vasculitis which is usually secondary to a previous systemic infection, particularly streptococcal infections. In this instance other clinical criteria such as mucosal petechiation are indicative of vasculitis. However, a skin biopsy will differentiate between true urticaria and vasculitis if necessary. See 'Vasculitis' in Chapter 8: 'Blood disorders'.

Physical urticarias

Physical urticarias are poorly documented in the horse. The situation may be complicated by food or drug allergies which predispose to physical urticarias. *Dermatographism* is a type of pressure urticaria which manifests as wheals in areas of pressure, e.g. under tack. *Cholinergic urticaria* and/or pruritis results from the local release of acetylcholine and is believed to be associated with an increase in core body temperature, e.g. hot baths, exercise or emotional stress. *Exercise-induced urticaria* and/or pruritis is specifically exacerbated by exercise.

Changes in hair growth

Alopecia

The term 'alopecia' is commonly used to indicate hair loss associated with any skin lesion, but it is used here to denote arrested growth or loss which occurs in the absence of an obvious inflammatory lesion.

Drug associated alopecia

Drug associated alopecia is rare and appears as a widespread loss of hair which occurs 3–5 weeks after drug administration. The effect is produced by a large number of hair follicles entering the resting phase of the hair growth cycle (telogen) together. A state of telogen is diagnosed by biopsy.

Hypothyroidism

Hypothyroidism in horses is probably rare but has the potential to be associated with a variety of clinical manifestations. It is an extremely rare cause of alopecia in which there is a progressive, patchy hair loss unassociated with pruritis or skin ulceration. Biopsy reveals inactive hair follicles in the absence of an inflammatory reaction. Functional hypothyroidism is confirmed by demonstrating the poor response of plasma triiodothyronine (T_3) and thyroxine (T_4) concentrations to injection with thyroid stimulating hormone (TSH). See Chapter 5: 'Endocrine diseases'.

Alopecia areata

Alopecia areata is a rare cause of extensive non-pruritic hair loss in horses. The aetiology is unknown but it is reported that biopsy reveals lymphocyte infiltration within and around the hair follicle.

Comments
- When submitting biopsies from areas of alopecia, it is important to look at the stages of the lesion. Samples should be obtained from normally haired skin, an area of moderate alopecia, and an area of marked alopecia.
- Dermatophytosis (ringworm) can present as focal or generalized hair loss in the absence of obvious crusting. For this reason, it is well worth submitting hairs from the periphery of an alopecic area for fungal culture (see later).

Hirsutism

A profuse, unkempt, curly coat is one of a number of clinical signs which is characteristic of *hyperadrenocorticism* in horses. Diagnosis is based on dynamic tests which demonstrate the presence of a functional pituitary tumour. See Chapter 5: 'Endocrine diseases'.

NB Systemic infections are associated with the immunosuppressive effects of hyperadrenocorticism and these sometimes include dermatitis.

Pigmentation changes

Leukoderma

Leukoderma is a loss of pigment from focal areas of skin. In most cases it is the sequel to melanocyte destruction as a result of contact reactions, local trauma, surgery, or cryosurgery. The hair is often affected too (leukotrichia). The associated history may be diagnostic.

Melanoderma

Melanoderma is a hyperpigmentation of skin which is rare in horses. It may occur at sites of inflammatory reactions to fly bites. The associated patch of hair is also darker (melanotrichia).

Arabian fading syndrome

This progressive depigmentation of the skin and hair is peculiar to Arab horses, usually between 1–2 years of age. It occurs particularly around the commissures of the lips and the muzzle, periorbital skin and eyelids. These areas of depigmentation are non-pruritic, non-painful and non-crusting.

Congenital skin disorders

Congenital abnormalities of the skin are uncommon in the horse. Diagnosis is based on their appearance.

Dermoids

Dermoids are areas of normal skin tissue, frequently haired, growing on the conjunctiva.

Dermoid cysts

Dermoid cysts are nodules occurring in the dorsal midline. Each consists of a fibrous wall lined with stratified epithelium and containing hair follicles, sweat glands and sebaceous glands.

Epitheliogenesis imperfecta

Epitheliogenesis imperfecta is the congenital absence of an area of skin, usually on a distal limb.

Cutaneous asthenia

Cutaneous asthenia is a condition where focal areas of skin are hyperextensible and easily torn by minor trauma. Biopsy shows disordered collagen in the dermis.

Hypotrichosis

Hypotrichosis is a condition in which the normal amount of hair is reduced. The hair is brittle and may fall out as the horse gets older.

II. Practical techniques

Skin scraping

Skin scraping is used primarily for the demonstration of mites, of which *Chorioptes* are the most important in horses. If the region is haired it should be lightly clipped before scraping, but no other preparation is necessary.

A scalpel blade is held at right angles to the skin and stroked swiftly to and fro under light pressure (Fig. 17.1). Multiple scrapings covering a large area of the affected region should be undertaken. Deep scraping is appropriate where demodicosis is a differential concern. In this instance the scraping must be deep enough to produce capillary ooze. A little mineral oil rubbed into the site prior to scraping produces a better sample for the examination of mites. Scrapings are taken into a sterile container for transfer to the laboratory.

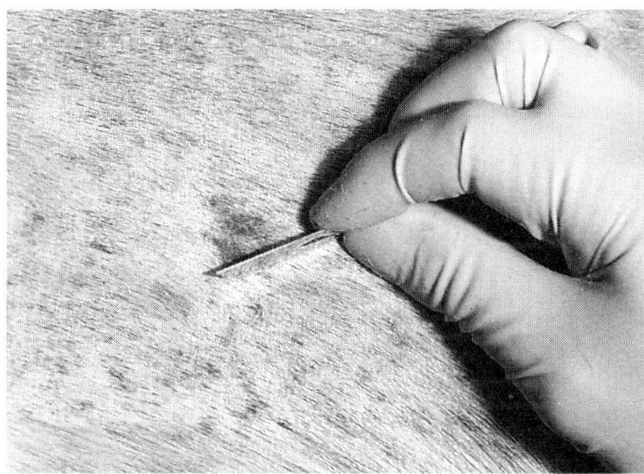

Figure 17.1   Skin scraping.

In the laboratory, the sample is placed on a glass slide and dispersed in a few drops of mineral oil before overlaying a cover slip. The specimen is scanned under low power for useful fields and then scrutinized under high power.

Comment

- The identification of *Demodex* in scrapings is not consistent with a diagnosis of demodicosis unless very large numbers are present.

Fungal culture

Dermatophyte culture is of the greatest value in horses with focal or generalized hair loss, with or without crusting. Lesions should be wiped gently with 70% isopropyl alcohol to remove as many bacterial and saprophytic contaminants as possible and allowed to dry. Broken hairs, scales and lightly crusted lesions should be sampled from the periphery of lesions using sterile forceps and placed in a sterile container for transfer to the laboratory.

Culture kits for dermatophytes are now available to the practitioner and consist of a pre-poured culture plate. The medium is an amber coloured Sabouraud's dextrose agar containing a pH indicator and antibiotic/ antimycotic agents to inhibit growth of contaminants. Samples are taken with sterile forceps and pressed onto (but not into) the medium. Most dermatophytes of importance to the horse grow at room temperature, but the colonies are slow to develop and appear soonest after 2 days. Cultures should be allowed to incubate for up to 12 days before being declared negative.

The dermatophyte colony is typically a white powdery growth (Fig. 17.2). It produces alkaline metabolites which turn the medium indicator red. It is essential to check the plate on a daily basis (from 2 to 12 days if necessary), to ensure that the white colony growth and the colour change occur within a similar time course to one another. Contaminant colonies are either brown, grey or green cultures which at first do not alter the colour of the medium. Ultimately, they too will produce an alkaline colour change and for this reason red colouration after 12 days in association with a non-white colony should be regarded as contaminant growth. In cases of doubt the sample should be submitted to a diagnostic laboratory for specific identification.

Comments

- It is important to ensure sample collection from the periphery of lesions, where dermatophytes are actively expanding the infection.
- Rapid microscopic identification of hyphae is possible using sample preparations cleared in 40% potassium hydroxide. However, this

requires experience, and false negatives are possible. Culture is always the most reliable technique.

- In difficult cases, biopsy sections submitted for staining with periodic acid–Schiff may demonstrate purple dermatophytes.

Identification of bacteria

Dermatophilosis

In a suspected case of dermatophilosis, if a crust is lifted and there is suppuration beneath, an impression smear may be made on a glass slide. This is then heat fixed for Gram stain. The characteristic appearance under the microscope is of Gram-positive rows of cocci arranged in branching, filamentous tracks (Fig. 17.3).

If stained preparations are negative or the lesions are limited to dry crusts, a minced crust preparation is necessary. A hairless crust is selected and chopped finely with a scalpel blade on a glass slide. The preparation is mixed with a few drops of water and allowed to soften for several minutes. It is then crushed with a glass rod, the excess debris is removed and the slide allowed to air dry. This is followed by gentle heat fixation, Gram stain and microscopic examination.

If microscopic preparations are negative, diagnosis should not be ruled out without submitting crusts to a microbiology laboratory for culture on blood agar.

Other bacterial lesions

Horses harbour a large number of commensal bacteria on the surface of their skin. To prevent contamination and overgrowth of cultures, lesions should be gently shaved, washed with antiseptic soap and dried with sterile gauze prior to sampling.

Pustules may be opened gently with a sterile scalpel blade and some of the contents transferred from the blade to a sterile culture swab. It is better to avoid swabbing the skin directly since non-pathogenic bacteria will be

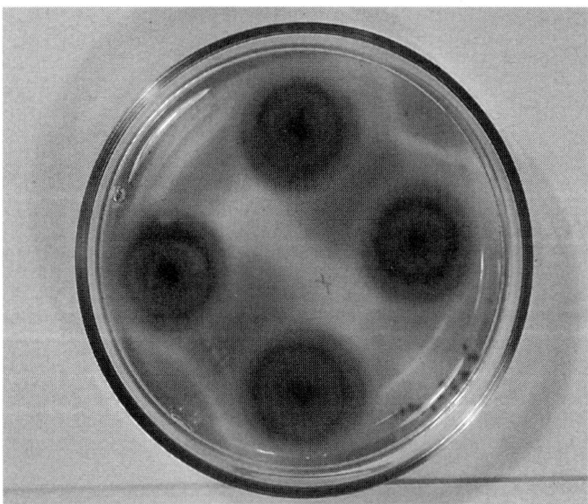

Figure 17.2 Typical dermatophyte colony on Sabouraud's medium.

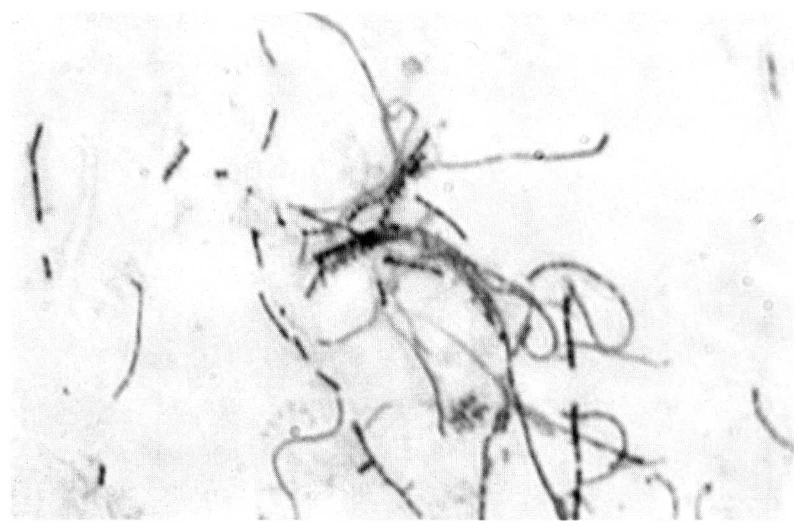

Figure 17.3
Photomicrograph showing the characteristic filamentous pattern of cocci in a dermatophilus smear.

cultured inadvertently. An alternative technique is to aspirate pustular contents with a 22 gauge sterile needle and transfer these to the swab. Microscopic preparations of pustular material may be made by heat fixing smears, followed by Gram stain.

When bacterial folliculitis/furunculosis is suspected in the absence of convenient pustules, a 6 mm punch biopsy of skin may be submitted for maceration and culture. In this instance the skin is prepared surgically, using povidine–iodine and spirit, to remove surface contaminants. Once obtained, the biopsy is placed in transport medium for submission to the laboratory.

Comment

- Culture of ulcerated lesions should be avoided, since isolates are likely to be opportunists rather than primary pathogens.

Skin biopsy

The interpretation of skin histopathology requires considerable experience and it is advisable not to take biopsies before being sure that they can be examined by a competent pathologist. Though often not specifically diagnostic, biopsies can rule out certain diseases and thereby narrow the range of differential diagnoses. A concise history, the distribution and features of the lesion, together with the site of sampling and the potential differential diagnoses should accompany the biopsy. This information enables the pathologist to make a better interpretation of the findings and consider the use of special stains, etc.

Biopsies should be undertaken in any condition which does not respond to appropriate treatment or where there is persistent ulceration, or suspected neoplasia. Exceptions to the latter are sarcoids, where it is preferable to submit a whole excised lesion for histopathology (see above under 'Neoplastic nodules').

Selected lesions should be fully developed primary lesions. Chronic lesions are not diagnostically useful. If possible, several biopsies should be taken to increase the chances of obtaining a diagnostic sample. These should include one representative lesion of the general condition and the remainder should be primary lesions. Care should be taken to avoid areas over superficial nerves, blood vessels, joint capsules or bony prominences.

Site preparation

Surgical preparation of the site is contraindicated. It may be soaked in 70% isopropyl alcohol but should not be scrubbed with antiseptics since this removes crusts and epithelial tissue that may be important in reaching a diagnosis. An exception to this principle is where a biopsy is to be submitted for maceration and culture (see above under 'Identification of bacteria'). Cutaneous infection as a consequence of biopsy is rarely encountered.

Most biopsies can be obtained under local anaesthesia, with sedation if required. For punch biopsies, a 25 gauge needle is inserted beneath the skin at the margin of the lesion until its bevel is buried in the subcutaneous tissues beneath the lesion. Half to 1.0 ml of adrenaline-free lignocaine hydrochloride is then injected. For larger excisional or elliptical biopsies, a ring block is performed in the subcutaneous tissues around the periphery of the sample. Dermal or epidermal infiltration of anaesthetic should be avoided, since this introduces artefactual changes into the sample. After infiltration, 5 minutes should be allowed before proceeding.

Excisional biopsy

If the lesion to be sampled is a single nodule, then excisional biopsy both removes the lesion and provides a histopathological diagnosis. It is particularly useful for suspected verrucous sarcoids.

Punch biopsy

The 6 mm disposable punch (Stiefel Laboratories, UK) is useful for most skin biopsies and can usually be used to obtain 2–3 biopsies before the edge is dulled. The punch is placed over the lesion and rotated in a clockwise direction under light pressure until the blade enters the subcutaneous tissue (Fig. 17.4). This is associated with a slight but palpable relief of resistance to pressure. On removal of the punch, the sample should be free of its adjacent dermis and remain loosely attached by connective tissue to the underlying subcutaneous tissue. The section is elevated by grasping the subcutaneous portion with fine rat-tooth forceps and it is cut free with fine, sharp scissors (Fig. 17.5). Care should be taken

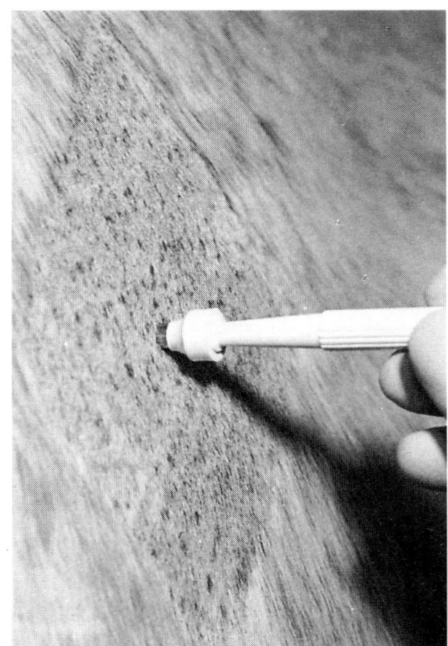

Figure 17.4   Use of the biopsy punch.

to avoid squeezing the sample with the forceps during this procedure. The sample is placed immediately in 10% buffered formalin for submission to the laboratory. The biopsy site may be closed with a single interrupted suture of 2-0 nylon, but this is not always necessary.

Elliptical biopsies

Elliptical biopsies are the method of choice for vesicular or bullous lesions, in which the biopsy can encompass the entire lesion; or for ulcerated lesions, in which the axis of the biopsy should include abnormal tissue, the edge of the lesion and the normal tissue beyond. The edge of an ulcerated lesion is the most rewarding in terms of histopathological diagnosis.

The site is anaesthetized by a ring block and a full thickness of skin is cut with the scalpel. The ellipse of skin is then undermined with narrow, curved scissors (Metzenbaum scissors) and the wound closed with 2-0 nylon in an interrupted pattern. Elliptical biopsies should be mounted with the dermis side pressed lightly down onto a piece of card or wooden strip (e.g.

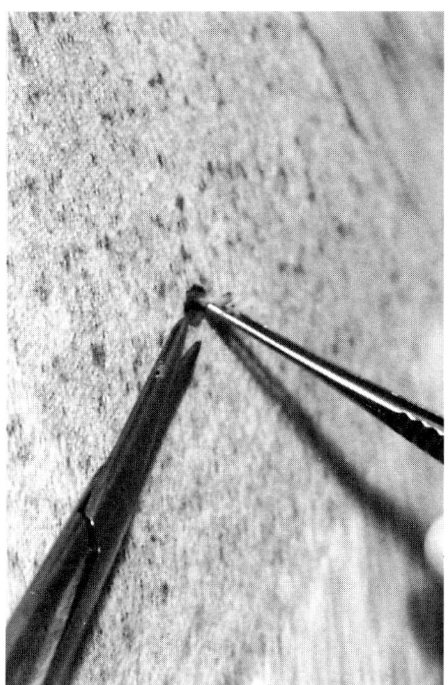

Figure 17.5   Releasing the punch biopsy sample from the subcutis.

a piece of tongue depressor) before immersion in 10% formalin, otherwise they curl during fixation.

Biopsy for immunofluorescence

In rare cases of suspected immune-mediated disease, such as pemphigus foliaceus, immuno-fluorescence testing is an adjunct to conventional histology. The purpose is to detect immunoglobulins or complement deposits in the epidermis or at the dermoepidermal junction. So far as the practicalities of obtaining a biopsy are concerned, the only difference is the need for a special citrated sulphide fixative which should be obtainable from the referring laboratory (Michel's fixative).

Comments

- In the laboratory, the success of immunofluorescence is influenced by the method employed (direct or indirect), the quality of the antisera reagents used, and the familiarity of the technician with the

technique. A negative result does not rule out the diagnosis and histopathology should always be undertaken in tandem.

NB Michel's fixative is unsuitable for routine histopathology and consequently a minimum of two samples are required for complete analysis; one in Michel's fixative and the other in 10% formalin.

Biopsy for onchocerciasis

Onchocerciasis is a rare clinical problem. In such cases biopsy may demonstrate foci of parasites surrounded by an inflammatory reaction. An alternative is to split the biopsy sample, submit one half in formalin for histopathology and the other in saline moistened gauze for live parasite examination. In the laboratory the section is placed on a glass slide and minced in a few drops of saline with a scalpel. It is then left for 30 minutes at room temperature and examined under the microscope. The slide is scanned at low power along the margins of tissue debris looking for indications of 'whiplash' movement. The microfilariae are then identified at high power. However, the simplest diagnosis is arguably the response to ivermectin (see above under 'Ectoparasites').

Hypersensitivity tests

Intradermal tests

In theory, intradermal sensitivity tests can be used to identify inhaled or insect allergens which are associated with immediate and/or delayed type hypersensitivities. These tests are offered by some specialist clinics but their technical limitations should be realized:

- Specific diagnosis depends upon the availability of the appropriate environmental antigen, of which there are hundreds, if not thousands.
- Each potential allergen needs to be titrated to an optimum dilution for sensitivity in test.

- Although a positive reaction indicates that the horse has a local antibody (IgE or IgG) which recognizes the antigen, it does not prove a clinical allergy, i.e. horses without clinical signs of allergy can have positive reactions.
- False negatives may be caused by concurrent medication with corticosteroids or antihistamines. Drug treatments which may interfere with the test should be withdrawn for at least 7 days beforehand.

Test procedure. An area of skin at the side of the neck, approximately 20 x 30 cm is clipped and marked out in 2.5 cm squares with a felt tip pen. Depending upon temperament, sedation may be necessary. Aqueous dilutions of specific antigen are injected intradermally into each square in volumes of 0.1 ml using a tuberculin syringe. A positive control (1:100 000 histamine), and a negative control (saline) are included. Any resultant swelling is recorded at 30 minutes, 4 hours, 24 hours and finally 48 hours later. The standard score for saline is 0 and for histamine ++++. All test reactions are graded relative to these controls. Reactivity greater than ++ is considered positive for a particular antigen.

ELISA

Allergen-specific serum immunoglobulin (antibody) can be detected and measured in horses by an allergen-specific enzyme-linked immunosorbent assay (ELISA). The test may be used to identify serum IgE antibodies to inhalent, food or insect allergens, but is offered by specialist laboratories only.

The test antigen is coupled to a plate and reacted with the horse's serum. Any antibody which attaches is then measured by a subsequent enzyme–substrate reaction. Just as in the case of the intradermal test, this assay relies on the availability of the appropriate potential allergens. However, unlike the intradermal skin test it is not influenced by the presence of any current medications which may be in use.

Comment
- The clinician is strongly advised to check the suitability of the panel of potential allergens offered by a laboratory before submitting a serum sample.
- The reliability of serum antibody tests and their correlation to the incidence of specific hypersensitivities have yet to be demonstrated in horses.

Acetate tape preparations

Acetate tape preparations are used primarily to diagnose *Oxyuris equi* infections. A piece of acetate tape (e.g. 'Sellotape') is pressed over several areas in the anal and perianal region and then placed adhesive side down onto a glass slide coated with mineral oil. Under the microscope oxyuris are recognized as oval eggs with a cap (operculum) located at one end.

Acetate preparations may also be used to diagnose superficial mites such as *Chorioptes*, but skin scraping is more usual.

Elimination tests for irritants and allergens

Environmental irritants are the usual cause of contact dermatitis, with or without urticarial lesions. The pragmatic approach to diagnosis is by changing the horse's management or environment to eliminate the irritant. Consideration should be given to everything that comes into contact with the horse's skin — for example: tack (including tack cleaners/ treatments); topical medications; bedding; timber treatments; foodstuffs; other livestock and their parasites (e.g. poultry fleas).

Less commonly, contact dermatitis is allergic in nature and allergic reactions to food, drugs or inhaled allergens are occasionally associated with the development of urticaria. If allergy is suspected, and the problem occurs indoors, then management at pasture may quickly resolve the problem. Alternatively, the horse should be stabled in an empty box devoid of bedding. Everything subsequently introduced into the stable environment should be considered for its potential irritant/allergic properties.

In relation to feed-associated allergies the diagnostic process is extended to elimination diets. If the problem occurs at grazing, the horse should be brought indoors or transferred to an alternative pasture. If the problem occurs indoors, the diet should be changed to a grass hay not previously fed to the horse. Most commercial feeds have the same basic constituents and changing from one brand to another is unlikely to demonstrate a difference. It is therefore advisable to withold concentrates and offer a bulk feed not previously used. Because food products can persist within the body for extended periods of time, feed trials should occupy a minimum of 4 weeks and arguably much longer. If the problem subsequently resolves, then individual parts of the old diet may be reintroduced at weekly intervals as a test challenge.

In respect of airborne allergens, the use of a different bedding, spore-free prepacked 'hayage' feed products and the elimination of animal dander (e.g. roosting birds), should all be considered.

Comment

- The diagnosis of irritant or allergen exposure can be a frustrating and time consuming process. The clinician should therefore be satisfied that all other potential causes of the lesion have been considered and tested before embarking on irritant and/or allergen elimination studies.

Further reading

Pascoe RR (1990) *A Colour Atlas of Equine Dermatology*. London: Wolfe Publishing Ltd.

Pascoe R.R. (1991) Equine nodular and erosive skin conditions: the common and not so common. *Equine Veterinary Education* **3**: 153–159.

18 Post-mortem examination

It is invariably difficult to conduct a thorough post-mortem examination under practice conditions because the time, facilities and practical experience are often lacking. In addition, there is the considerable and increasing problem of carcase disposal.

When it is known that the results of a post-mortem examination will have implications for other horses in a group, or that an insurance claim or litigation are contemplated, the advisability of transporting the carcase to a referral centre should be considered. In this instance, however, the following points must be appreciated by the owner and all interested parties:

- The carcase must be submitted as soon as possible; autolysis begins immediately after death.
- The pathologist will require details of the animal's management, its clinical history and the time and circumstances of its death.
- The procedure is expensive.
- There is no certainty that the cause of illness or death will be determined.

Most usually, circumstances will dictate a compromise in which a partial examination is undertaken at the premises of a licensed slaughterer (knackerman) or a hunt kennels. This chapter describes a technique for a full post-mortem examination under practice conditions, which may be adapted to individual circumstances.

Requirements

The floor area to be used as an examination surface should be entirely washable, with suitable drainage, and there should be adequate lighting and washing facilities. The requirement for protective clothing includes overalls, gum boots, a rubber apron and gloves.

The necessary investment in equipment is not prohibitive and includes: a hand saw; rib shears; a selection of knives with a sharpening steel; scissors; forceps; a scalpel; tissue containers with fixative, and various sterile equipment (syringes, needles, swabs and transport media) to sample fluid and other tissues for microbiology (Fig. 18.1).

Preliminary information

The animal's management, clinical history and the circumstances of its death should be considered carefully before post-mortem examination. If there is an insurance interest in the animal, the company should be informed since they may require their own agent to be present at the examination

Throughout the examination, written or taped notes should be kept and ideally any lesion of significance should be photographed. Pathological changes in tissues should be recorded in terms of their location, colour, size, shape, consistency and the appearance of a cut surface.

A number of variations to the technique described below are possible, but the aim should always be to proceed in a systematic manner ensuring that no organ is overlooked, rather than seizing at the first potential lesion and being misled.

The animal will probably be in lateral recumbency and for the technique described here should be rolled onto its right side, i.e. the examination proceeds from the left side of the horse.

External examination

Those distinguishing marks that would identify the animal in life should be recorded. This is especially important where there is an insurance interest or prospect of litigation. If possible, photographs of distinguishing features are an additional advantage.

External examination should include the skin, noting any abrasions which suggest either struggle or other trauma, or the presence of burns (e.g. 'lightning strike'). The mucous membranes, sclerae, hooves and coronary bands should all be inspected for abnormalities.

Opening the carcase

A ventral midline skin incision is made from the mandibular symphysis to the region of the prepubic tendon. The skin overlying the upper half of the body is dissected free and reflected back as far as possible (Fig. 18.2). In the male, the skin incision is carried around the penis and prepuce and both are reflected caudally. In females, the mammary gland can be undermined and removed with the skin.

The foreleg is freed by cutting its medial muscular attachments, dissecting into subscapular tissues and folding it dorsally. The

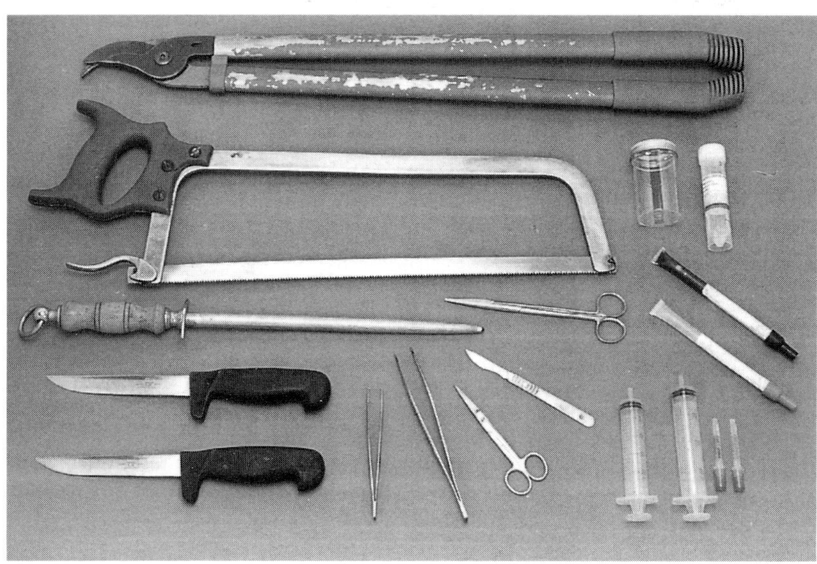

Figure 18.1 Basic kit for post-mortem examination.

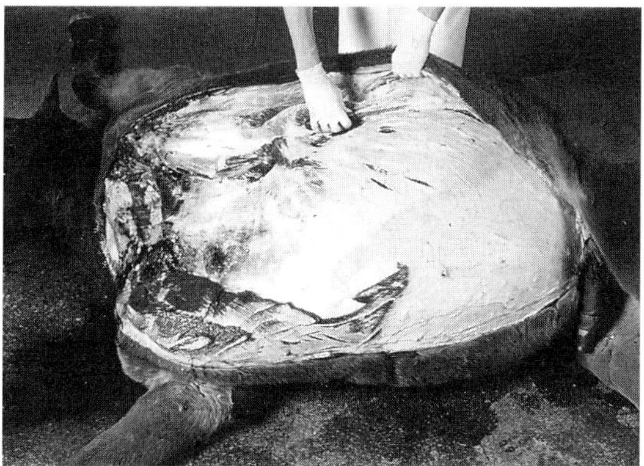

Figure 18.2   Reflecting the skin from the uppermost half of the body.

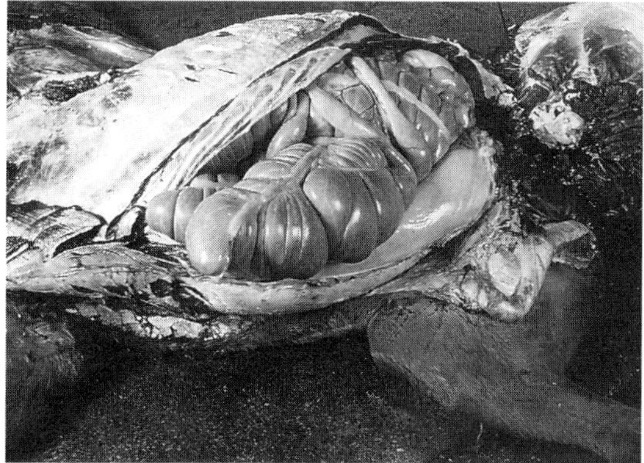

Figure 18.4   The abdominal wall reflected.

hind leg is treated similarly, but requires the capsule of the hip joint to be opened and the round ligament at the head of the femur to be cut (Fig. 18.3).

The abdominal wall is folded back in a ventral direction after incising along the costal arch and around the flank. Care must be taken not to cut into the underlying organs (Fig. 18.4).

The diaphragm is punctured near the sternum, at which time there should be an audible aspiration of air as the lung collapses, indicating intact negative pleural pressure. The cut is continued dorsally to release the diaphragm from the costal arch.

Using shears, the ribs are cut at their dorsal and ventral attachments and the thoracic wall is removed (Fig. 18.5).

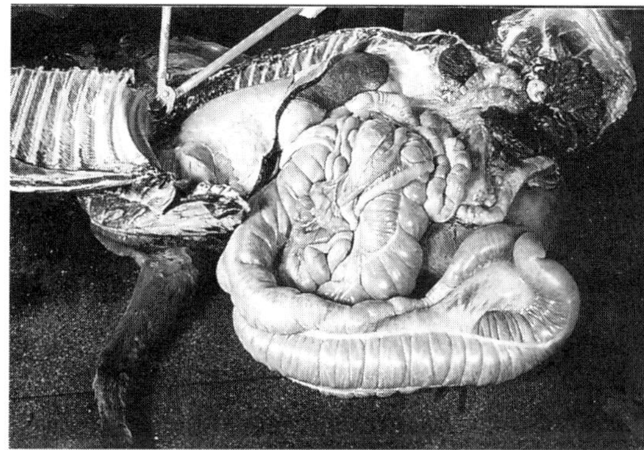

Figure 18.5   Opening the ribcage.

Inspection and removal of abdominal viscera

The abdominal viscera are first examined *in situ* for any gross abnormalities. Organs of the intestinal tract should be checked to ensure their correct anatomical position with respect to one another. The volume, colour and turbidity of peritoneal fluid is noted and, if appropriate, sampled for cytology (EDTA), biochemistry (plain tube), or culture (sterile container).

The pelvic flexure is lifted out and placed ventrally (Fig. 18.6). The spleen is cut free and removed, followed by the left kidney. The kidney should be freed from its perirenal fat and its arterial supply cut close to the renal pelvis. It is then removed with its ureter intact.

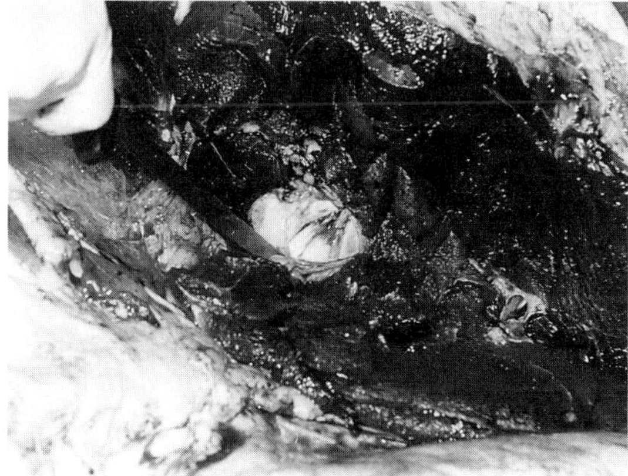

Figure 18.3   Cutting the round ligament at the head of the femur to enable the hindleg to be folded back.

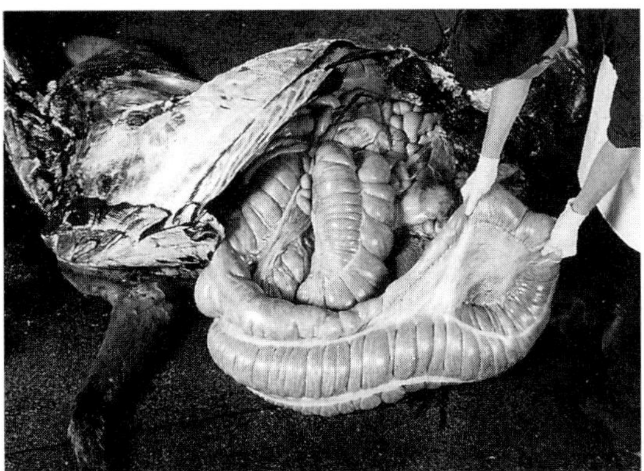

Figure 18.6 Removing the intestine. The pelvic flexure is lifted out first.

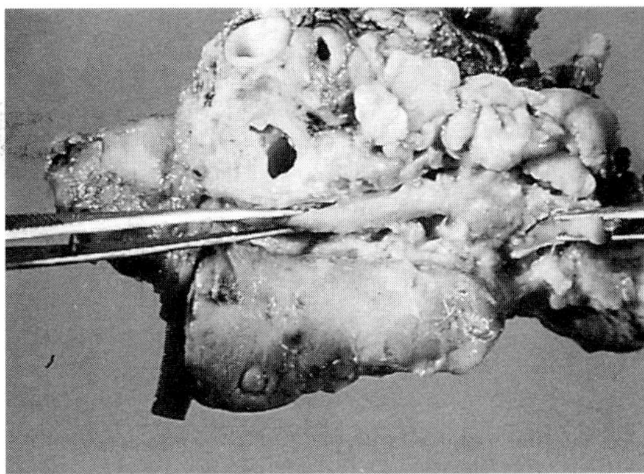

Figure 18.7 Dissection of the coeliacomesenteric ganglion from fixed (formolized) fat between the reflected adrenal gland (bottom of the picture) and the aorta (hidden underneath). The renal artery is seen at bottom left.

Access to the coeliacomesenteric ganglion

The adrenal gland which is adjacent to the kidney should still be attached by its vasculature, fat and fascia to the aorta at the point where the renal artery was cut. Between the adrenal gland and the aorta lies the coeliacomesenteric ganglion which is required for definitive histopathological diagnosis of *grass sickness*. This fusiform structure is about the width of a pencil, some 4–5 cm long in the adult horse, and has fibrous nerve attachments at each end. However, being soft and white it is often extremely difficult to differentiate this structure from the surrounding fat. Consequently, the adrenal gland, together with its adjacent segment of aorta, vena cava and the attached fat, should be removed *en bloc* and fixed in formalin. After fixing for 24 hours, the ganglion becomes harder and is more easily distinguished once the overlying adrenal gland has been dissected away (Fig. 18.7). Its cross-sectional appearance has the typical creamy white colour of nerve tissue. Other sympathetic ganglia will provide evidence for the diagnosis of grass sickness, but none will provide such large amounts of readily accessible tissue.

The small colon is cut free as far within the pelvic region as possible. At the other end of the gut the small intestine is stripped from its mesenteric attachment. The stomach is then cut free and exteriorized with the small intestine.

The caecum and colon are freed of their attachments, thus enabling the whole intestine to be removed intact (Fig. 18.8). Depending upon the available facilities, it may be more convenient to ligate sections of the alimentary tract with string and remove them for further examination as more manageable units.

The opposite kidney is then removed as described above. If necessary, a second attempt to retrieve a coeliacomesenteric ganglion can be made on this side. The bladder is drawn over the pelvic brim and opened *in situ*. In the mare, the uterus and ovaries are removed by drawing the tract forward and sectioning behind the cervix. If necessary, the pelvic organs may be removed, but this requires cutting the bones of

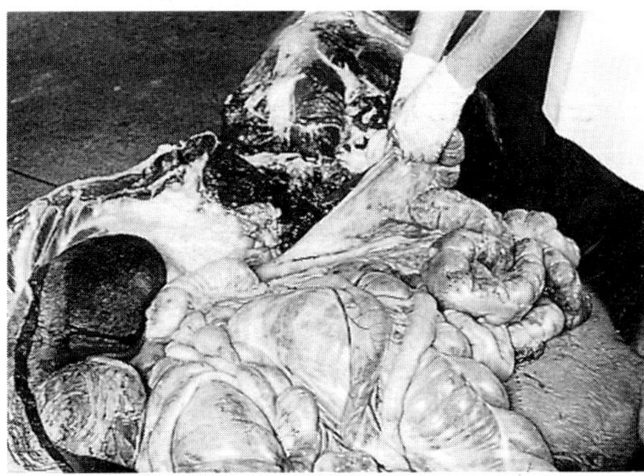

Figure 18.8 Removal of the whole intestine.

the pelvic cavity using the hand saw, or splitting the pelvis with an orthopaedic chisel.

The liver is removed by cutting its attachment to the diaphragmatic crura.

Inspection and removal of oral, cervical and thoracic viscera

The contents of the thoracic cavity, including the volume, colour and turbidity of pleural fluid, are examined. The tongue, pharynx, larynx (including adjacent thyroids), trachea, lungs, heart and oesophagus are then removed as one unit. This is achieved by freeing the tongue from its attachments with the oral cavity. Working from the underside of the jaw, a hand saw is used to cut across the rami of the mandible just behind the incisor region. The rami are prised apart and the tongue's attachments are cut on either side, parallel to each mandibular ramus (Fig. 18.9). Its base will also need to be freed from the stylohyoid apparatus by cutting through the cartilaginous attachment on either side. The whole is then pulled through the intermandibular space and further cuts medial to the stylohyoid apparatus will free the larynx, cranial trachea and oesophagus. The trachea and oesophagus are then dissected free from the neck as far as the thoracic inlet (Fig. 18.10). The pericardium is released from its sternal attachment and the dorsal mediastinum is cut along its length. This enables the entire thoracic contents to be

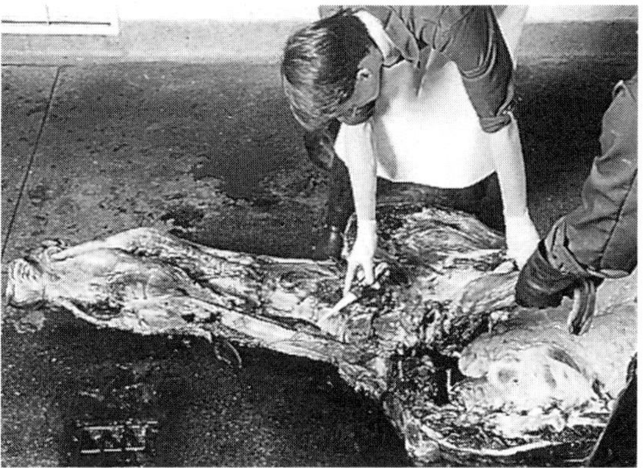

Figure 18.10   Separation of the trachea and oesophagus from the neck.

removed once the aorta and oesophagus are severed from the diaphragm (Fig. 18.11).

The parietal pleura is checked for evidence of inflammation or adhesion. The aorta can be examined by opening along its length and into its tributaries with scissors, starting at the thoracic end. If the examination procedure has been followed as described, the arterial system within the mesentery should still be intact for inspection.

The appearance of each individual organ is then assessed and recorded separately.

Inspection of removed organs

Abdominal contents

The stomach is opened along its greater curvature and the small intestine is opened along its length using scissors (Fig. 18.12). The

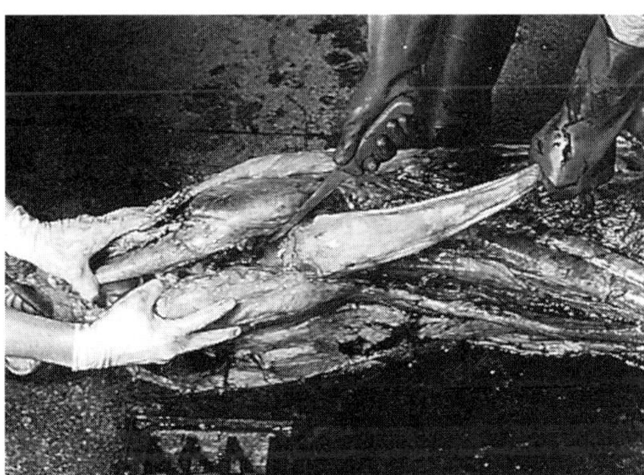

Figure 18.9   Cutting the tongue free of its attachments through the intermandibular space.

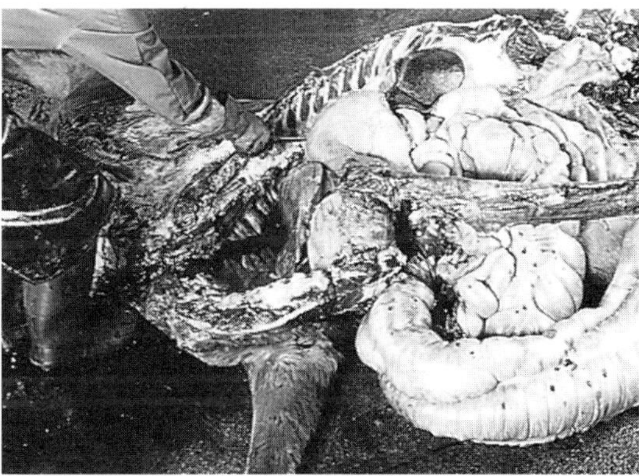

Figure 18.11   Removal of the thoracic contents.

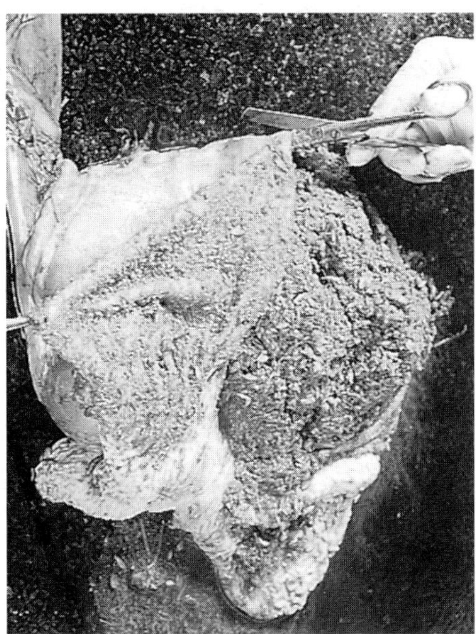

Figure 18.12   Opening the stomach and small intestine.

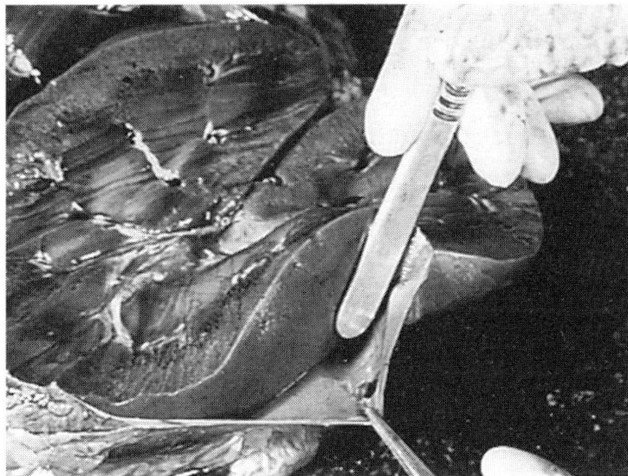

Figure 18.13   Peeling back the kidney capsule.

volume and nature of the gastrointestinal contents are noted and the mucosa is examined after rinsing with water. The large intestine is examined in like fashion. The size and colour of the colonic and mesenteric lymph nodes should be noted.

The liver, spleen, kidneys and adrenal glands should be sectioned and the cut surfaces examined for any abnormality of colour, content or shape. The kidneys should be cut lengthwise from the outer surface towards the pelvis and the capsule should be peeled back to check for any pathological change at the cortical surface (Fig. 18.13).

Oral, cervical and thoracic contents

The tongue is examined and sectioned, the oesophagus is opened along its length for inspection and then removed from the trachea. The thyroid glands are identified and examined in cut section. The cervical parathyroids are difficult to identify because of their small size, variable location and similar appearance to cervical lymph nodes. A larger pair of caudal parathyroid glands is located on the ventrolateral aspect of the trachea, close to the level of the first rib.

The pharynx, epiglottis, larynx and retropharyngeal lymph nodes are examined and the trachea is opened along its length to the bronchial tree (Fig. 18.14). This is facilitated by prior removal of the heart from the pericardium and its vascular attachments. An excess of pericardial fluid or other pathological change should be noted. The lungs are then palpated to detect any changes in consistency and are sectioned at several sites to check for small internal lesions and the presence of abnormal fluid or exudate (Fig. 18.15).

In cases of sudden death, particular attention should be paid to examination of the heart and its associated vessels. Ideally, the heart should be opened in such a way that the valves and their attachments can be examined intact before pathological evidence is lost by

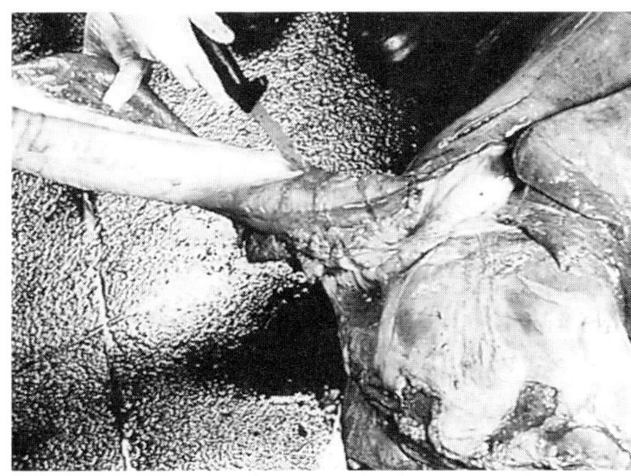

Figure 18.14   Opening the trachea.

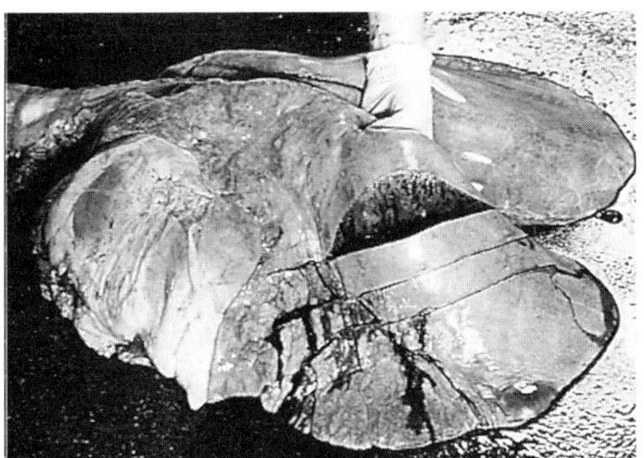

Figure 18.15   Sectioning the lungs to detect gross lesions and assess fluid content.

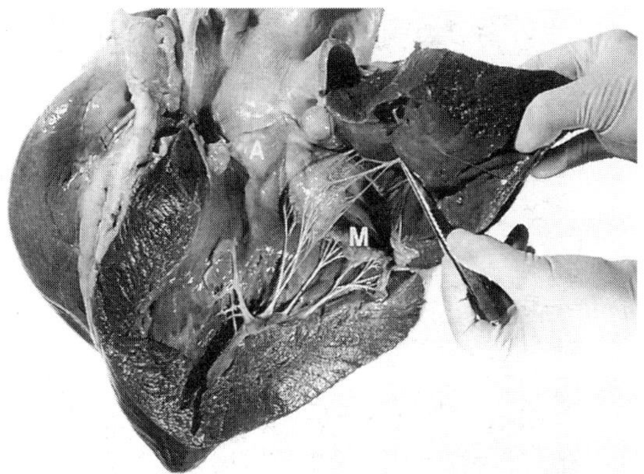

Figure 18.16   The left side of the heart opened for gross examination. The aortic (A) and mitral (M) valves are clearly exposed.

dissection. This can be accomplished using the following procedure.

Left side of the heart. The aorta is separated from the overlying pulmonary artery and is cut open so that the aortic valve can be inspected from above. A downward incision is then made through the valve into the left ventricular wall, opening up the aortic vestibule. This enables a limited view of the mitral valve and its attached chordae from below. The left atrium is then opened by extending a cut through the pulmonary vein to expose the dorsal surface of the intact mitral valve for inspection. A downward incision is then made through the valve and into the left ventricular wall as far as the apex. A third cut to join the two incisions in the ventricular wall allows the left chamber to be opened to full view (Fig. 18.16).

Right side of the heart. The right atrium is opened by joining incisions into the anterior and posterior vena cavae. The intact tricuspid valve is then inspected from above. The pulmonary artery is cut open to expose the pulmonary valve from above. An incision is then made down through the valve, opening the wall of the right ventricle as far as the apex. This provides a limited view of the tricuspid valve from below. A final cut is made through the tricuspid valve to open up the front of the right ventricle and join the pulmonary artery incision at the apex, thus exposing the right chamber to full view (Fig. 18.17).

Submission of samples

At this stage appropriate samples should be considered for histopathology, culture, serology, biochemistry and toxicology. Tissue samples of major organs and all observed lesions can be collected for routine histopathology in 10% buffered formalin. The fixative to tissue ratio should be at least 10 to 1 by volume to ensure adequate penetration. Serology and serum biochemistry may be achieved by retrieving heart blood from the right ventricle if ante-mortem samples are not available. In cases of suspected poisoning, liver, kidney, fat, stomach or intestinal contents, urine and heart blood should be frozen down

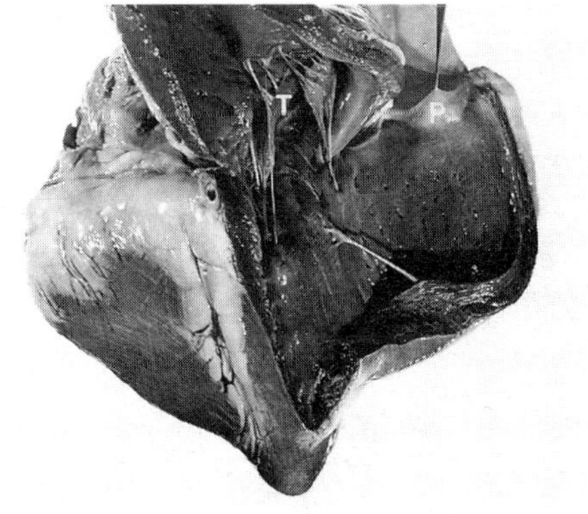

Figure 18.17   The right side of the heart opened for gross examination. The pulmonary (P) and tricuspid (T) valves are clearly exposed.

as soon as possible (see 'Causes of fatal poisoning' in Chapter 19: 'Sudden and unexpected death'). In ideal circumstances, sufficient material should be retained to enable duplication of tests, or alternative testing if required.

Examination of the locomotor system

Joints should be examined if indicated by the clinical history. Prior to opening a joint it may be necessary to aspirate synovial fluid for cytology, biochemistry or culture. Contaminant free culture is facilitated if the joint is first skinned. Normal fluid is scant, straw coloured and viscous.

Cases of laminitis should be examined by cutting off the foot above the coronary band and cutting the whole in longitudinal section (Fig. 18.18).

Skeletal muscle should be examined in cut section and submitted for histopathology if appropriate.

Examination of the head and brain

The head is removed from the neck at the atlanto-occipital joint (Fig. 18.19).

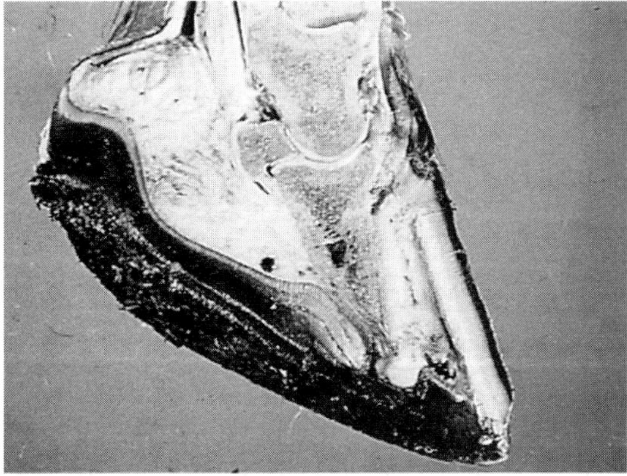

Figure 18.18 Longitudinal section of a laminitic foot. Note the displacement of the pedal bone and the accumulation of exudate between its dorsal edge and the hoof wall.

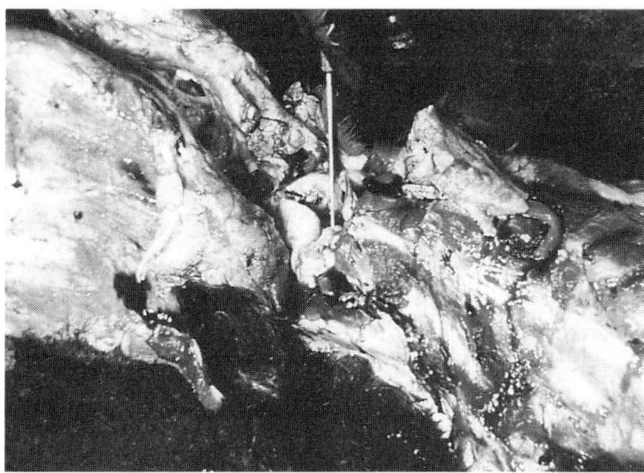

Figure 18.19 Removal of the head by section of the atlanto-occipital joint.

Access to the brain is obtained by stripping back the skin over the poll and removing the temporal muscles overlying the dome of the skull. An oscillating circular saw is ideal to open the bony cranium, but a hand saw can be used. The head must be held tightly for this procedure, preferably in a vice. A cut is made across the head through the frontal bones at a point just caudal to the zygomatic arches. Two further cuts are then made at right angles, with the line of the blade passing just medial to the occipital condyles (Fig. 18.20). The bony plate is then carefully prised off in a caudal direction whilst separating the meningeal attachments beneath (Fig. 18.21).

For removal, the brain is supported in one hand and the cranial nerves, meningeal and vascular attachments are cut whilst an assistant

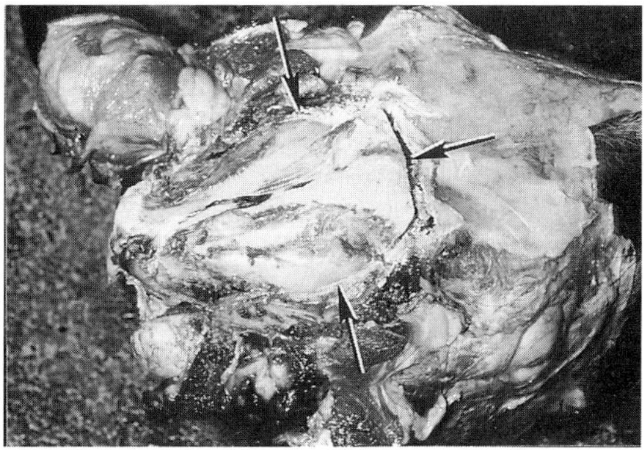

Figure 18.20 Dorsal view of saw cuts in the cranium prior to removal of the bony plate.

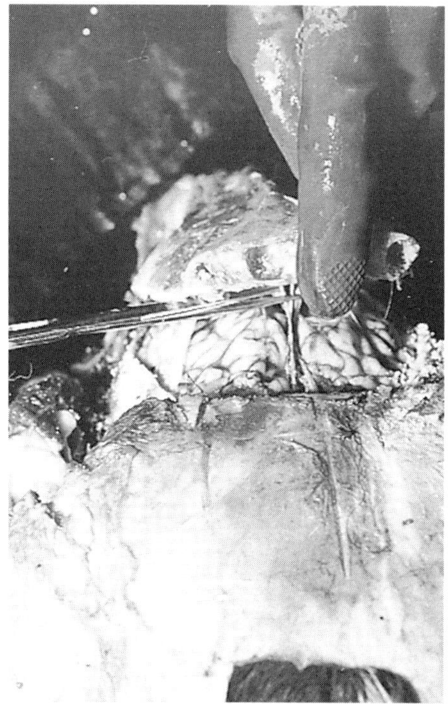

Figure 18.21   Separating meningeal attachments as the cranial plate is prised open.

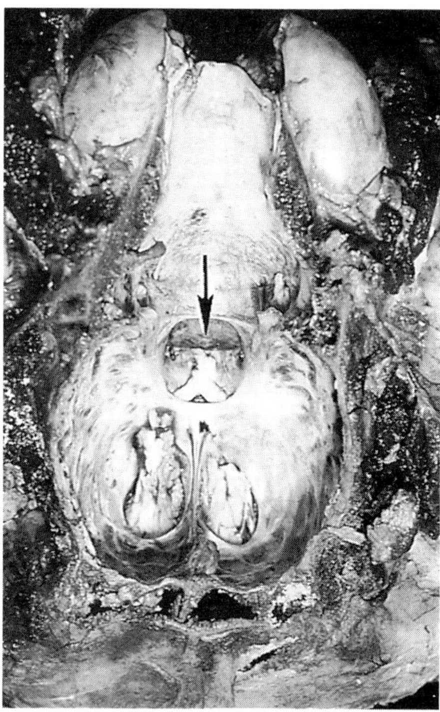

Figure 18.22   Dorsal view of the pituitary *in situ* (arrowed).

tilts the head back. Once the brain is removed, the pituitary gland is seen from above (Fig. 18.22) and can be lifted up by forceps and cut free of its fossa. In cases of pituitary adenoma, the optic chiasma should be checked for evidence of distortion and the adrenals should be examined for cortical hypertrophy.

If necessary, the whole brain may be immersed in 10% formalin, but a week is then required for complete penetration of the fixative.

The eyes are removed by cutting through the periorbital skin and dissecting through the tissues of the orbit with curved scissors, using much the same procedure as for surgical enucleation.

The mandibles can be separated from the upper jaw by cutting through the soft tissues of the cheeks in a line towards the temporo-mandibular joints. The mandible is held steady and the upper jaw is pulled up and away to disarticulate the joint. The head can then be sawn longitudinally to reveal the nasal passages and paranasal sinuses.

Examination of the spinal cord and peripheral nerves

The removal of an intact spinal cord is both difficult and extremely time consuming (several hours). The exercise demonstrates how well the organ is protected under ordinary circumstances. It is usually acceptable, and certainly faster, to remove short sections of the cord from a cut-down vertebral column. If appropriate, post-mortem radiographs can be used to locate a site of cord compression.

The spinal column is freed from the limbs, ribs and its superficial muscle attachments. It is then transected into several convenient segments by sawing through vertebral bodies. The siting of the cuts must be chosen to avoid the direct area of interest. Further cuts are then made through the arches and bodies of the vertebrae adjacent to the supposed clinical location of the lesion; these cuts should avoid the intervertebral joints.

In each short segment the spinal cord is removed by grasping the dura with forceps and

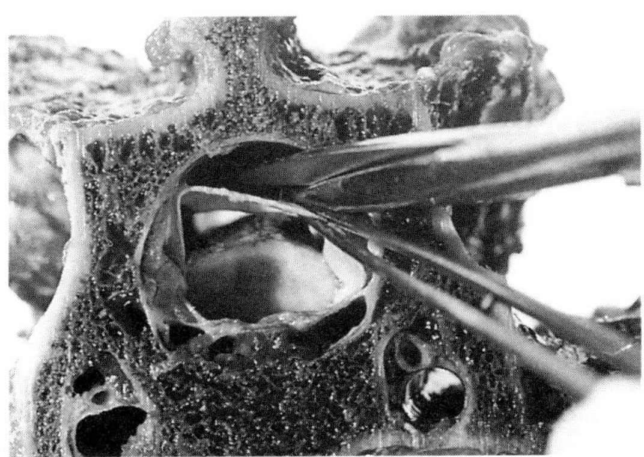

Figure 18.23   Removal of the spinal cord from a cut segment of the vertebral column.

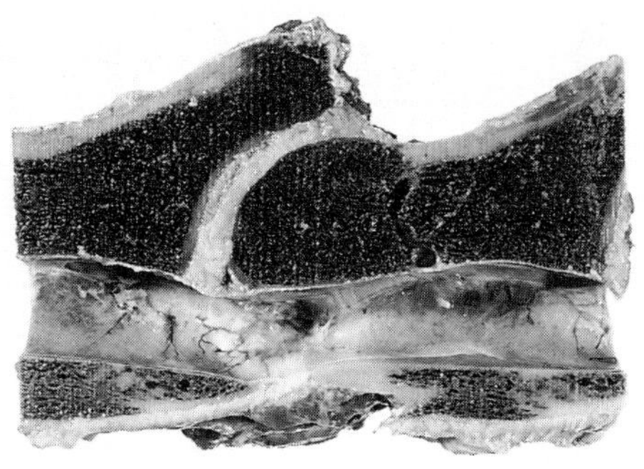

Figure 18.24   Longitudinal section of a vertebral segment exposing the spinal canal and intervertebral articulation.

cutting through the spinal nerve roots with a pair of scissors (Fig. 18.23). Appropriate cord sections can then be cut into short lengths (1 cm) for immersion in fixative. The associated sections of vertebrae can then be cut again in longitudinal section to examine the spinal canal and the intervertebral articulation (Fig. 18.24).

Further reading

Buergelt CD and Young A (1992) Necropsy procedures in practice. I: The initial examination. *Equine Veterinary Education* 4: 167–171.

Buergelt CD and Young A (1992) Necropsy procedures in practice. II: Special procedures. *Equine Veterinary Education* 6: 273–276.

19 Sudden and unexpected death

When a horse is seen to die suddenly it is usually an unexpected event. When a horse is found dead it may also be unexpected, but in that instance death may or not have been sudden. The distinction is important because the implicated causes are often different. Sudden death is frequently associated with exertion, but horses found dead may have suffered a disease process of several hours' duration. However, in either case the approach to investigation is the same.

A detailed history is required and the animal's environment must be examined carefully. These parts of the investigation assume paramount importance because there will be few, if any, clinical signs to indicate a cause. Detailed notes are essential and a photographic record is preferable in cases of potential litigation or insurance claim.

History

The previous veterinary history is required together with details of the horse's management. Any changes in the feeding or exercise practice should be noted and the current health of any other horses in a group is relevant. The clinician should be aware that in some circumstances the handler may withhold vital information for fear of exposing negligence.

Recent drug administration should be considered with respect to an adverse response or overdosage. All drugs have the potential to provoke an adverse response. Fatal responses often take the form of a systemic hyper-sensitivity (anaphylactic response) within a short time of intravascular injection. Penicillin preparations are often incriminated. Where a reaction has followed a supposed intravenous injection, the possibility of accidental intra-carotid injection should also be considered.

The horse has a marked susceptibility to overdosage with certain drugs such as warfarin and phenylbutazone. Current therapy with either should be checked. Warfarin is used therapeutically for the treatment of navicular disease. Unless carefully monitored, the rate of blood coagulation is critically extended and minor traumas can produce fatal haemorrhages. In the case of phenylbutazone, prolonged use at the upper therapeutic limits results in ulceration of the alimentary tract and a protein-losing enteropathy. Most usually the result is intractable colic, but extensive submucosal oedema of the large intestine can precipitate shock.

Poisoning as a cause of sudden and unexpected death in horses is often suspected, but is rarely substantiated. Potential sources of poison should be considered within the history and the examination of the environment.

Examination of the environment

If possible this should be undertaken with the carcase *in situ*. There may be signs of recumbency and struggling before death, or a significant amount of haemorrhage may be seen. Following a recent storm, a horse found dead under a tree suggests lightning strike. Alternatively, the animal may be found near power lines suggesting electrocution. Signs of struggling indicate a protracted death, as in a gastrointestinal catastrophe, whereas electrocution causes sudden death without struggle.

Owners often seize on poisoning as the explanation of sudden and unexpected death, but in reality it is an extremely uncommon cause. Nevertheless, the possibility should be investigated by considering the animal's feed and the possibility of industrial or agrochemical pollution.

Potential sources of poison

Feedstuffs

Poisonous plants. A huge number of native plants are potentially poisonous but they are seldom eaten by grazing horses unless driven by hunger or, significantly, they are trimmed, cut down or treated with herbicides. At this time horses seem positively attracted to the wilting plant. Hedge, ditch, shrub, tree or weed material which is cut and dumped within the grazing area should be viewed with great suspicion. Samples should be held over for identification and further analysis.

Plant poisoning in horses most usually follows the chronic intake of plants whose toxic principles survive the hay making process (e.g. ragwort, horsetail, bracken, St. John's wort). Consequently, there are usually signs of toxicity long before death supervenes and sudden unexpected death is extremely unlikely. *The singular exception is yew, which is attractive to horses and exceptionally poisonous.*

Adulterated feed. Horses are exquisitely susceptible to ionophore toxicity. Ionophore antibiotics (e.g. monensin, salinomycin) are included in compounded livestock feeds as growth promoters or coccidiostats. The finished material has the appearance of a horse or pony cube and may be fed accidentally, or maliciously, resulting in a generalized myopathy which includes cardiac myodegeneration with consequent dysrhythmia. The clinical course is usually chronic but sudden death may occur within 24 hours of intoxication. Reports occur from time to time of horse feeds which have been inadvertently contaminated at the feed mill.

Forage poisoning. Horses are particularly susceptible to botulism and the most usual source is big bale silage. Ingestion of the preformed toxin results in a generalized flaccid paralysis, the severity of which is directly proportional to the amount of toxin consumed. Death follows respiratory failure but the clinical course is usually extended over several days. Access to big bale silage on the premises should alert suspicion.

Industrial and agrochemical pollutants

Industrial emissions. Factory emissions are controlled by modern legislation, but the proximity of industry should be noted. Old industrial processes such as lead mining or smelting may have left dangerous amounts of residue in the topsoil. The course of lead poisoning in horses is usually chronic. Nevertheless, asphyxiation associated with laryngopharyngeal paralysis continues to be recorded in horses following chronic lead poisoning. On enquiry, it is likely that the locality is known to be a source of lead poisoning in horses.

Agrochemicals. Herbicides, fungicides, pesticides and fertilizers may either be ingested from the grazing and/or contaminated water courses, or inhaled as a drifting aerosol spray. The use of agrochemicals within the grazing area should be checked and the possibility of rain 'wash off' from land into adjacent water courses should be considered.

Post-mortem examination

Once the history and examination of the environment are completed, the need for a post-mortem examination is considered. If other animals are at risk, or there is an insurance interest and/or prospect of litigation, the advisability of referring the carcase to a specialist centre should be considered. However, the potential costs of post-mortem investigation must be kept in perspective, together with the realization that most surveys of sudden and unexpected death in adult horses show that 30% or more are unexplained, despite careful and extensive post-mortem study.

If post-mortem examination is elected but is not to be undertaken at a specialist centre, then the following notes on potential causes of sudden and unexpected death may prove helpful during the examination. However, the cause should not be prejudged by lists of possibilities such as these, and the clinician should resist the temptation to seize at a convenient diagnosis. In all cases a systematic examination should be undertaken as outlined in Chapter 18: 'Post-mortem examination'.

Causes of sudden death (death observed)

During great exertion, as in racing, sudden death is often associated with haemorrhage into the lungs, thorax, abdomen or brain. That said, many instances of death during exertion are unexplained and in the particular instance of racehorses a toxicological examination is required, emphasizing again the need for specialist facilities and experience. Sudden unexpected death at rest is less common. It may be associated with an iatrogenic cause, i.e. an anaphylactic response to administration of a drug. Alternatively, lightning strike, electrocution or poisoning are possible.

Some of the causes of sudden death are considered below by organ system.

Cardiovascular system

Massive internal haemorrhage. This is the commonest cardiovascular lesion causing sudden death in horses and usually follows the rupture of a major vessel at exercise. The pulmonary vessels are commonly involved and the usual result is a profuse nasal haemorrhage, although a vessel will occasionally rupture into the pleural space. Less commonly, increased intra-aortic pressure predisposes to tears in the aorta and the resultant haemorrhage into the pericardium can produce extreme pressure on the heart (cardiac tamponade). Haemorrhage from an aortic rupture may enter the thoracic cavity or dissect along the aorta into the abdominal cavity. Older breeding stallions occasionally succumb to rupture of the aorta during sexual activity. Haemorrhage may also be associated with bone fracture and laceration of an adjacent major vessel.

Rupture of the mitral chordae tendinae. The obvious post-mortem finding is extensive pulmonary oedema. Examination of the heart requires careful dissection, otherwise the primary lesion is easily overlooked. See Chapter 18: 'Post-mortem examination'.

Fatal dysrhythmia. This is not detectable at post-mortem examination and is therefore a speculative conclusion. Visible abnormalities of the myocardium warrant histopathology.

Respiratory system

Exercise-induced pulmonary haemorrhage. Severe engorgement of pulmonary vessels with haemorrhage into the alveoli, airways, interstitium and subpleural tissues are obvious post-mortem findings, but the aetiology is controversial. The condition may be predisposed by chronic lung disease.

Pneumothorax. This is rare and is usually associated with trauma or penetrating wounds. It is easily missed at post-mortem examination since the normal lung will also collapse as soon as the diaphragm is opened.

CNS

Trauma. Running into solid objects may be associated with trauma and intracranial haemorrhage; with or without fracture of the skull.

Adverse drug responses

Acute respiratory distress as a result of pulmonary oedema or bronchospasm is often a feature of adverse drug reactions in horses. The gross post-mortem findings can be unremarkable, but there may be froth in the airways and histopathological evidence of acute pulmonary oedema.

The accidental injection of a medication into the common carotid artery, rather than the jugular vein, is likely to cause sudden severe signs or death. These circumstances may then be mistaken for an anaphylactic response. In such cases a haematoma is usually present at the puncture site. The site itself may be low in the neck, because the carotid is more superficial there and the accident is therefore more likely to occur at that point.

Poisoning

See later.

Causes of unexpected death (found dead)

Horses unexpectedly found dead may have suffered a more protracted death. In these circumstances it might be anticipated that a post-mortem examination will be more revealing, but this is not necessarily the case. The causes of unexpected death can be the same as those of sudden death, but with additional possibilities. In this group, gastrointestinal lesions tend to be the commonest finding. It should be emphasized that 'unexpected death' assumes that the owner's opinion of previous good health is accurate and that some prior disease process has not been overlooked.

Gastrointestinal tract

Gut rupture. Rupture and peracute peritonitis usually follow an abdominal catastrophe.

Torsion and strangulation of the hindgut. This produces an overwhelming toxaemia which is rapidly fatal.

Gross tympany of the hindgut. This may or not be associated with torsion and strangulation (above), but the extensive tympany causes dyspnoea and circulatory failure.

Peracute enteritis with endotoxic shock. This is a rare form of *salmonellosis*. There may be oedema and petechiation of the large bowel wall. Caecal and colonic tissue should be submitted for culture.

Cardiovascular system

Slow exsanguination. This may be the result of damage to a medium sized vessel following fracture or trauma. An example of the latter is rupture of the middle uterine artery during parturition in older brood mares.

Rupture of the internal carotid artery. The horse is found dead in a pool of blood discharged from its nostrils. The lesion is associated with guttural pouch mycosis.

Poisoning

See below.

Investigating causes of fatal poisoning

The post-mortem examination in cases of poisoning is usually non-specific and selection of tissues for histopathology and/or toxin analysis relies heavily upon conclusions drawn from the history and environmental examination. If possible, it is extremely useful to obtain guidance from a veterinary toxicologist before undertaking the post-mortem examination.

It is a wise precaution to hold over samples suitable for toxicological analysis for as long as the investigation is pursued. Samples collected for toxin analysis should include: liver, kidney and fat (at least 200 g of each); stomach or intestinal contents (400 g); urine (100 ml), and serum from heart blood (20 ml). Consideration should also be given to storing samples from suspected sources of poison: feed; baits; soil or crop dressings; water and plants. Clean glass or plastic containers that can be tightly sealed are ideal. Each should be labelled with the owner and animal identification, the date, and the type of tissue or specimen contained. The samples are then frozen. If they are eventually to be submitted to a specialist laboratory, every attempt should be made to deliver the material quickly and in a frozen condition.

The laboratory analysis of tissues for specific toxins is highly specialized. The concept of 'screening' for poisons is unrealistic. If pursued, it would be prohibitively expensive and in all probability unrewarding. The most practical approach is to discuss the history, environmental and post-mortem findings with a veterinary toxicologist and then decide upon the most worthwhile tests to pursue. Before submitting material it is of the utmost importance to discuss the case with the toxicologist as follows:

- Report fully the history, environmental and post-mortem findings.
- Decide in discussion the specific toxin test(s) to be undertaken.
- Check which tissues/specimens are required, in what bulk, and how they should be packaged and dispatched.
- Always warn the laboratory of any possible litigation, since the handling of samples and recording of results may need to be scrutinized.

NB The isolation of a potentially poisonous substance in tissues is proof of exposure but not necessarily proof of poisoning, unless the amounts found are consistent with toxicity. For example, all horses grazing areas known to contain lead will have lead in their tissues, but not necessarily in toxic amounts. The interpretation of laboratory results must therefore be undertaken with the full guidance of the referral laboratory.

Feedstuffs

Poisonous plants

The stomach contents should be checked for evidence of recent ingestion. In horses, plant material reaches the stomach in a well masticated condition and will be difficult to identify. A specimen of contents should be put by in case further investigation is required.

Yew is exceptionally poisonous, so much so that leaves may still be found in the mouth. As little as 100–200 g is fatal in horses.

Adulterated feed

Sudden death from the ingestion of ionophore containing feeds is likely to produce non-specific signs, unlike the chronic situation where myopathy would become recognizable. If suspicious, samples of gut contents and a specimen of feed should be collected.

Forage poisoning

Post-mortem findings in cases of botulism are non-specific and diagnosis is based on the identification of toxin in the serum, feed, liver or faeces. The toxin is extremely labile and samples should be frozen and submitted for assay as soon as possible. To date, the most sensitive assay is still the mouse inoculation test, but this is undertaken by a very limited number of laboratories. A negative result from this bioassay does not disprove botulism in horses. Evidence of secondary fermentation in big bale silage (ammoniacal smell and/or alkaline pH) indicates conditions favourable to the growth of *Clostridium botulinum*.

Industrial and agrochemical pollutants

Lead

Post-mortem findings are likely to be non-specific. Food debris in the trachea, or aspiration pneumonia, suggest ante-mortem dysphagia. In known areas of lead contamination, liver and kidney samples should be submitted for analysis; concentrations of at least 15 ppm support a diagnosis.

Agrochemicals

If a particular product has been implicated during the the history and environmental investigation, it is worth contacting a hospital-based regional poison centre. These centres are an excellent source of up to date information concerning the likely effects of poisoning with commercially available products. This enables a more focussed post-mortem examination and helps to define the tests which should be undertaken by the veterinary toxicologist.

Further reading

Brown CM and Mullaney TP (1991) Sudden and unexpected death in adult horses and ponies. *In Practice* (supplement to the Veterinary Record) **13**: 121–125.

Index

*Entries in **bold** type indicates where the main discussion occurs*